Fish's
OUTLINE OF PSYCHIATRY

Fish's Outline of Psychiatry

for Students and Practitioners

Revised by

MAX HAMILTON
MD, FRCP, FRCPSYCH, FBPsS

Emeritus Professor of Psychiatry, University of Leeds
Formerly Honorary Consultant to General Infirmary
at Leeds
St James's (University) Hospital, Leeds
Stanley Royd Hospital, Wakefield

FOURTH EDITION

BRISTOL
WRIGHT
1984

Published by
John Wright & Sons Ltd, 823–825 Bath Road, Bristol BS4 5NU, England.

First Edition 1964
Second Edition 1968
Third Edition 1978
Reprinted 1980
Reprinted 1983
Fourth Edition 1984

British Library Cataloguing in Publication Data

Fish, Frank
  Fish's outline of psychiatry for students and practitioners.—4th ed.
  1.   Psychiatry
  I.   Title   II.   Hamilton, Max
  616.89   RC454

ISBN 0 7236 0797 4

Library of Congress Catalog Card Number: 84–50682

Typeset by
Severntype Repro Services Ltd,
Market Street, Wotton-under-Edge, Glos.

Printed in Great Britain by
John Wright & Sons (Printing) Ltd
at The Stonebridge Press,
Bristol BS4 5NU

PREFACE TO THE FOURTH EDITION

In the seven years since the last edition appeared published researches have been of relevance even to an introductory text. This is partly because of the renewed interest in clinical phenomena and in the classification of mental disorders. In consequence, most of the chapters have required some revision. The changing pattern of psychiatric work justifies the increased space given to anorexia nervosa in Chapter 6 and the new material on drug dependence in Chapter 8. Chapters 8 and 9 also reflect new ideas on anxiety states and affective disorders. The somewhat out of date section on Pavlov in Chapter 3 has been changed to give an account of Behaviour Therapy. The new Mental Health Act has required the rewriting of Chapter 15. Finally, References and Further Reading have been updated.

The teachings of Adolph Meyer were the basis of the first edition of this book. They emphasized the importance of the uniqueness of the individual and his experiences in determining the features of his illness and the details of treatment, but they led to a neglect of the need for proper diagnosis. The renewed interest in diagnosis has arisen, on the theoretical side, from the work in psychiatric genetics and, on the practical side, from the development of effective treatments. General psychiatry has become much less Meyerian and much more neo-Kraepelinian. This edition reflects that change.

I would like to thank my personal assistant, Mrs J. M. Brierly, for her indefatiguable help with the preparation of the materials, checking of references and proof reading.

May 1984   M.H.

v

PREFACE TO THE FIRST EDITION

This book is the result of ten years' experience in the teaching of psychiatry to undergraduate and postgraduate students. Every effort has been made to describe signs and symptoms carefully and to separate fact from theory. No attempt has been made to deal with child psychiatry or mental deficiency, because neither of these subjects can be adequately presented in a short chapter of a general psychiatric textbook. I hope that this book will provide the undergraduate and the general practitioner with the fundamentals of psychiatry and that it will give the postgraduate a framework around which he can organize his knowledge.

The general orientation of this book is best described as 'neo-Meyerian'. In other words, I believe that in any given case all the factors which may *possibly* be relevant should be considered and the appropriate measures, based on empirical knowledge, psychoanalytic theory, sociology, or common sense, should be applied.

The responsibility for the views expressed in this book is, of course, entirely mine, but I would like to take this opportunity of expressing my grateful thanks to my former teachers, especially to Sir Aubrey Lewis, D. L. Davies and Robert Orton. However, perhaps this book owes most to my Chief and friend Alexander Kennedy, whose untimely death three years ago was a great loss to British psychiatry. Although our ideas about psychiatry often diverged, he always encouraged me to express my own point of view and never attempted to impose his views on me. I hope that this book will encourage the development of psychiatric education in Britain—a cause to which Alexander Kennedy devoted his life.

F.J.F.

Department of Psychological Medicine,
University of Edinburgh,
January, 1964.

ACKNOWLEDGEMENTS

Thanks are due to the following: Cassell & Co. Ltd, for permission to quote from *Emotion and Personality,* by M. B. Arnold; the Editor of the *British Journal of Psychiatry,* for permission to quote from an article by J. Inglis (1959) *J. Ment. Sci.* **105,** 440; The Williams & Wilkins Company, Baltimore, for permission to quote from *The Measurement of Intelligence,* by D. Wechsler; Professor G. M. Carstairs, for permission to print the case-taking scheme used in the Department of Psychological Medicine, University of Edinburgh; Professor Karl Leonhard and VEB Verlag Volk und Gesundheit for permission to use material from *Differenzierte Diagnostik der endogenen Psychosen, abnormen Persönlichkeitsstrukturen und neurotischen Entwicklungen;* and William Heinemann Medical Books Ltd, for permission to quote from *Heredity and Environment in the Functional Psychoses,* by E. Kringlen.

CONTENTS

Chapter		Page
1	Aetiology and General Principles	1
2	The History of Psychiatry and the Development of Modern Clinical Psychiatry	8
3	The Schools of Psychiatry	23
4	General Symptomatology	36
5	Abnormal and Psychopathic Personalities	68
6	Psychogenic Reactions, Personality Developments and Neuroses	76
7	Psychosomatic Disorders	92
8	Drug Dependence	100
9	Affective Psychoses and Manic-Depressive Illness	113
10	Schizophrenia and Paranoid States	135
11	Psychiatric Organic States: General Principles	151
12	Psychiatric Organic States: Specific Illnesses	161
13	Sexual Disorders	184
14	The Treatment and Management of Psychiatric Disorders	199
15	Psychiatry and the Law	228
16	Method in Psychiatric Case-Taking	251
	References	259
	Further Reading List	262
	Glossary	265
	Index	287

'Il faut aimer les aliénés pour être digne et capable des les servir.'—ESQUIROL

Chapter 1

Aetiology and general principles

THE NATURE OF PSYCHOLOGICAL THEORIES

Explanatory Psychology

In natural science an attempt is made to establish causal connections. By means of observations and experiments rules are discovered and with further investigations laws are established which, in the end, can be expressed in the form of a mathematical equation.

In morbid and normal psychology the same sort of investigations are carried out: for example, we know that stimulation of the brain can cause hallucinations or forced movements. This type of psychology can be called 'explanatory psychology'.

Empathic or Understanding Psychology

We are all able to empathize with our fellows to some degree. When we do this we feel our way into the situation of the individual and understand his behaviour. In this way we establish an understandable connection between psychological events. Thus we understand that the man who is attacked physically or verbally will become angry and defend himself in some way.

Interpretative Psychology

Simple understanding of our fellows soon develops into interpretations of their behaviour in terms of some ideas borrowed from folk-lore, science, or philosophy. The psychotherapist is forced to organize his experiences of the behaviour of patients in some way. Thus, different varieties of interpretative psychology have arisen which are dependent on the background and personality of the originator.

The Nature of Psychological Explanations

In any discussion of psychopathological phenomena one must be sure of the type of psychology which is being used and not confuse ideas taken from explanatory psychology with those from understanding and interpretative psychology.

THE CAUSATION OF PHYSICAL DISEASE

Often false concepts of the causation of physical disease are carried over into psychological medicine. Thus an infectious disease such as pulmonary tuberculosis is regarded as being caused by the tubercle

1

bacillus, but if this were so, then all of us who have been exposed to infection would develop pulmonary tuberculosis. This does not explain the increased incidence of the disease in certain age-groups and races. While the tubercle bacillus is the essential cause of the illness, a large number of other factors, such as the inherited constitution, the endocrine balance, the diet, overcrowding, and so on, may determine the onset of the illness.

THE CAUSATION OF MENTAL ILLNESS

There is no reason to suppose that the causation of mental illness is different from that of physical illness. As we are uncertain of the essential cause of many nervous illnesses, it is necessary for the psychiatrist to take into account all factors which could possibly have played a part in the production of the illness under consideration. Mental illness should be regarded as the response of the individual to his life situation. When we see a mentally sick person we must ask the threefold question: 'Why did this person break down, in this way, at this time?' The answer is to be found in:

1. The Immediate Situational Stress
   a. Living conditions.
   b. Family relationships.
   c. International relationships outside the home.
   d. Occupational adjustment.
   e. General social conditions such as economic crises, war, etc.
   f. Physical illness.

2. The Constitution
This is the sum total of all the physical and psychological predispositions of the individual and is determined by:
   a. Genetic factors. Sometimes this aspect of the constitution is meant when the word is used. In this case the term 'genetic constitution' should be used.
   b. Physical damage to the nervous system caused by intra-uterine and postnatal disease and trauma.
   c. Psychological influences during development.

GENETICS OF MENTAL DISORDER
Methods of Study
1. *Family Histories of Mental Disorder*
In mental disorders in which psychological factors may play a part, the increased incidence in the children of patients may be due to the psychological effect of parent on child, thus giving a false idea of the genetic basis of the illness.

2. *Incidence of Cousin Marriages in a Given Illness*
If the condition is inherited as a Mendelian recessive, then there will be an excess of cousin marriages among patients with the illness.

3. *Uniovular Twin Studies*
Since both uniovular twins have the same genetic inheritance, they should both suffer from an inherited disease if one of them develops it.

4. *Adoption Studies*
Children adopted early in life will develop mental illness like that of their biological parents, if there is a genetic basis, and like that of their adoptive parents if the main influence is upbringing.

The Importance of Genetics in Mental Disorders
There is no doubt that genetic factors are important in the causation of mental disorders, but so also are environmental ones. It is a mistake to regard them as alternatives. Some psychiatrists neglect the genetic aspects of their work because they feel that, if the illness is inherited, treatment is useless. This is not so, since even inherited biochemical defects can be treated.

It is equally one-sided to deny the importance of psychological factors in the causation of mental illness, since neglect of such factors may lead to inadequate psychotherapy or even to a recurrence of the illness.

COARSE BRAIN DISEASE AND MENTAL ILLNESS
(*See also* Chapter 11)

Mental illness can be caused by damage to the brain due to inflammations, anoxia, wounds, ischaemia, and so on. These usually produce non-specific syndromes, but schizophrenic or manic-depressive clinical pictures can occur (*see* p. 156).

Mild brain damage occurring before birth or in early childhood may not produce mental deficiency as severe damage does, but may make the child more liable to childhood behaviour disorders or, in the presence of genetic factors, to schizophrenia. The disturbance of normal psychological development produced by such mild brain damage may produce a grossly abnormal personality.

There may be a complicated interplay between the direct psychological effects of brain damage and the psychological difficulties due to the disturbance of the environment by the symptoms produced by the coarse brain disease. Thus, in epilepsy, the fits may make it difficult for the sufferer to find work and may cause a revulsion on the part of fellow employees, while the epileptic personality change leads the epileptic to antagonize his fellows. It may be difficult to attribute the degree of the responsibility of the different factors in the epileptic's maladjustment.

PSYCHOLOGICAL INFLUENCES DURING DEVELOPMENT

Parental Attitudes

The child's first environment is its mother. Later, father and siblings may influence the child, and still later the school and the neighbourhood. The influence of the mother on the child is determined by the mother's attitude and the child's constitution. It has been claimed that a dominant, over-possessive mother may produce different disorders in different children, e.g. a passive child who cannot protest, or an overactive child with low tolerance to frustration.

Maternal Deprivation

It has been claimed that maternal deprivation leads to the development of an affectionless character but this has been disputed. There is some evidence that loss of mother before the age of 11 years may predispose to depressive illness.

SOCIAL ENVIRONMENT

Distribution of Schizophrenia and Other Psychoses

Schizophrenics are found in excessive numbers in urban areas characterized by poverty or social isolation. Evidence has accumulated to indicate that this is due to a 'downward drift' by such individuals, probably in the early stages of their illness. This does not apply to manic-depressive disorders. It has been found that the incidence of schizophrenia is higher in Norwegian seamen than in the general population. This may be due to the higher incidence of abnormal personalities among seamen.

Occupation

Chronic mental illness always lowers a person's working capacity, but there is no evidence that particular occupations tend to produce mental illness. Certain workers are at risk for alcoholism, e.g. those in the drink trade, commercial travellers, actors and business executives.

War

Mental hospital admissions decline during major wars, and it is claimed that 'endogenous psychoses' do as well, so that these psychoses are not truly endogenous but partly produced by stress. This is probably fallacious, since mental hospital admissions do not necessarily directly reflect the incidence of psychoses in wartime.

Prison

True prison psychoses ('stir crazy') occur in abnormal personalities who react badly to prison.

Schizophrenia in prison may be the clear appearance of the illness, the prodromal symptoms of which led the person to commit a crime.

STRESS AND REACTION

Stress

If this word is used to mean all the difficulties with which the person is faced, then stress is not a matter of all or nothing, but of degree. Given enough stress, anyone will break down.

The liability to breakdown depends on the nature of the stress for the person as well as on the intensity.

The significance of the stress cannot be estimated in a rational way or in terms of the psychiatrist's own attitudes, which may themselves be irrational in a different way.

Attitudes and ambitions are often illogical, but if they are frustrated then the subject may become profoundly disturbed. There is always the difficulty of understanding too much and attributing causal significance to events which have been produced by the abnormal behaviour which is an essential part of the disease.

Reaction

This word has five different meanings in psychiatry:

1. An active, but mild mental illness may be made worse by some event.

2. An individual with a defective personality caused by mental illness may respond to his environment in an unusual way.

3. A mental illness may be provoked by severe environmental stress.

4. A mental illness may be regarded as an organic reaction, viz. a response of the brain to a physical pathogen.

5. A mental disorder may be a reaction to the environment in the Newtonian mechanical sense that action and reaction are equal and opposite.

Reactive Illnesses

Arguments about reactive illnesses are due to misunderstandings of the use of the word 'reactive'.

If the word is used in the sense of 5 above, then the illness conforms to Jasper's criteria for a reactive illness, as follows:

   a. The content of the mental symptoms has an understandable relation with the experience which caused the illness.

b. The illness would not have occurred without the experience.

c. The course of the illness is dependent on the experience. Thus if the experience could be reversed or cancelled out, the illness would disappear.

If these criteria are accepted, then severe mental illnesses are rarely reactive. The anxiety states in battle are the clearest example of this kind of reactive illness.

However, illnesses do occur in which some event appears to have played a causal role, but the subsequent course of the illness is independent of the causal event and dependent on the individual's personality or his inherited predisposition to a mental illness.

Thus some typical 'endogenous' depressions appear to be touched off by some environmental upset such as losing a job, moving house, or a bereavement, but the further course of the illness is autonomous (independent of the environment). These are reactions in the sense of 3 above, and were called 'provoked depressions' by Lange.

It is best not to distinguish sharply between reactive and endogenous illnesses, but in any given case one should try to estimate the extent to which reactive factors and constitutional predispositions play a part.

PHYSICAL FACTORS

Apart from the direct damage to the brain, there are various physical factors which may provoke or modify mental illnesses. These are age, sex, endocrine changes (including pregnancy), exhaustion, operations, climatic conditions and seasonal variations.

1. Age

Mental illnesses appear to be commoner during puberty and adolescence and also during the involutionary period (females, 40–55 years; males, 50–60 years). Endocrine changes are occurring at both these times, but psychological difficulties are also present. Rigidity increases with age, so that the rigid person tolerates change less as he grows older. All intellectual abilities decline with age, so that the marginally adjusted person may have additional difficulties with age. Decline in immediate memory becomes obvious in the forties. This may cause occupational difficulties.

2. Sex

Some illnesses, such as depression and senile dementia, are commoner in females, while epilepsy and sexual disorders are more frequent in males.

3. Physiological Endocrine Changes

PREMENSTRUAL TENSION

Some women become extremely tense in the week before menstruation and may even be very depressed, with suicidal thoughts, and may attempt suicide. Usually they improve after the first day of menstruation. The tension is sometimes relieved by oral progesterone compounds. Violence, unpleasant behaviour, fits in epileptics, and poor performance in intellectual tasks are more frequent in women just before or during menstruation.

PREGNANCY

Some chronic neurotic women say that the only time that they feel fit and well is during pregnancy. This is also true for those women who suffer from premenstrual tension or dysmenorrhoea. Normally, once the sickness of the first 3 months has died away the next 6 months of pregnancy are not stressful. On the whole, suicide and mental illnesses are rare in pregnancy and if they occur are more often reactions of abnormal personalities to an unwanted pregnancy, in particular an illegitimate one, than major functional psychoses.

PUERPERIUM

A stressful prolonged labour may give rise to a mild organic syndrome, with depression, emotional lability and anxiety. Mild depressions, sometimes accompanied by much anxiety, are much commoner in the post-puerperal period than has been hitherto realized. Schizophrenia may appear during the puerperium, but in some cases there is evidence that symptoms first developed much earlier. Depersonalization may be a prominent symptom in the more severe depressions.

4. *Exhaustion*

Physical exhaustion, particularly when associated with lack of sleep, may produce transient confusional states in which paranoid delusions as well as visual and auditory hallucinations may occur.

5. *Operations*

Psychoses following operations may be produced by exhaustion, lack of sleep, biochemical disorders, infection, or combinations of these factors. Sometimes the operation has been performed on a patient who has hypochondriacal delusions due to depression; the patient is no better despite the removal of an offending viscus, but the psychological basis of the illness is then obvious.

6. *The Climatic Conditions and Seasonal Variations*

Some patients seem to be sensitive to changes in the weather. Gjessing claimed that attacks of periodic catatonia might be brought on by cold fronts and other weather conditions.

The peak period for mental hospital admissions and suicides is the spring. A minor peak occurs in the autumn. No satisfactory reason has been given for this.

Chapter 2

The history of psychiatry and the development of modern clinical psychiatry

THE VALUE OF THE HISTORY OF MEDICINE

The history of our subject allows us to understand the wider aspects of psychological illnesses, to realize the uncertainty of our present-day concepts, and to learn from our predecessors' mistakes by realizing that we are, just as they were, victims of our social and cultural heritage. This will allow us to preserve what is best in the body of knowledge which has been handed down to us, and to discard hampering traditional ideas.

THE ANCIENT WORLD

Hippocrates (*c.* 460–355 B.C.) took a rational and empirical attitude towards disease and claimed that epilepsy was due to natural causes and was not 'The Sacred Disease'. He attributed madness to increased humidity of the brain. He described depression, which he regarded as due to an excess of black bile—hence the term 'melancholia'. He also described delirium, which he called 'phrenitis', and hysteria, which he believed was due to the womb (*hysteros*) wandering about in the body.

Galen (*c.* A.D. 131–200) was a Greek physician practising in Rome, who systematized previous medical knowledge. By this time most physicians believed the theory that all diseases were due to a lack of balance between the four humours out of which the body was composed. Galen claimed that depression was due to an excess of black bile, but that if there was also an excess of yellow bile or if the excess of black bile became overheated the melancholia might develop into mania. This is one of the earliest suggestions that mania and depression are connected. It should be remembered, however, that until the end of the nineteenth century melancholia often meant any kind of insanity in which severe mood changes occurred. Both Galen and Aretaeus the Cappadocian (*c.* A.D. 100) described epileptic personality changes and dementia.

The treatment of the insane varied; on the whole they were treated with drugs such as hellebore, and diversion. However, some doctors recommended beatings, confinement in dark rooms, and general rough handling of the patients in order to bring them to their senses.

8

Psychotherapy: Temple Sleep

Magical treatment was carried out in the temples. The patient went to the priest with a votive offering and slept the night in the temple. Apollo appeared to the patient while he was asleep and cured him.

THE EARLY CHRISTIAN WORLD AND THE DARK AGES

Possession by evil spirits as a cause of disease was a standard belief in the Sumerian civilization (2000 B.C.). It is probable that the Jews took over this belief from the Babylonians. By the time Christianity became an official religion this demoniacal theory of disease was an essential part of the faith. After the fall of Rome, medicine in the Western world was dominated by magical and religious beliefs.

The revival of rational and empirical medicine in the Arab world (tenth and eleventh centuries A.D.) had little effect on psychological medicine, because the Arabs believed in the demoniacal causation of disease. However, Avicenna (980–1037) described the effect of emotions on the pulse-rate.

THE MIDDLE AGES AND THE RENAISSANCE

Witchcraft

It has been alleged that witchcraft existed as a form of devil worship and pagan practices among the European peasantry and was the remains of pre-Christian religion. True or not, witchcraft was regarded by the Catholic Church as a heresy to be rooted out. With the Reformation the Church became more active in its fight against heresy, including witchcraft. The Protestants based their beliefs on the Bible, so that anyone who denied that witches existed was denying the Holy Writ. Thus both Catholic and Protestant hunted for witches.

This belief in witchcraft led to the mentally ill being called witches on account of their strange behaviour. Thus most of the cases of Huntington's chorea in New England are descendants of two brothers from Bures, Suffolk, who emigrated to America in 1630 after their mother had been burnt as a witch. Many schizophrenics believed that they were witches or that they were bewitched. Little was known about the causation of disease, so that the death of humans and animals from natural causes was often attributed to witchcraft.

In Germany, Johannes Weyer (1515–88), and in Britain, Reginald Scott (1538–99), pointed out that witches were mentally ill. However, King James I of England firmly believed in witches and wrote a book in support of this belief.

In France, St Vincent de Paul (1576–1660) claimed that many witches were really mentally disordered and founded the mental hospital of St Lazare. He wrote: 'Mental disease is no different from bodily disease. Christianity demands of the humane and the powerful to protect and of the skilful to relieve the one as well as the other.'

THE FOUNDATION OF MODERN PSYCHIATRY

One of the great breaks in the humoral theory of disease came from the work of Thomas Sydenham (1624–89) who put forward the concept of the natural history of disease and the idea that diseases could be regarded as entities and not as a lack of balance of the humours. In the following years many different classifications of disease were put forward. In 1971 G. B. Morgagni (1682–1771) published *De sedibus et causis morborum per anatomen indagatis,* in which he correlated post-mortem findings with the clinical pictures of disease. At the same time many large new hospitals were being founded and doctors had the opportunity of studying large numbers of patients with the same sorts of illness.

In psychiatry, developments lagged fifty to one hundred years. Philippe Pinel (1745–1826) began in 1793 the humane treatment of the insane when he was appointed as Chief of the Bicêtre, a large institution in Paris for the custodial care of the insane. Just about the same time William Tuke, a York merchant and a member of the Society of Friends (Quakers), was horrified by the death of a Quaker woman in York Asylum. He persuaded the York meeting of Quakers to found a hospital for the humane care of the insane. This hospital was called 'The Retreat' and set a standard which helped to raise the institutional care of the insane throughout the world.

The increase in the numbers of institutions for the care of the insane led to the development of clinical psychiatry, while the rediscovery of hypnotism by Franz Anton Mesmer (1734–1815), and its more practical use by Braid and Charcot in the nineteenth century, led to the development of psychotherapy and psychodynamics.

THE MENTAL HOSPITALS AND THE 'NON-RESTRAINT' MOVEMENT

In Britain after 1800 many private and public mental asylums were built, and in England after the English Lunacy Act of 1808 the local authorities had a legal obligation for the care of the insane. Many of these asylums used physical restraint in the form of handcuffs, strait-jackets and chains. In 1835 Dr Gardiner Hill began to remove mechanical restraints in Lincoln Asylum, and in 1839 Dr John Conolly abolished all mechanical restraint in Hanwell Asylum, Middlesex. This led to a decline in the use of mechanical restraint throughout Britain, Europe and the USA. This is usually referred to as the 'non-restraint movement'. It has been alleged that to some extent physical restraint was replaced by chemical restraint, and also that non-violent patients suffered from the lack of restraint of the violent ones. Thus, a mentally ill clergyman in Hanwell Asylum wrote:

> We have in this asylum, Sir, some doctors of renown,
> With a plan of non-restraint which they seem to think they own;
> All well-meaning men, Sir, but troubled with the complaint,
> Called the monomania of total non-restraint.

THE DEVELOPMENT OF MODERN CLINICAL PSYCHIATRY

The Problems to be Solved

The nineteenth-century psychiatrists were faced with two puzzling problems: (1) the relationship between coarse brain disease and mental symptoms; and (2) the relationship of delusions to insanity.

1. *The Relationship between Coarse Brain Disease and Mental Symptoms*

This was clarified by post-mortem studies, but the solution of this problem was difficult, because most coarse brain diseases produce non-specific clinical pictures (*see* pp. 14, 151) which are more related to the extent and tempo of the disease process than to the specific nature of the disease (*see* p. 151). An additional complication was that delusions and other psychiatric symptoms occurred in patients with coarse brain disease and in those whose brains were normal at post-mortem.

2. *The Relationship of Delusions to Insanity*

Some patients, such as manics, are not deluded but are nevertheless insane, while in others delusion is an essential feature of the madness. It was these non-deluded patients whom Prichard (1786–1848) classified as cases of moral insanity. The other problem was the prognostic significance of delusions. Some patients, severe depressives in our current classification, were very deluded but recovered, while others, whom we now call schizophrenics, were just as deluded and never recovered.

The French School

Since Pinel examined and made clinical notes on the large number of patients under his care, it is natural that the first school of clinical psychiatry was in Paris. Pinel's most outstanding pupil, J. E. D. Esquirol (1772–1840), was the founder of modern psychiatry. He introduced the term 'hallucination' as a *perception sans objet* and distinguished it from illusion. He made simple statistical investigations of the causes of mental illness, which are to be found in his two-volume book on mental disorders published in 1838. In 1805 he pointed out that paralysis was a common complication of insanity.

In 1822 A. L. J. Bayle presented a thesis in the University of Paris in which he attributed the mental symptoms, delusions, intellectual enfeeblement and exaltation, to the same disease of the coverings of the brain which produced the paralysis. In 1824 J. B. Delaye claimed that general paralysis was due to a disease of the white matter of the brain. Calmeil (1798–1895), Baillarger (1809–90) and Falret (1794–1870) all helped to establish general paralysis of the insane (GPI) as a disease entity. Kraft-Ebing (1840–1903) proved the syphilitic origin of the disease.

This discovery of the somatic basis of a mental illness led many psychiatrists to expect that a physical basis would soon be found for all psychological disorders.

The French school also laid the basis for the classification of the so-called functional psychoses. J. P. Falret was interested in suicide and found that some depressives improved and then passed into a state of elation, and some elated patients became depressed. He called this closed emotional cycle *la folie circulaire*. Baillarger, a great neuro-pathologist and clinical psychiatrist, studied hallucinations and realized that sometimes they were produced psychologically. He also described melancholic stupor, when previously all stupors were regarded as organic. He confirmed the existence of Falret's *folie circulaire* and called it *folie à double forme*.

B. A. Morel (1809–73) was interested in the concept of degeneration and considered that mental illnesses were hereditary weaknesses. In 1860 he described mental deterioration in a previously bright boy of 14 years of age, and called this *démence précoce* (dementia praecox).

The German School

The Germans further developed French work and German psychiatry expanded rapidly. From 1864 to 1889 ten chairs of neuropsychiatry were founded in German-speaking universities. In comparison, the first English Professor in Mental Diseases was W. Bevan Lewis, appointed in Leeds in 1908, and the first permanent chair in psychiatry in Britain was established in Edinburgh in 1919.

The first outstanding German psychiatrist was Wilhelm Griesinger (1817–68). He was convinced that mental disorders were disorders of the brain and believed that all psychoses were merely different expressions of one common disease (*Einheitsfsychose*). His successor, Westphal, described and defined obsessions and also made observations on homosexuality and phobias.

The first step in the classification and understanding of 'functional' mental disorder was made by K. L. Kahlbaum (1828–99) and his lifelong friend and colleague E. Hecker (1843–1909). Kahlbaum suggested that any disease entity must conform to the following two criteria: (1) the whole course of the illness must be taken into account;

and (2) the total clinical picture must be adequately delineated. On this basis, he described a severe motor disorder consisting of strange attitudes, odd movements and postures, together with stupor and mental deterioration, in a monograph, *Catatonia or Tension Insanity*, published in 1874. He also coined the words 'verbigeration' and 'symptom complex' and later introduced the term 'cyclothymia' when writing about circular insanity. Hecker, in 1871, described a rapid mental deterioration occurring during puberty and called it 'hebephrenia'.

Emil Kraepelin (1855–1926) is probably the most outstanding psychiatrist who ever lived. In the English-speaking world, where much of his work has never been well known, there is a tendency among some so-called dynamic psychiatrists to use his name as a synonym for useless dry-as-dust pedantry in psychiatry. Nothing could be farther from the truth. He qualified in 1878 and became an assistant to Gudden in Munich. In 1882 he moved to Leipzig to work in Flechsig's clinic, but left there fairly soon to study experimental psychology under Wundt. In 1883 he published a *Compendium of Psychiatry*. At about the same time he also wrote a brochure against capital and corporal punishment and the determinate sentence, as he believed that criminal law should have the purpose of betterment and rehabilitation of the law-breaker. The *Compendium* was later republished as a textbook in nine different editions, the last appearing the year after his death. He was called to the Chair in Heidelberg in 1891 and thereafter he developed his classification of mental disease very rapidly, using Kahlbaum's two principles of common symptomatology and common course of illness. In 1893, in the fourth edition of his textbook, he brought together Morel's dementia praecox, Hecker's hebephrenia, Kahlbaum's catatonia, and paranoid illnesses with deterioration (dementia paranoides) as psychological degeneration processes. In the next edition of this book in 1896, he called this group 'processes of mental deterioration' and included them in a larger group of metabolic disorders. In the sixth edition of his book he called all these illnesses 'dementia praecox', although by then he knew that these illnesses did not always occur in adolescence and did not always lead to deterioration of the personality.

In 1893 he grouped depressive and manic illnesses together as 'periodic mental illnesses', but in 1899 he grouped together recurrent depressions, recurrent mania, and circular insanity as manic-depressive insanity. He claimed that these patients showed mild mood abnormality when well and from time to time developed severe affective illnesses. He pointed out that, apart from clear states of mania and depression, 'mixed states' occurred in which manic and depressive symptoms were present at the same time.

Apart from his clinical work, he and his pupils carried out many psychological experiments on patients and he can be regarded as the founder of clinical psychology. In 1904 he returned to Munich as the Director of the Psychiatric Research Institute and remained there until his death.

Kraepelin's great rival was Carl Wernicke (1848–1905), whose early work on aphasia led him to look for discrete lesions as the cause of mental illnesses. He did not accept Kraepelin's division of the major functional psychoses into two main groups, but tried to isolate many different clinical pictures. This careful delineation of different functional psychoses was carried further by his pupil Karl Kleist (1879–1960). Wernicke explained all psychiatric phenomena in terms of 'sejunction', viz., the breaking of connections between different centres in the brain. He was the first to use the term 'autochthonous ideas' and to differentiate between disorders of impressibility (registration) and retention in memory disorders. He also defined overvalued ideas and distinguished between primary delusions and explanatory delusions.

Karl Bonhoeffer (1868–1948), Wernicke's most outstanding senior assistant and later Professor of Neurology and Psychiatry at Berlin University, investigated the mental disorders associated with coarse brain disease and in 1910 published his classic monograph in which he showed that on the whole the type of mental disease produced by coarse brain disorders was dependent on the site, extent and tempo of the morbid process rather than on the specific nature of the brain disease.

Before turning to the problem of neuroses we must consider the last of the great German-speaking founder psychiatrists, Eugen Bleuler (1857–1939). He was the first clinical psychiatrist to apply Freud's ideas to the study of psychotic symptoms. He did this with his assistant, C. G. Jung, who himself carried out verbal association experiments on the psychologically ill. In 1911 Bleuler wrote his classic monograph *Dementia Praecox, or the Group of Schizophrenias*. He coined the word 'schizophrenia' in order to get away from the implications of the term 'dementia praecox', viz., that the condition always occurred in adolescence and led to intellectual impairment. He used the term 'schizophrenia' because he believed that the functions of the mind were split off from each other in this disease. Although the importance of this book was quickly recognized by English-speaking psychiatrists, it was not translated into English until 1955.

THE DEVELOPMENT OF PSYCHOTHERAPY AND THE THEORIES OF THE NEUROSES

Hypnotism

Hypnotism and suggestive psychotherapy have been used from time immemorial. In the late eighteenth century Franz Anton Mesmer practised hypnotism, which he called 'animal magnetism'. He made exaggerated claims, was to some extent a charlatan, and brought the subject into disrepute. Later, in 1837, John Elliotson (1791–1868) practised hypnotism in University College Hospital, where he was Professor of Medicine. This caused so much resentment among the physicians and surgeons there that he was forbidden to practise hypnotism within the hospital, and resigned in protest.

James Braid (1795–1860), a Scot who practised in Manchester, coined the term 'hypnotism'. He showed that animal magnetism and similar theories were nonsense, but that the phenomena were real.

Liébault (1823–1904) was a family doctor in Nancy who used hypnosis to treat his patients. Later Professor Bernheim taught hypnotism in the same town.

J. M. Charcot (1825–93), the founder of modern neurology, was Professor of Pathological Anatomy in Paris from 1867 and was appointed in 1882 to a Chair in Diseases of the Nervous System, specially created for him in the University of Paris. He was very interested in hysteria and hypnotism and can be said to have made the latter a respectable subject. This French school of neurologist-psychotherapists produced many outstanding psychiatrists, including Pierre Janet.

Freud

Sigmund Freud (1856–1939) was interested in mild nervous disorders, and in 1885 he studied under Charcot in Paris and also visited Bernheim in Nancy. It was when Freud saw a case with Bernheim that he first had an inkling of the idea of the unconscious.

Freud had practically no training in psychiatry and this was at one and the same time his strength and his weakness. At this time neurotic illnesses were regarded by most psychiatrists as constitutional disorders mainly due to inherited predisposition to degeneration. This view was clearly expressed by J. L. A. Koch (1891) in his monograph *The Psychopathic Inferiorities*. Freud, following the Nancy School, regarded the minor nervous disorders as illnesses susceptible to treatment. He was first a neurologist and his investigations into aphasia and infantile hemiplegia were fundamental contributions to this specialty. In the course of his work he met with many mild non-organic nervous disorders, which at first he tried to treat with hypnosis. He found that this was not of much use, since the patient tended to forget any material which was recalled during hypnosis.

He developed the technique of psychoanalysis, in which the patient was encouraged to allow his thoughts to proceed without any conscious direction. It was assumed that the thought would then be directed by unconscious processes and important material would emerge which would be responsible for the patient's symptoms. By bringing this unconscious material into consciousness the patient would be relieved of

his symptoms. Gradually Freud realized that this simple idea of a
neurosis as due to some hidden conflict in the unconscious was a gross
oversimplification. He then developed his theory of infantile sexuality
and the development of the sexual drive or libido during childhood.
Difficulties in family relationships and constitutional factors led to
conflicts at certain points in childhood sexual development, and
reactivation of such conflicts by disappointments later in life produced
neurosis (see p. 27). Later, Freud and his followers realized that in
some individuals the mental disorder could be regarded more as a part
of the total character abnormality and called such states 'character
neuroses'. Freud and his followers popularized psychotherapy and
helped untold numbers of neurotics directly and indirectly. However,
they tended to overlook the simple fact that the psychological
determination of a symptom is not necessarily the same as the
causation of the symptom. Or, to put the problem in another way, what
determines the content of the symptom is not necessarily its
cause.

Two of Freud's early pupils, Alfred Adler (1870–1937) and
C. G. Jung (1875–1961), disagreed with him and formed separate
schools of individual and analytical psychology (see pp. 29–31).

THE DEVELOPMENT OF PSYCHIATRY IN BRITAIN
AND THE USA

The outstanding British contributions to psychiatry were the humane
care of the insane and the 'non-restraint' movement. In clinical
psychiatry Anglo-American medicine has contributed little.

John Haslam (1764–1844) described a case of GPI in his
Observations in Insanity in 1798. Pinel thought very highly of his work
and in his own book *Sur l'Alienation Mentale,* published in 1800, he
refers to Haslam's work more than to any other author. Haslam was
Apothecary to Bethlem Hospital under the physician Monro. In 1816 he
was dismissed from his post with Monro because of scandals concerning
the management of patients.

J. C. Prichard (1786–1848), who introduced the term 'moral
insanity', was physician to the Bristol Royal Infirmary, a pioneer in the
field of ethnology, and a man of great erudition, but he added nothing but
confusion to psychiatry.

In Scotland, the Royal Edinburgh Asylum, Morningside, was founded
in 1809. Sir Alexander Morison started a systematic course of lectures
in Edinburgh in 1823, since when psychiatry has been taught systemati-
cally to the present day.

David Skae became Physician Superintendent of the Edinburgh
Royal Asylum in 1846 and was the founder of the Edinburgh School of
Psychiatry, which was the only psychiatric postgraduate teaching centre

in Britain until the Maudsley Hospital opened in 1922. G. M. Robertson (1864–1932) was one of the first psychiatrists to introduce round-the-clock nursing of acutely mentally ill male patients by female nurses. He campaigned to change asylums into hospitals and it was largely due to him that Jordanburn Nerve Hospital was opened in 1929 as a public hospital for mild nervous diseases, which was quite outside the Lunacy Acts, so that patients could be admitted and discharged without any legal formality.

In London, Bethlem Hospital improved as the nineteenth century wore on, and came under the direction of George Savage, an enlightened man and a good clinician. The Retreat came under the direction of Daniel Hack Tuke, the great-grandson of William Tuke, the only psychiatrist produced by the family of the man who pioneered the humane care of the mentally ill.

Henry Maudsley (1835–1918) was one of the outstanding psychiatrists in Britain in the late nineteenth and early twentieth centuries. He gave a large sum of money in order to found a university teaching clinic in London from which came the Maudsley Hospital, now associated with the Institute of Psychiatry of the University of London. He was sceptical of most forms of treatment current in his day. He classified mental illnesses into effective and ideational groups.

One of the most influential psychiatrists in the English-speaking world in recent times was Adolf Meyer (1866–1950), a Swiss, who became Professor of Psychiatry at the Johns Hopkins University, and Director of the Henry Phipps Clinic at the Johns Hopkins Hospital in 1910.

He regarded mental illness as a reaction of a person to environmental difficulties, so that when faced with a patient the psychiatrist should ask the following questions: (1) What are this person's available resources? (2) What are his faults and failings? (3) What are his assets? (4) What was he like at his best? (5) How can his various difficulties be modified?

He stressed the need for a longitudinal study of the life of each patient because it would help in prognosis, diagnosis, and treatment. All possible factors—social, environmental, sexual, and somatic—must be considered in relation to the life of the individual. A complete estimate of potential assets is essential for adequate treatment and prognosis. He considered that Kraepelin's system was too rigid and allowed the unwary to neglect the role of the patient's life situation in the causation, continuation and treatment of the illness. He encouraged the growth of psychiatric social work and occupational therapy. Unfortunately, although his vague and all-embracing concept of 'psychobiology' encouraged an interest in the individuality of the patient, it gave very much less direction on what to do about him.

DEVELOPMENTS IN TREATMENT
The Malarial Therapy of GPI
The year 1917 is one of the most important in the history of psychiatry, because in that year Wagner-Jauregg, Professor of Psychiatry in Vienna, showed that malaria could cure GPI. This was the first successful treatment of a mental disease by physical means and raised great hopes for the future.

Insulin Coma Therapy
Sakel of Vienna introduced this treatment following the successful use of insulin in the treatment of withdrawal symptoms in drug addicts. He published his results of insulin coma therapy in 1933. This treatment received enthusiastic support but fell into disuse after the introduction of the phenothiazines. Only one controlled trial of this treatment was ever carried out, by Ackner and his colleagues (Ackner, Harris and Oldham, 1957; Ackner and Oldham, 1962), and the results gave no indication that the treatment was any better than a dummy treatment. It is still used in the more backward parts of the psychiatric world. The lack of evidence in favour of a treatment has never deterred enthusiasts from carrying it out, whether within psychiatry or without.

Convulsion Therapy
About A.D. 45 Scribonius Largus, a Roman physician, recommended that as a cure for a headache the Mediterranean torpedo fish should be placed across the brows of the sufferer. This fish develops an electrical potential of 100–150 Volts. In the late eighteenth and the nineteenth centuries are were scattered references to insanity being cured by fits induced by large doses of camphor.

After the isolation of schizophrenia the belief that schizophrenics did not suffer from epilepsy was expressed by many German psychiatrists. This was sometimes expressed in another way, i.e. schizophrenia and epilepsy are opposite diseases. Working on this theory, von Meduna of Budapest decided in 1933 to give schizophrenics epilepsy. He used intramuscular injections of 20 per cent camphor and some of his schizophrenics recovered. However, since camphor was uncertain in its action, it was suggested to him that an artificial convulsant, pentamethylenetetrazol (cardiazol), be used instead. This treatment was then widely used in schizophrenia.

Ugo Cerletti, a neuropsychiatrist and neuropathologist, had for many years investigated the effect of electrically produced fits in dogs in an attempt to determine whether the changes found in Ammon's horn in epileptics were primary or a secondary effect of the anoxia during fits. His collaborator, Bini, took part in this work and devised the electrical apparatus. After von Meduna introduced convulsive therapy Cerletti thought that electrically produced fits would probably be just as effective, but he was deterred by reports that passage of an electric current through the human head was fatal. Shortly after he was called to the Chair of Psychiatry and Neurology in Rome, he was told that pigs were killed by electricity in the Rome slaughterhouses, but he found that the pigs were stunned by the passage of electricity through the head and then the throat was cut. He obtained permission to kill pigs by electricity and found it was only possible to do this if the current passed through the chest, but not if it passed through the head. He therefore felt justified in passing an electric current through a patient's head in order to produce a fit. He did this in 1938 and found it to be an effective and safe treatment.

As convulsive treatment became widely used it was realized that it was a much more effective treatment for depression than for schizophrenia.

Leucotomy (Lobotomy)

In 1874 Leopold Goltz, of Strasbourg, reported that large ablations of the cerebral hemispheres in dogs led to striking changes in behaviour. G. Burckhardt, medical director of a small Swiss mental hospital, inspired by this work of Goltz, carried out ablations of the temporo-parietal cortex in four agitated mental patients, with improvement in only one case. The publication of his results led to a storm of criticism of his unethical behaviour.

At the International Congress of Neurology in 1935, Fulton and Jacobsen described the behaviour of chimpanzees after ablation of the frontal cortex. Unlike normal chimps, these animals did not become upset when they failed on psychological tests and did not develop 'experimental neuroses' when overtrained. This led Egas Moniz to persuade his neurosurgical colleague Almeida Lima to destroy the connections of the frontal lobes in mentally ill patients. This treatment was successful in anxious and tense patients. Lima and Moniz published their work in 1936. Since the introduction of the phenothiazines and the thymoleptic drugs, it has been largely abandoned, though it has some limited use for severe chronic treatment-resistant depressions, anxiety and obsessional states.

The Modern Drugs

Amphetamine was introduced for the treatment of narcolepsy in 1935 and was later used in psychiatry as a euphoriant. It is now of very little value in psychiatry and should be regarded as obsolete in this branch of medicine.

Reserpine, the active principle of the Indian plant *Rauwolfia serpentina,* was introduced in the early fifties for the treatment of disturbed schizophrenics, although it had been used in the treatment of mental disease by the indigenous practitioners of India for centuries.

The phenothiazines were introduced into medicine as antihistaminics, but it was soon realized that they tended to produce drowsiness. This led to the use of chlorpromazine as a tranquillizer in mania and schizophrenia. Since then many other phenothiazines have been introduced and also other classes of compounds. Several of these have an antidepressive effect.

In 1951 isoniazid was found to be an effective antibiotic in tuberculosis and to have a euphoriant side-effect. Later, iproniazid, an isomer of isoniazid, was found to be an antidepressant. As this drug tends to produce severe jaundice, other drugs were introduced which, like iproniazid, inhibited the activity of mono-amine oxidase.

PROBLEMS OF CLASSIFICATION OF MENTAL DISORDERS

The work of the morbid anatomists of the eighteenth and nineteenth centuries led to a fundamental distinction between those disorders which were associated with evidence of damage to the organs of the body and those which were not. The traditional classification of mental disorders starts with this dichotomy. The organic group of disorders are then further subdivided in accordance with their aetiology. The functional group are subdivided into psychoses and neuroses. The former includes schizophrenia (including the paranoid conditions) and manic-depressive disorder. The latter includes anxiety neuroses, obsessional neuroses, hysteria and anorexia nervosa. The personality disorders, sexual anomalies and disturbances, and drug addictions are sometimes included among the neuroses but are often considered to be a separate group.

The distinction between psychoses and neuroses is usually based on the following criteria:

1. Insight
The neurotic has insight, but the psychotic has not.

Objection
Some hysterics have no insight, while some depressives (autonomous dysthymics), some young intelligent schizophrenics and quite a number of arteriosclerotic dements realize that they are mentally ill.

2. Involvement of the Personality
In neurosis the personality is only partly involved, but in psychosis the whole personality is distorted by the illness.

Objection
Some hysterics and obsessional neurotics have personalities which are totally involved in the illness, while some manic-depressives manage to live with their illness.

3. Social Adaptation
The neurotic makes a fair social adjustment, but the psychotic is unable to do so.

Objection
Hysterics may be unable to work, while some depressives and paranoid schizophrenics can.

4. The Reality of Subjective Experiences
The neurotic can distinguish between his subjective experiences and reality while the psychotic cannot.

Objection
Some hysterics live in a world of fantasy, while some depressives can distinguish between their inner experience and reality.

5. The Reality of the Environment
The psychotic constructs a false environment, but the neurotic does not.

Objection
Some hysterics and obsessional neurotics live in fantastic environments of their own creation, while delusional reconstruction of the environment does not necessarily occur in severe depression.

6. Disorder of Drives
In psychosis there is a gross disorder of drives including that of self-preservation, whereas this does not occur in the neuroses.

Objection
Some neurotics commit suicide and patients with anorexia nervosa starve themselves to death.

7. Understandability
A psychosis is a mental illness in which a marked personality change occurs, which cannot be interpreted as an understandable development of the personality to psychological trauma.

Comment
It is clear that, with the exception of the last criterion, understandability, the distinctions between psychoses and neuroses are unsatisfactory. The value that this classification had when it was first made has now diminished considerably as can be seen in the confused discussions in the literature on the alleged differences between psychotic and neurotic depressions.

The distinction between psychosis and neurosis only too often signifies the difference between schizophrenia and other mental disorders. Sometimes 'psychotic' is used to mean severe in contrast to 'neurotic', which means mild, but it is inexcusable to use obscure jargon instead of plain words with a clear meaning. Those who do so are either trying to impress their hearers or have never really seriously tried to clarify their thinking. However, it is customary to use 'neurosis' to cover those functional conditions other than the schizophrenic and affective disorders. This is similar to the distinction between 'organic' and 'functional' mental disorders where, although modern research has blurred the boundary, it is still convenient to use 'organic' for a group of disorders with clearly recognized pathological bases.

Psychiatric disorders can conveniently be classified into three major groups:

1. Organic states, where the illness is the result of a demonstrable brain disorder.

2. 'Functional psychoses', in which a definite break has occurred in the life pattern, which cannot be understood as a reaction or a development of the personality. These illnesses—schizophrenia and the affective psychoses—are probably the result of special disorders of the brain.

3. Variations of human existence, which deviate from the mean quantitatively but not qualitatively, and which produce subjective disturbances or disrupt interpersonal and social relationships. They can best be regarded as psychogenic reactions or personality developments, which are understandable responses of normal, accentuated, or abnormal personalities to stress.

Chapter 3

The schools of psychiatry

PSYCHOANALYSIS: FREUD AND HIS PUPILS

Psychoanalysis was originally used to designate the technique of free association which Freud used in psychotherapy. Later it also came to mean the theory which Freud constructed to explain the material which emerged in psychotherapy. This can be considered from three different points of view: (1) the theory of mental structure; (2) the theory of libidinal development; and (3) the economics of the mental dynamics.

The Unconscious

Freud originally divided the mind into the conscious and the unconscious. The latter consisted of the representations of the instinctual forces which were always striving for expression in consciousness, and also of representations which had been conscious but because of their conflict with the person's general attitudes had been unconsciously forced into the unconscious or repressed. According to Freud, unconscious processes were non-logical and ignored the concepts of space and time. Contradictory ideas and feelings could exist together. Unconscious processes make use of various mechanisms (*see* pp. 125–127).

The Structure of the Mind

Freud divided the mind into three dynamic systems: the id, the superego, and the ego.

1. *The Id*

This is the fundamental source of all psychic energy, since it consists of all the instinctual needs striving for fulfilment. It includes the instinct of aggression as well as the sexual instinct.

2. *The Superego*

Roughly this is the conscience. In the Oedipal stage (*see* p. 25) the child identifies with his parents and incorporates their standards of right and wrong. This introjected parental image acquires energy from the id and forms the superego, which is partly unconscious. Since the parental image of the child of 4 or 5 years of age is capricious, illogical, and even destructive, the superego may show these traits.

3. *The Ego*

This has the task of balancing the demands of the real world, the id and the superego. It has no energy of its own and has to borrow energy from the other two systems.

This structure of the mind develops *pari passu* with the development of infantile sexuality and the ability to relate to objects.

The Instincts and Libidinal Development

Freud derived all drives from two major instincts—Eros, or the group of self-preservation drives, and Thanatos, or the self-destructive, aggressive group of drives. The latter group has not been accepted by all his followers. The sexual instinct, which has a somatic basis, is the main source of psychic energy, and is called the libido.

When Freud used the words 'infantile sexuality' and referred to the infant having libidinal satisfaction, he was using the word 'sexual' in a very wide sense, to include all kinds of pleasure that the child obtains from his bodily sensations.

The activities of the child at different stages of its development are focused on different mucocutaneous junctional areas of the body. Thus there are the oral, anal and phallic stages of libidinal development. The infant desires gratification of the instinctual needs connected with the given stage. If these needs are under- or over-gratified, or there is a constitutional bias, then the conflicts usually present at the particular stage are not resolved. The child passes on to the next stage, but a weak spot in the libidinal organization is left behind, which may allow the reactivation of the conflicts at this stage under stress in adult life. This is a *fixation point*. The stages of development are:

1. *Primary Narcissism*

Against all the evidence, it is held that the neonate cannot distinguish between himself and his environment and is unable to relate to objects. He gets attention when he is dirty or hungry by crying and the regular association between his actions and the response of the environment leads to a sense of omnipotence and a belief that he has unlimited powers over his environment.

2. *The Oral Stage*

This begins at birth and can be divided into:

a. THE EARLY ORAL STAGE
Here the infant gets pleasure from sucking.

b. THE LATE ORAL STAGE
Teeth have now appeared and the child gets pleasure from biting. Aggressive impulses can be expressed by biting and this stage is therefore called the *oral sadistic* stage.

The world now consists of objects which can or cannot be swallowed; the only object relation possible at this stage is therefore incorporation.

3. The Anal Stage

This begins in the second year, when the child gets pleasure from defecation. Passing and retaining faeces are easily connected with aggression so that this is the *anal sadistic stage*. This stage can be divided into:

    a. The early anal stage: Here the child gets pleasure from eliminating and pinching off the faeces.

    b. The late anal stage: Here he experiences pleasure from retaining faeces. Thus the child behaves in a contradictory way, as he wants both to retain and expel his faeces. This ambivalence (*see* p. 58) is associated with anal eroticism. Partial love of objects with ambivalence is possible in this stage.

4. The Phallic Stage

By the fourth year the libido is centred on the genitalia, and sexuality is connected with a special love object. The little boy loves his mother, regards father as a rival, and wishes him dead. This is the Oedipus complex. The boy attributes to his father the same sort of wishes that he himself has towards his father. He realizes the anatomical difference between the sexes and regards females as castrated males, so that it seems possible to the boy that his father's supposed aggression towards him might take the form of castration. This crisis is solved by the boy identifying with his father and introjecting parental attitudes as they appear to him, i.e. the superego is formed. In the girl sexual sensation is experienced in the clitoris, but she soon realizes that she has no penis; this gives rise to penis envy and she wants to get a penis from her father. The penis is equated with a child and she now loves her father and wishes her hated rival, her mother, dead. This is resolved by identification with the mother. In both sexes the Oedipal situation is resolved by identification with the parent of the same sex, or partially dealt with and then repressed.

5. The Latency Period

Sex drive subsides after the sixth year and reappears at puberty.

The Economics of the Mind

The ego has to control the unacceptable instinctual drives in such a way as to suffer the least discomfort and to achieve the greatest possible degree of coherence with the minimum amount of effort. This is done by defence mechanisms which (1) emerge at different stages of libidinal development; (2) have different relationships with consciousness; (3) vary in flexibility; and (4) may be more often associated with one or another of the instinctual drives. These mechanisms are: repression, reaction formation, displacement, aim inhibition, sublimation, projection, introjection, identification, isolation, undoing and regression. These will now be discussed individually, but they are usually all at work at the same time.

Repression

All ideas have a charge of energy or cathexis which produces the emotion appropriate to the idea, when the idea becomes conscious. Some ideas give rise to anxiety when conscious because the associated instinctive drive is not approved of by ego or superego. If this occurs, the unwanted idea is unconsciously pushed out of consciousness by the mechanism of repression in which there is a withdrawal of cathexis from the idea and a charging of opposing ideas with cathexis, so-called countercathexis. The repressed idea may obtain indirect representation in consciousness, but if this causes anxiety it may be repressed as well. This is secondary repression.

Reaction Formation

The disturbing ideas are kept unconscious by the presence of the opposite ideas in consciousness. Thus excessive prudery can be a reaction formation against powerful sex drives.

Displacement

The cathexis is transferred from the unacceptable ideas to other associated ideas which can appear in consciousness without causing anxiety. This is a more flexible means of defence than reaction formation. Displacement is closely linked to symbolization.

Aim Inhibition

The aim or goal of the instinctive drive is modified, but the original drive is satisfied to some extent. Thus a desire in a child for sexual relations with a parent may be changed into an attitude of love and respect in which there is no overt sexual element.

Sublimation

The original aims of a drive are permanently and totally changed and are gratified by the new aim. Thus infantile sexual drives are desexualized and the libido is transferred to a new goal-directed activity which is decided by the ego and approved by the superego.

Projection

Repressed ideas are attributed to others. The unpleasant affect which such ideas would arouse in consciousness is blamed on the ideas and attitudes of others.

Introjection

The object is, as it were, ingested by the mind, so that the psychic energies of the ego appear to be organized as if they were under the control of the introject.

Identification

The person adopts the ideas and attitudes of an object, but still maintains a relation with the object which, unlike the introject, does not function only as if it were part of the ego.

Isolation

The impulse to action, thought, or act is isolated from the associated affect and the wider associations connected with it. The thought, for example, is conscious without the distressing associations or affect. This defence is found in obsessional neuroses.

Undoing

The disturbing thought or action is allowed to occur and is then followed by the opposite thought or act, which cancels out the effect of the first thought or act in a magical way. This mechanism is especially seen in obsessions and compulsions.

Regression

The mind returns to an earlier stage of libidinal or ego organization, so that there are both libidinal and ego regressions. The degree of regression depends on the fixation points (*see* p. 24). Regression in normals occurs in dreams, daydreams and fantasy. Fantasy is a means of defence since it often allows the ego to balance the demands of the id and the environment.

Introversion*

This occurs when a person withdraws from environmental contacts and indulges in excessive fantasy. This is usually followed by marked regression.

The Freudian Theory of Neurosis

1. *Release of Libido*

A loved object is lost, e.g. a friend or relative dies, and this means that the libido invested in that object is set free. This causes regression and reactivation of the conflicts at the fixation points. A neurosis occurs if the amount of free libido is excessive and if the infantile conflicts at the fixation point were not solved or partially solved by pathological mechanisms.

*This should not be confused with the Jungian concept of introversion (*see* p. 31).

2. *Failure of Repression*

Unconscious ideas, related to the reactivated infantile conflict at the fixation point, acquire enough psychic energy to force themselves into consciousness and give rise to anxiety. Other defence mechanisms such as displacement and projection then come into action in order to camouflage the ideas painful to the ego. This leads to a symptom which is a conscious but distorted expression of the unconscious conflict. The major defence mechanism at work in any given mental illness depends on the stage of libidinal development at which the fixation point occurred.

Character Neurosis

In many neurotics the defence mechanisms have modified the ego and superego. In this case the patient acts out his difficulties and is suffering from a character neurosis. It is, therefore, possible to refer to the character in terms of the fixation point, so that one can have an anal character or an oral character, and so on (*see* pp. 24–25).

Freud's Theory of Dreams

As Freud and his followers often used dreams as a starting point in analysis, Freudian dream theory is of considerable importance.

1. *Manifest and Latent Content*

Freud believed that the dream as it was reproduced in the waking state (its manifest content) could be traced back to its origins (latent content). The change from latent to manifest content was the product of dream work in which condensation, displacement and symbolization played a great part. One can always find in the latent content material from the previous day and from childhood.

2. *The Dream as 'Wish-fulfilment'*

Freud claimed that the dream was always the fulfilment of a wish, although, because of the effect of the dream work, the wish might be grossly distorted. The dream was an attempt on the part of the unconscious to express this wish-fulfilment and it was represented in a pictorial way, since this is the primitive way of thinking in the unconscious. Those unconscious wishes which cannot be tolerated by the conscious are rendered relatively innocuous by the dream work.

Klein's Modifications of Freudian Theory

Klein believed that mental organization developed rapidly in the first year of life and that the ego existed from birth. The neonate experiences being wet and dirty as persecution, but when his wants are satisfied he has the feeling of love.

The Paranoid Position

The mother is at first the child's whole world and his hate and love are directed solely towards her. The ego protects itself by the mechanisms of introjection, projection and splitting. Thus object relations exist from birth. The lack of cohesion of the early ego leads to a splitting of impulses into good and bad; in particular the mother image is good and bad. In the first 3–4 months the chief features of mental life are feelings of omnipotence and persecution and the mechanism of splitting. This is the *paranoid schizoid position.*

The Depressive Position

The integration of the ego increases and the splitting decreases, so that the good and bad aspects of introjects and objects can be synthesized. The superego begins to function at the end of the fifth and sixth months. The child fears the effect of his aggressive impulses and greed on his loved objects. Since a wish and an act are the same thing to him he feels guilty, and feels compelled to make some compensation for the harm he believes he has done. This leads to an anxious depression or the *depressive position.* This is slowly worked through as the child's knowledge of the world increases. Depressive and persecutory anxieties are never completely mastered and may return when internal or external pressures become intense.

The fundamental criticism of the Kleinian views is that they assume a degree of perceptual organization and intellectual ability which is not in keeping with the facts about the infant's abilities in the first year of life.

Bowlby's theory of depression as an adaptation to loss is derived from Klein. The theory describes three phases: (1) the phase of protest, with an urge to recover the lost object; (2) the phase of disorganization; and (3) recovery, with a capacity to set up new relationships to new objects.

Other Deviations from Freud

Space forbids discussion of the views of Horney, Fromm, Erikson, Hartmann, Sullivan, and others. The interested reader should consult the reviews of their work which are to be found within books in the reading list.

This summary is indeed short. When Freudian theories are compressed into this closely packed form, one can comment only that they have to be seen in order not to be believed. Spread out thin they sound much better.

ALFRED ADLER AND INDIVIDUAL PSYCHOLOGY

Adler broke away from Freud partly because he could not accept the rigid discipline of belief which Freud imposed on his followers, and partly because his own work had led him to a point where he could not accept the Oedipus complex as the basis of all neuroses. He never gave a complete and systematic description of his theories, and it is difficult to give a straightforward account of them since they have to be picked out from his writings. This is made even more difficult because, as with Freud, his theories underwent considerable development.

Development of the Child

The child's fundamental problem is the recognition of his weakness and helplessness in relation to the world. In consequence, he strives constantly to find some way of controlling his environment in order to achieve his needs. This is done by acquiring skills, but it can also be achieved by dominating adults and others who would then serve him, rather than the other way round.

Position in the Family

The mode in which the striving occurs is strongly influenced by the early life experiences in the family. Thus the only child, who is the centre of attention, will try always to maintain his position. If other children appear, they may be seen as rivals. The youngest child, who is always the weakest and most helpless in the family, is always trying to catch up with the others. These patterns of behaviour persist into adult life and become the 'life style'.

Organ Inferiority

Another feature which plays an important part in the development of the life style is the recognition of bodily weaknesses and deficiencies of personality. The individual may strive to overcome these deficiencies directly, by developing the weakness until it becomes a strength, or indirectly by compensation. It was the recognition of these bodily deficiencies, which Adler termed 'organ inferiority', which actually served as the starting point for the development of his work.

Masculine Protest

In Western society, women occupy an inferior position in the family and in the community. A girl may attempt to overcome this inferiority by trying to emulate men and adopt masculine roles, or by developing a masculine style of life. This was called the 'masculine protest'. In men, the 'masculine protest' appears as a recognition that inferiority is equivalent to feminity and this is overcome by striving for a super-masculinity.

Theory of the Neuroses

If the goals of the striving are socially approved and successful, then the life style is appropriate. If these goals are impossible or fail, then the individual takes refuge in external difficulties, in symptoms or neuroses. In this manner, the inferiority becomes an 'inferiority complex' and the individual's life style is directed towards a 'fictive goal'. The inferiority complex was central to Adler's theory of neurosis in the same way that Freud's Oedipus complex was central to his theories.

A modern Adlerian would point out that this theory is much more in accord with present-day psychological outlook. Adler abandoned the theory of a driving sexual instinct as the basis of all human behaviour and replaced it with the notion of man as a social being, influenced by and acting on human society. The theory of repression of an 'unconscious' mind, with its special mechanisms and its universal sexualization, are thrown out as redundant. The unconscious becomes merely subliminal awareness and thinking. Thus the overriding importance of early experiences is diminished, and the theory makes room for later experiences to play their part in the pattern of life. Psychotherapy is one such experience but it must be part of active social life.

Freud's comment on Adler was that humanity would accept anything when tempted with 'ascendancy over sexuality' in order to be relieved of the burden of its sexual desires. This tells us more about Freud than about Adler. Adler's theory never became as popular as Freud's, because social striving is much less interesting than sex, and anyway the time was not ripe. Neurotic illness is not less common even though the twentieth century has largely overcome the sexual inhibitions of the nineteenth century. Finally, cultural anthropology has made clear the tremendous importance of social factors in determining behaviour, even sexual behaviour, rather than the other way round.

C. G. JUNG AND ANALYTICAL PSYCHOLOGY

Jung did not reject the idea of the unconscious, but regarded it as composed of individual repressed material and the inherited collective unconscious.

Personality Types: Extrovert versus Introvert

The introvert turns his libido inwards and lives more in his own inner life, while the extrovert turns his libido outwards to the world around him, makes relationships easily with others, and is active and confident. The opposite attitude is to be found in the unconscious. The more pronounced the conscious attitude the more marked the unconscious one.

The Four Functions

These help the person to orientate himself. They are: sensation, intuition, feeling and thinking. These work in harmony in the normal individual and process the information he receives, but if one function is exaggerated there is a personality type. Sensation and intuition form one set of opposed pairs, and thinking and feeling form another. Thus sensation and intuition are different ways of dealing with perception, and thinking and feeling are different ways of evaluating situations. As a rule, two of the functions are prominent in consciousness, while the opposing pair are more important in the unconscious.

The Persona

This is the aspect of the self which is deliberately presented to the environment. If it is too well organized, then attitudes which do not fit in are repressed and conflict may occur. If it is badly organized the environment will easily modify it and the person will feel insecure because he is unsure of his role in life.

The Unconscious

This is made up of a personal and a collective part, in both of which symbols are used. Thought processes in the personal unconscious are often the reverse of those in the conscious mind. The 'shadow' is the reverse side of the conscious mind, comprising all the unpleasant aspects of the conscious psyche. This is partly collective as well as personal and is often represented symbolically as a devil or witch.

The Archetypes

These occur in the collective unconscious and each corresponds to some basic aspect of the individual's existence. The anima and animus are archetypes equivalent to the 'soul' of primitive man. Every man has an unconscious anima or female soul, while each woman has an animus or male soul. Other important archetypes are the wise old man and the great mother. The self may appear as an archetypal image in the form of a small child, a hermaphrodite, or a flower.

Theory of the Neuroses

There is a conflict between a conscious tendency and a complex or an affect-laden group of unconscious ideas. The attitude to life is one-sided, so that what could not be integrated has been repressed. The complex may be due to childhood difficulties or a change in the life situation which renders previous attitudes non-adaptive. A neurosis is not only an illness, but an attempt at adjustment.

During psychotherapy the patient becomes a complete personality and finds his true self as an integral part of humanity. This is 'individuation' and occurs when the analysis has helped the patient to encounter and understand the different archetypes.

The notion of 'individuation' indicates that Jungian theories may be regarded as a precursor of existentialist psychotherapy. The later developments of Jung's theories indicated that he had given up an attempt to develop a scientific theory of neuroses for a preoccupation with pseudoreligious moralizing. The theoretical basis of Jungian psychotherapy seems to have only a tenuous connection with the actual practice. The treatment given by some Jungian psychotherapists can best be described as a sort of bowdlerized psychoanalysis.

BEHAVIOUR THERAPY

As the abnormal behaviour which constitutes mental disorder is not inherent but acquired, it can be regarded as learned behaviour, and what can be learned can be 'unlearned' or extinguished. From this point of view, 'neurosis' is merely learned maladaptive behaviour. The relevance of learning theory to neuroses was first seen when experiments on conditioning dogs to make fine discriminations beyond their capacity led to them 'breaking down' and showing disturbed behaviour such as refusal to eat, incontinence and struggling against entering the experimental room when previously it had been welcomed.

Most learning can be regarded as occurring through:
   a. Pavlovian or respondent conditioning;
   b. operant or instrumental conditioning;
   c. imitation or observational learning.

Respondent or classical conditioning is associated with the name of Pavlov. A reflex is a particular inherent response which appears on the occurrence of a particular stimulus. These are described as the unconditional response and stimulus. When the latter occurs in association (either temporal or spatial) with another neutral stimulus, the response begins to appear when the associated stimulus occurs by itself. The associated stimulus thus becomes a 'conditional stimulus' and the response a 'conditioned response'. The conditioned response will also occur to stimuli resembling the conditional stimulus, i.e. it is 'generalized'. The unconditional stimulus must occur sufficiently often after the conditioning has been established; if it does not, then the conditioned response fades away, i.e. is 'extinguished'. The presence of the unconditional stimulus is necessary to 'reinforce' the conditioning.

Operant conditioning is associated with the name of Skinner. It refers to the process whereby the strength or frequency of a particular behaviour is modifed by the consequences of that behaviour. When the consequences strengthen the behaviour, they are 'positive reinforcers'. When the removal of a reinforcer leads to the strengthening or increased frequency of a particular behaviour, it is a 'negative reinforcer'. When reinforcement is removed, extinction occurs.

Behaviour can be 'shaped' by reinforcing approximations to the desired behaviour and allowing everything else to be extinguished.

Observational (cognitive or modelling) learning is of great importance, particularly in children. It includes not only the acquirement of new

behaviours but also extinguishing by observing the negative consequences. The same principles of discrimination and generalization apply
as to other forms of learning. It depends very much on characteristics of
the model and the relationship between model and learner, e.g.
dependency of the latter on the former.

The first step in applying the principles of learning to a given
behavioural problem is a detailed 'functional analysis'. This examines
the problem in terms of 'excesses' (unwanted responses), 'deficits'
(appropriate responses being absent) and 'assets' (the background of
behaviour and experience on which appropriate adaptive behaviour can
be built).

The problem situation has to be clarified as to the factors leading to
occurrence of the maladaptive behaviour, especially its stimuli and
reinforcements. These have to be related to the individual's social
circumstances, previous background and development. On this basis,
various methods are available for replacing maladaptive behaviour.

Operant Conditioning (Token Economy)

This has been much used for rehabilitation of deteriorated chronic
schizophrenic patients. The patients are given tokens which they may
spend in the hospital shop for whatever they want. Once the patients
have become accustomed to them, the tokens are then used as positive
reinforcers to shape their behaviour in the direction of greater self-
care and higher social behaviour. In practice, the tokens are
supplemented as reinforcers by social approval from the staff and
others.

Systematic Desensitization

This method is also known as *reciprocal inhibition* or *counter-
conditioning*. It is particularly useful when maladaptive anxiety is
produced by a recognizable stimulus or situation, e.g. phobias. The
subject learns how to relax at will, sometimes helped by hypnotism or the
use of sedative drugs, and then the stimuli which produce anxiety are
introduced either in imagination or in reality. It is essential that the
stimuli should be introduced in a graded hierarchy, starting with those
producing the least anxiety and moving on to the next step only when
anxiety-reaction becomes controlled (extinguished). Much depends on
the skill with which the hierarchy is constructed.

Flooding

In the method of flooding, the patient is rapidly exposed to the full
anxiety-provoking situation, either in imagination or in reality, until the
response fades. The latter method is more effective. Flooding requires
that the patient be fully motivated and adequately understands the
procedure.

Other Methods

These are much used for interpersonal fears and social anxiety. They are:

1. Specific instructions from the therapist. The patient is given specific instructions on how to deal with a particular situation.

2. Behaviour rehearsal or role playing. The patient enacts what his role should be in a given anxiety-provoking situation.

3. Modelling. The therapist or other will go through the role first.

The techniques have moved some distance from the original simple application of learning theory; for example, role playing is akin to psycho-drama. To the credit of behaviour therapists, they have constantly attempted to evaluate and improve their techniques by controlled trials.

Chapter 4

General symptomatology

INTRODUCTION

In this chapter individual symptoms will be discussed in isolation, as disorders of different functions of the mind. This is merely a convenient fiction, useful for ordering facts. They will be dealt with as disorders of: (1) perception; (2) thought; (3) memory; (4) consciousness; (5) emotion and feeling; (6) intelligence and personality; (7) motor behaviour; and (8) speech and writing.

DISORDERS OF PERCEPTION

These can be divided into: (1) sense deceptions and (2) sense distortions.

1. Sense Deceptions

These in turn consist of illusions and hallucinations.

a. Illusions

These are misinterpretations of a real stimulus, e.g. a shadow is taken to be a man. The causes are: set or attitude, intense emotions (normal and abnormal) and lack of perceptual clarity. Illusions are therefore common in delirium since perception is poor, anxiety and perplexity are prominent, and a paranoid attitude is usual.

The depressed, guilty patient may mishear what people are saying and it may be difficult to decide at times whether the patient has illusions based on set or is attributing hallucinatory voices to people in the environment.

b. Hallucinations

These are perceptions without an object or mental impressions of sensory vividness without an adequate external stimulus.

i. PSEUDOHALLUCINATIONS

Here the hallucination lacks the vividness of a true percept and does not appear to be substantial and in perceptual space. Hypnagogic and hypnopompic hallucinations, which occur on falling asleep and waking up respectively, are usually pseudohallucinations and are not uncommon in normals. Similar hallucinations are found in fatigue, exhaustion and sleep deprivation.

ii. TRUE HALLUCINATIONS
Here the hallucination has perceptual clarity. They can be suggested to normals or may arise from self suggestion, e.g. someone expecting a telephone call may hear ringing.

c. Causes of Hallucinations

i. AFFECT
Very depressed self-reproachful patients may hear reproaching voices. This is a vivid 'voice of conscience'.

ii. DELUSIONS
The false belief leads to misinterpretation of the environment and expected words may be hallucinated.

iii. SUGGESTION
Hysterics may describe hallucinations and pseudohallucinations, but one is not compelled to believe them.

iv. DISORDER OF A PERIPHERAL SENSE ORGAN
Ear disease or eye disease may produce hallucinations, but often some central change is also present. Negative scotomata occur in delirium tremens and may be partly responsible for the visual hallucinations.

v. SENSORY DEPRIVATION
If the amount of incoming sensation is reduced to a minimum then hallucinations will occur after a few hours. This may be an additional factor in producing hallucinations when there is some disorder for the eye or ear.

vi. BRAIN LESIONS
Focal lesions of the central nervous system, lesions in the brain-stem, midbrain and cortex may cause hallucinations. Temporal lobe epilepsy is often associated with visual and auditory hallucinations.

vii. NO CLEAR CAUSE
Hallucinatory voices are very common in schizophrenia but the reason is not clear. In some instances it has been possible to detect 'sub-vocal' speech corresponding to the voices.

d. Hallucinations of Individual Senses

i. HALLUCINATIONS OF HEARING
These can be divided into: (α) elementary, and (β) organized hallucinations (hallucinatory voices).

α. *Elementary hallucinations:* These consist of noises and music. They occur in schizophrenic and organic psychoses.

β. Hallucinatory voices: These may be clear, or unclear and vague. They may talk to the patient and give him orders—so-called imperative hallucinations which the patient may carry out or ignore. They may talk about the patient in the third person and may even give a running commentary on his acts. Usually they are abusive, but occasionally they are friendly and reassuring. The abuse is commonly of a sexual nature, women being called whores, etc., and men homosexuals and so on.

Sometimes the content is senseless and may even contain neologisms (*see* p. 49). Some patients can reproduce the content of the voices without difficulty, while others can only give a very vague idea of what the voices say. The patient's attitude to the voices varies considerably. Some complain about their content, but others complain more of the phenomenon itself. In some cases the voices may cease if the patient directs his attention to some form of occupation, while in others the voices are continuous and interrupt all mental activity. The sudden onset of voices often causes intense anxiety and depression which may lead to suicide. When the phenomenon becomes chronic the patient may accept the voices with resignation or may continue to protest about them, or, realizing that others do not believe him, he may deny hearing voices and only talk about them to someone whom he trusts. Patients attribute their voices to various sources, such as witchcraft, telepathy, radio, television, atomic rays and so on. Some claim that the voices are from real people in their environment and may assault innocent bystanders from whom the voices appear to come. Thoughts heard aloud and functional hallucinations are special kinds of voices.

Thoughts heard aloud: Here the patient hears his own thoughts spoken aloud as he thinks them. In chronic patients this may take the form of other people speaking his thoughts aloud or replying to his thoughts before he speaks them. There is no accepted English term for this symptom. F. Fish used the term 'thought-echo' for it.

Functional hallucinations: Here the voices occur only if there is some external source of noise. This is not an illusion, since both the noise and the hallucination are heard at the same time.

Elementary auditory hallucinations occur in schizophrenia and organic psychoses. Odd words may be heard in organic states but continuous voices are not common. Depressives may hear reproachful voices, but these are somewhat repetitive and disjointed, consisting of odd words and phrases reviling the patient or instructing him to commit suicide. In schizophrenia the voices are usually more continuous and if they revile the patient he usually resents it, whereas the depressive feels that the voices, which say such things as 'Miserable sod', 'Rotten bugger', and so on, are making justified reproaches.

ii. HALLUCINATIONS OF VISION

These may be elementary, consisting of flashes of light; organized, in which case they may be organized figures seen against the normally perceived environment; or scenic, when whole scenes are hallucinated. All varieties of visual hallucination are common in organic psychoses, when consciousness is clouded, but they can occur, though rarely, in acute and chronic schizophrenia. Small animals are often seen in delirium, especially in delirium tremens. Usually they are associated with extreme fear or terror. Scenic hallucinations are probably most common in epileptic attacks and psychoses. Sometimes a memory appears with perceptual clarity, so-called hallucinatory flashback. Some epileptics have visions of fire and religious scenes, such as the Crucifixion.

Occasionally in organic states Lilliputian hallucinations occur; the patient sees little men and women. This is usually associated with pleasure; for example, one patient with delirium tremens saw a German band made up of tiny men playing on her counterpane, and enjoyed the experience.

Autoscopy (Doppelgänger): This is a special type of visual hallucination in which the subject sees himself and realizes that it is he. This tends to occur in lesions of the parietal lobes, which are most often due to cerebral thrombosis.

Mass hallucinations: Some chronic schizophrenic patients see and hear scenes of mass butchery and violence.

Extracampine hallucinations: The person has a hallucination which is outside the perceptual field; for example, a patient sees a hallucinatory object behind his head, or hears a voice speaking in London when he is in Edinburgh and is fully aware of his situation.

iii HALLUCINATIONS OF OLFACTION

Hallucinations of smell occur in many different disorders, but it is not always easy to be sure whether the patient is complaining of a hallucination, an illusion, or a delusion. Some acute schizophrenics and organic psychotics complain that they are being gassed and can smell the poisonous gas. Some depressives and schizophrenics are certain that they emit an unpleasant smell, while others believe that they do not stink but that other people think that they do. Attacks of temporal lobe epilepsy are often ushered in by a hallucination of a very unpleasant smell, such as that of burning paint or rubber.

iv. HALLUCINATIONS OF TASTE

Hallucinations of taste do occur, but cannot always be distinguished from secondary delusions. Thus the schizophrenic feels utterly changed physically and mentally, which leads him to assume that he is being poisoned.

v. HALLUCINATIONS OF TACTILE SENSATION

Hallucinations of touch and, in particular, the feeling of animals crawling over the body are not uncommon in organic states. They are particularly well marked in cocaine toxicosis, where they are known as the 'cocaine bug'.

Sexual hallucinations can be regarded as a special variety of tactile hallucinations. Some male schizophrenics complain that erections and orgasms are forced on them and that semen is extracted from their penises. Female chronic schizophrenics complain of rape and sexual sensations; occasionally they have an almost continuous hallucination of a penis in the vagina.

vi. HALLUCINATIONS OF DEEP SENSATION

Some patients, usually schizophrenic, have hallucinations of twisting and tearing pains and electric sensations which may be expressed in a bizarre way. In the absence of coarse brain disease all bodily hallucinations clearly experienced as due to external influence are schizophrenic in origin. However, care must be taken to be sure that the patient really experiences the bodily sensation as due to outside influences and is not saying that it is 'as if' this was the source of the sensations.

vii. HALLUCINATIONS OF VESTIBULAR SENSATION

Some patients, usually with organic states, have vestibular sensations and have the experience of flying through the air or being twisted and turned.

e. Reflex Hallucinations

In some schizophrenics a stimulus in one perceptual field will produce a hallucination in another. This is known as a reflex hallucination.

f. Patient's Attitude to Hallucinations

Occasionally in organic states the patient is not troubled by his hallucinations, but usually there is terror and he may try to escape from his supposed persecutors; in so doing he may injure or kill himself by jumping out of windows, etc. Most hallucinating depressed patients consider the remarks justified, but some blame their depression on the persecution. In the acute shifts schizophrenics are frightened by the voices and may attack the alleged source. This attitude may continue in the chronic stage, but many chronic patients are on the whole little troubled by their voices and may treat them as old friends. Such persons often refer to them as 'the voices' and can distinguish them from real voices.

Hallucinations are, of course, only a part of an illness and the patient's attitude is determined by the change in the personality produced by the disease.

g. Hallucinatory Syndromes

Schröder described four common hallucinatory syndromes: confusional, self-reference, verbal and fantastic hallucinosis. Their features have already been described.

i. CONFUSIONAL HALLUCINOSIS

Consciousness is clouded and visual hallucinations are prominent, while auditory hallucinations, if they occur, consist of music, noises, or odd words; connected sentences are rarely hallucinated.

ii. SELF-REFERENCE HALLUCINOSIS

The patient hears voices talking about him. Often it is difficult to decide if phonemes are present or if the patient is merely mishearing real conversations. He cannot give the actual words used, but only a rough idea of what is being said.

iii. VERBAL HALLUCINOSIS

Clear voices are heard, talking about the patient, and he is able to reproduce their content accurately. The voices are attributed to real or imaginary people or machinery.

iv. FANTASTIC HALLUCINOSIS

The patient reports weird fantastic experiences, based on auditory, bodily and visual hallucinations. It is impossible to disentangle the hallucinations from delusions and sometimes it seems that dream experiences are also involved.

2. Sense Distortions

a. Visual Distortions: Dysmegalopsia

Distortion of the retinal image can be produced by lens abnormalities and may also occur in lesions of the posterior temporal and occipital lobes.

In micropsia objects in the visual field appear smaller or farther away than they actually are. In macropsia or megalopsia the opposite occurs. These terms have also been used to designate the size of objects in hallucinations and dreams.

Attacks of dysmegalopsia, usually with marked anxiety, may occur in focal lesions, such as tumours of the temporal-occipital cortex and scars in the same region due to disease or injury. Similar attacks occasionally occur as an aura or an equivalent of an epileptic fit, but macropsia seems to be more common than micropsia in epilepsy. Acute

organic states due to alcohol, bromides and infectious fevers
sometimes cause dysmegalopsia and if micropsia occurs Lilliputian
hallucinations are also usually present. Dysmegalopsia is, of course,
extremely common in psychoses due to mescaline and LSD (*see* p.
214). This disorder is sometimes seen in schizophrenia, hysteria and
disturbed adolescents. In these illnesses the patient usually complains
that people look distorted, in particular that their heads are too
small.

b. Distortions of Hearing

Local ear conditions can cause hyperacusis, while anxiety from any
cause can increase sensitivity to noise. In acute organic states noises
may seem to come from an extreme distance and if the examiner takes
care to speak slowly, loudly and distinctly, the patient can accept
reassurance. The delirious patient is less influenced by incoming
sensations, but more influenced by free-rising fantasy than the normal.
Some anxious, preoccupied depressives experience all sound as if it were
coming from a long distance away and have great difficulty in
concentrating on what is being said. This experience can be regarded as
the auditory equivalent of micropsia.

c. Distortions of Bodily Sensation

Each individual has an unconscious model of his body, which serves as
a standard against which the posture, movements and other motor and
sensory functions can be assessed. This is the body image or schema.
Lesions of the parietal lobe may produce disorder of the body schema
for the opposite half of the body. The patient may say that the limbs on
the side affected feel as if they are not there, or he may actually deny
that they are his own limbs, saying that they belong to the person in the
next bed. Very rarely the patient has the experience of reduplication, i.e.
that he has two arms or legs on the same side of the body. Disorders of
the body schema due to lesions in the minor hemisphere are usually
produced by damage to the cortex and subcortical white matter of the
supramarginal and angular gyri. In the major hemisphere lesions of the
angular gyrus and the adjacent occipital lobe produce Gerstmann's
syndrome, consisting of finger agnosia, right-left disorientation,
agraphia and acalculia (*see* p. 159).
    A hallucination which is best dealt with here is the 'phantom limb'. In
fact, any part of the body if removed can leave behind a phantom. The
patient experiences the limb as if it were still present, but usually it
shrinks with time. Sometimes it is excessively painful. Strange bodily
sensations which appear to be disorders of the body schema occur in
schizophrenics and some hysterics. Thus some schizophrenics complain
of alterations in the size of parts of their bodies.

THOUGHT DISORDER

General Observations

The word 'thinking' is used rather loosely in everyday English. Thus it may be used with the meanings of remembering, believing and attending carefully. If we exclude these three meanings there are another three which are legitimate uses of the word 'think'. These are:

1. Undirected fantasy thinking; autistic or dereistic thinking.

2. Imaginative thinking, in which the thought is dependent on the environment to some degree and the ideas do not go beyond the possible and the rational.

3. Rational thinking, or reasoning in which the material is organized in a rational way and an attempt is made to solve the problem facing the individual. This can be called 'conceptual thinking'.

Autistic Thinking

Some individuals indulge in excessive fantasy thinking. This may be a reasonable adjustment to an intolerable situation. Excessive autistic thinking occurs in schizophrenia and Bleuler suggested that this was due to the failure of logical thinking allowing the fantasy to go on unchecked by rational considerations.

Classification of Thought Disorder

For purposes of description, thought disorder can be considered as disorders of the stream of thought, the possession of thought, the content of thought and the form of thought. No attempt will be made to separate thought and speech disorders of the major functional psychoses except in so far as the speech act is obviously disordered. Aphasic disorders will be considered separately (*see* p. 65).

Disorders of the Stream of Thought

1. *Inhibition of Thought*

The progress is slowed down so that thought proceeds slowly and with difficulty. This occurs in depression.

2. *Pressure of Thought*

The patient feels compelled to think and his thoughts run away with him. Some anxious depressed patients cannot stop thinking about morbid topics and cannot concentrate on anything else.

3. *Flight of Ideas*

Thought is not determined by any overall directing tendency, but ideas follow each other in quick succession, the train of thought being determined by chance associations and clang associations. This occurs in mania, but is sometimes seen in excited schizophrenics and in organic states, especially those due to hypothalamic lesions.

4. *Thought Blocking*

The train of thought suddenly stops and a new one, totally unconnected with it, takes over. This is characteristic of schizophrenia, but some exhausted and anxious parents may show a rather jerky train of thought.

5. *Incoherence*

Here one thought follows another without any logical connection. This occurs in schizophrenia, delirium and severe mania.

6. *Circumstantiality*

Thought proceeds slowly with many unnecessary and trivial details, but the point of the discussion is finally reached. This occurs in epileptics, the feebleminded and in some obsessional personalities; it is normal in some cultures.

7. *Prolixity*

The prolix patient embellishes his thinking with arabesques, while the circumstantial patient gives many wearisome details, but never loses the goal of thought. Prolixity is the transitional stage between normal thinking and flight of ideas. It occurs in hypomania and in hyperthymic personalities.

8. *Perseveration*

This can also be considered to be a speech disorder. The same thought which was initially relevant to the discussion is repeated several times. Sometimes the exact words do not recur, but the patient is unable to break away from the theme, which is repeated in many different variations. This is perseveration of theme and could be regarded as a disorder of content. Both varieties of perseveration occur commonly in organic states, but are also found, though very rarely, in schizophrenia.

Disorders of the Possession of Thought

Normally we experience our thoughts as belonging to us, or there is a quality of 'my-ness' of our thoughts. Apart from this we feel in control of our thinking. Both the control and the possession of thought can be disturbed by mental illness. Thus the patient may be compelled to think his *own* thoughts against his will or he may experience his thoughts as alienated from himself in some way.

1. *Obsessions*

These are contents of consciousness which cannot be got rid of, although when they occur they are judged as being senseless or at least as dominating and persisting without cause. The basic feature is that the obsession is experienced as occurring against the patient's will, but it is the patient's own thought. If the obsession leads to an act, then it is called a compulsion.

The obsessional thought may occur alone in the form of ruminations, or it may be part and parcel of the obsessional act, or it may be followed by a compulsive act which is only indirectly associated with the preceding thought. Obsessive compulsive phenomena can be classified into: (a) obsessional ideas or mental images; (b) obsessional impulses; (c) obsessional fears or phobias (see p. 78); and (d) obsessional ruminations.

Obsessions may occur in obsessional neurosis, depression, schizophrenia and organic states.

2. Alienation of Thought

This takes three forms:

a. Thought withdrawal, or the experience that thoughts are taken away from the mind.

b. Thought insertion, in which a thought is experienced as being inserted into the patient's mind.

c. Thought broadcasting, in which the subject has the experience that everyone else is participating in his thinking.

All these experiences of thought alienation are characteristically schizophrenic.

Disorders of the Content of Thought

Definitions

A DELUSION
A false unshakeable belief which arises from internal morbid processes. It is easily recognizable when it is out of keeping with the person's educational and cultural background.

AN OVERVALUED IDEA
An idea that because of its feeling tone takes precedence over all other ideas. It may be true or false. If it is odd or persecutory in content it may not be easy to distinguish it from a delusion.

1. Primary and Secondary Delusions

A primary delusion is one that cannot be understood as arising from some other psychological phenomenon, while a secondary delusion can be understood as arising from some other psychological event, such as a depressive mood, a suspicious attitude and so on. Since some new meaning is becoming manifest in the primary delusion Conrad called this phenomenon 'apophany'.

a. PRIMARY DELUSIONAL EXPERIENCES (APOPHANY)
These occur in the early stages of schizophrenia, but similar phenomena occur in some cases of epilepsy. The new meaning may emerge in connection with many different psychological events. The older German psychiatrists differentiated a large number of such delusional experiences, but it is possible to reduce them to three important ones:

i. Delusional (apophanous) mood: This is a strange, uncanny feeling state, in which the subject feels that there is 'something going on' around him, which concerns him in some way, but he does not know what it is. A sudden delusional idea or a delusional perception may appear and then the patient has a primary delusion and the mood dies away. It may also cease without any delusion emerging.

ii. Delusional (apophanous) perception: A perception acquires an abnormal significance, usually in the direction of self-reference, and this abnormal meaning cannot be understood as arising from a mood state or an attitude. It should be noted that in delusional mood the emerging delusion cannot be understood as a natural sequence of the mood.

iii. Sudden delusional idea (autochthonous delusion): A delusion suddenly arises fully formed in the subject's conscious mind.

The diagnostic import of apophany: Delusional mood cannot always be differentiated from states of anxiety and perplexity which may occur in affective disorders and acute organic states or may be expected among some religious sects. Sudden delusional ideas can occur in abnormal personalities and in manic-depressives. Delusional perception is diagnostic of schizophrenia, as long as coarse brain disease can be excluded.

b. SECONDARY DELUSIONS IN DEPRESSION
Basic concerns of all human beings are about their own health, moral worth, financial status and relations with others. Delusions of bodily ill-health, guilt, poverty and persecution are understandable morbid exaggerations of these basic concerns.

2. Types of Delusion, according to Content
a. PARANOID DELUSIONS
The word 'paranoid' strictly means that there is a disturbance in the relation of the subject to the world, so that both delusions of grandeur and persecution are paranoid. However, when the word is used without qualification by English-speaking psychiatrists it usually means 'persecutory'. The delusional ideas found in this group are as follows:

i. Ideas of self-reference: The patient believes that people look at him, talk about him, and that his surroundings have a special significance for him. This may range from a vague feeling that this is so, which the patient recognizes as ridiculous, to a firm delusion. It occurs in depressive states, schizophrenia, organic states and in some abnormal personalities.

ii. Persecutory delusions: The subject believes that he is being persecuted by individuals, organizations, or racial groups, such as doctors, Communists, Jews, Catholics and Freemasons. These delusions are common in schizophrenia, but occur also in some depressions, organic states and in abnormal personalities.

iii. Grandiose delusions: The patient believes that he is some important person such as Napoleon, Jesus, or even God Almighty, or that he is connected with important people, such as the Royal Family. This occurs in schizophrenia, rarely in mania, and classically in GPI; although it is more common in this organic psychosis than in others, most cases of GPI do not have grandiose delusions.

b. HYPOCHONDRIACAL DELUSIONS
The patient believes that he has cancer, tuberculosis, syphilis, or some other dreadful disease. Very often hypochondriacal delusions and overvalued ideas are mistakenly referred to as phobias, such as cancerophobia and so on.

These delusions are very common in depressive illnesses, but can occur in schizophrenia and in abnormal personalities.

c. DELUSIONS OF GUILT
The patient believes that he is extremely wicked, has committed a terrible sin, and deserves punishment. He may even believe that such punishment is being prepared and that soon he will be seized by the police, tried, hanged or tortured. In extreme cases he believes that he is eternally damned and will be punished for all eternity. The unforgivable sin is usually that of masturbation or fornication, but occasionally it is some sexual perversion or real crime. Delusions of guilt mainly occur in depressive illnesses.

d. DELUSIONS OF POVERTY
The patient is convinced that he is utterly impoverished, despite documentary evidence to the contrary. This is a rare symptom which occurs mainly in depressives.

e. NIHILISTIC DELUSIONS
These occur chiefly in very severe depressions. The patient believes that he is dead and everything around him is dead or has stopped working.

Disorders of the Form of Thought

In formal thought disorder there is an inability to think abstractly in the absence of coarse brain disease, although there is evidence that the patient has had that ability in the past. Evidence that abstract thought was present in the past is the occurrence of words out of keeping with the low level of intellectual performance or information that there was a reasonable intelligence in the past. Formal thought disorder is characteristic of schizophrenia, where it occurs as: (1) negative formal thought disorder; (2) positive formal thought disorder.

1. Negative Formal Thought Disorder

The patient shows an inability to think abstractly, but does not produce any false concepts. This variety of the disorder cannot always be distinguished from that due to defective motivation, catatonic disorders of attitude, or inattention.

2. Positive Formal Thought Disorder

This is the disorder which is usually meant by such terms as 'schizophrenic thought disorder' and 'thought disorder' in the English literature. It has been described by many different workers, each with his own terminology of the same phenomena. Cameron's (1944) description and terminology are the most convenient, and are described under the following four headings:

a. ASYNDETIC THINKING

This means that there is a lack of genuine causal links in thinking. The patient uses clusters of more or less related sequences in place of well-knit sequences. There is a lack of ability to eliminate unnecessary material and focus on the task in hand.

b. METONYMS AND PERSONAL IDIOMS

The patient uses metonyms, which are imprecise approximations in which some substitute phrase or term is used instead of a more exact one. The patient uses his own private mode of speech which is full of personal idioms. The vagueness, sometimes called 'woolliness of thought', makes the patient's conversation so uninformative as to leave hearers completely baffled.

c. INTERPENETRATION OF THEMES

The patient's speech contains elements which belong to the current task interspersed in a stream of preoccupation which he cannot stop.

d. OVERINCLUSION

There is an inability to maintain the boundaries of the problem and to restrict operations within their limits. This means that the subject cannot narrow down the operations and bring into action the relevant organized attitudes and specific responses. The schizophrenic is therefore able to generalize and to shift from one hypothesis to another, but his generalizations are too involved, too inclusive and much too entangled with private fantasy.

Neologisms

These are new words invented by the patient or standard words to which a new meaning has been given. They may arise from formal thought disorder or have been invented by the patient to designate an experience which is outside the normal. Sometimes the new word is really a catatonic symptom, of the nature of a stereotypy or mannerism.

Disorders of Thinking mainly due to Disordered Attitudes

1. *Self-reference of Thinking*
Some patients, usually chronic schizophrenics, are unable to deal with any problem without referring it to themselves.

2. *Talking Past the Point (Vorbeireden)*
Here the patient deliberately gives the wrong answer and this is shown by the content of the wrong answer, which is a falsification of the correct one. This typically occurs in hysterical pseudodementia, but it also occurs in some young acute schizophrenics, who have a silly facetious attitude due to their illness. It is also seen in a few chronic catatonics.

DISORDERS OF MEMORY

The Essential Steps in Remembering

1. The material has to be perceived and understood. This usually takes place within the framework of schematized past experience.

2. The new material must be stored in a short term store which allows the material to be evaluated. If the material is relevant, it is fitted into the organized body of knowledge; if not, it disappears after a minute or so.

3. If it is fitted into the organized body of knowledge then some sort of permanent trace is formed.

4. The trace lasts until recall, but undergoes changes because of the effects of intervening activity.

5. A new situation requiring the utilization of the information stored in the trace has to be recognized.

6. The required information has to be isolated from the rest of the stored materials. This is the final stage in experiments on memory, but in everyday life we make use of the information we have recalled by using it in dealing with the current task.

It is obvious that memory is only one aspect of intelligent behaviour, so that isolated defects of memory, without any diminution in intelligence, are not likely to occur in coarse brain disease.

Total Amnesia

1. *Psychogenic Amnesia*

The memory for a period of time and often also for personal identity is more or less consciously repressed. Sometimes severe anxiety produced by some personal problem causes a restriction of the field of consciousness and inattention to the environment. This suggests the idea of amnesia, which is then unconsciously exaggerated. In many cases amnesia of this kind seems to be malingering rather than hysteria. When in doubt wait for the police to arrive with a complaint of criminal behaviour.

2. *Organic Amnesia*

Head injury, epileptic fits and acute organic states can produce total amnesia. Retrograde amnesia extends backwards in time from a given point. Anterograde amnesia begins at a given point and extends over a period, during which the subject appears to be fully conscious. Both these types of organic amnesia are not as complete as appears at first sight, because with hypnosis or intravenous sodium amylobarbitone some part of the forgotten material can be recovered.

Specific Memory Defects

1. *Minute Memory*

In some acute and chronic organic states new material cannot be integrated into the schematized past experience, so that it exists for a period of 50–60 seconds and then disappears. This is minute memory.

2. *Failure of Registration*

In the past it was customary to say that memory consisted of registration, retention and evocation, which was subdivided into recall and recognition.

It was claimed that a failure of registration was the outstanding feature of the amnestic of Korsakoff syndrome. This was sometimes expressed as a 'loss of impressibility' and from time to time it has been claimed that permanent complete loss of impressibility has been produced by acute coarse brain disease. In some patients with severe acute and subacute recoverable brain damage and in others with severe chronic progressive brain disease 'minute memory' occurs and the patient is unable to integrate new material into his schematized past experience, so that any new material is maintained briefly, after which it is replaced by some incoming stimulus.

3. *Failure of Recall*
This occurs in anxiety, fatigue, generalized coarse brain disease and in aphasia due to focal brain lesions.

Distortions of Recall. False Memories
Paramnesia
This is a morbid distortion of memory produced by an attitude or emotional state. It occurs in normals, paranoid personalities, depressives and sometimes in manics.

Retrospective Falsification
The past is falsified in keeping with the person's present attitudes and moods. Some depressed patients may falsify their past and assert that they have always been useless, incompetent people. This may lead the unwary examiner to believe that they are inadequate personalities. Some paranoid patients claim that their delusions have existed for years despite evidence from friends and relations that the delusion is of fairly recent origin.

Falsifications of Memory
Isolated memories are produced with unshakeable conviction, but are completely false.

Confabulation
Detailed descriptions are given of past events which are false. Usually they are plastic and can be modified to suit circumstances. They occur in the amnestic syndrome and if they are not produced spontaneously the patient can usually be provoked into confabulating. Confabulations also occur in some chronic schizophrenics and in pathological liars.

Delusional Memories
These may be apophanous in the acute phase of schizophrenia since a new meaning arises in association with the memory. In some cases the new significance is associated with a memory image; for example, a patient remembers that there was a crown on his fork when he was a boy and this means that he is of Royal descent. In other cases the memory contains the delusion, as when the patient remembers being told that he was of Royal descent.

Distortion of Recognition
Déjà vu and Déjà vécu Experiences
The subject has the impression that he has seen or experienced the situation before. This occurs in normals but may occur in attacks of temporal lobe epilepsy.

Delusional Misidentification

Some acute and chronic schizophrenics misidentify all the people in their environment. In the acute cases this may be a variety of delusional perception, while in the chronic cases it may be due to perceptions acquiring the sense of acquaintance, usually only possessed by memory images. Other patients refuse to admit that their friends and relations are really these people and insist that they are strangers (Capgras syndrome).

DISORDERS OF CONSCIOUSNESS

Definitions

Consciousness

This is a state of awareness of one's self and environment. It is usual to compare it to a stage on which images appear like actors; so that consciousness can be restricted or clouded or, to continue the simile, the actor may be spotlighted, or the footlights may be weak. When consciousness is diminished, various deficiencies can be found. They are related to:

1. GRASP OR COMPREHENSION

This is the ability to hold in consciousness all the relevant information in order to react to it. In mild disturbances an individual will be able to answer simple questions but not complicated ones, or to perform a simple action but not those requiring sequences of steps.

2. ATTENTION

This is the ability to bring a percept or concept into the forefront of consciousness, or to focus on a content of consciousness and to hold it. This may occur actively or passively, i.e. the subject can direct his attention to some content of consciousness or his attention may be attracted by some content without any active effort on his part. Fatigue and anxiety may make active attention difficult as does any disorder of consciousness. Passive attention may be affected in anxiety, in some excited schizophrenics, in manics and in some organic states where there is undue distractibility. Some hysterical personalities and overactive children are also unduly distractible.

3. RETENTION

Memory is impaired (*see* p. 49).

4. THINKING

This is slowed down and obviously requires greater effort than normal.

5. DIRECTED ACTIVITY (GOAL)

Because of these deficiencies, the individual is unable to maintain a coherent trend in thinking and behaviour. Conversation becomes desultory and activity is reduced to aimless wandering.

6. ORIENTATION

It is customary to describe orientation in terms of time, place and person, i.e. the patient knows the date and time, where he is and who he meets. Maintenance of orientation is in that order of decreasing difficulty. Orientation in time requires a continual maintenance of awareness of the passage of time and grasp of the information which indicates its changes. Orientation of place is easier because the individual's surroundings provide some clues. Orientation for persons is the easiest because they themselves provide the clues for identification. Disorientation is usually present in acute organic states with clouding of consciousness and in chronic organic states with memory disorders. It also occurs in hysterical fugues and rarely in acute paranoid schizophrenia, when delusions and hallucinations may produce a false orientation, although the patient usually knows the correct one if he can be induced to give it.

Types of Disordered Consciousness

Three stages can be described between full consciousness and deep coma. They are the generalized consequences of deterioration of cerebral function and are most commonly seen in toxic conditions, but may also occur as a result of cerebral damage. In the presence of a progressive condition, the patient sinks through these stages, finally ending in a state of coma and death; but if the patient recovers, then he ascends through these stages. The rate of progress will depend on the nature of the underlying pathological process. In some conditions, e.g. hypoglycaemia, the rate of progress is sufficiently slow for the stages to be clearly recognized, but treatment with intravenous glucose produces very rapid recovery. In concussion, coma occurs instantly but recovery is slower. Similar changes can be seen as a result of anaesthesia.

1. *Clouding of Consciousness*

All mental processes are slowed. Thinking is difficult and attention cannot be maintained. Grasp is reduced. The patients are lacking in initiative and easily become fatigued. In mild cases, the condition fluctuates and may not be easily detected. The patient can answer simple short questions but not difficult or long ones. He cannot maintain a conversation because of the lack of grasp and retention. He is not fully in touch with his surroundings but can be aroused if encouraged. Because of fatiguability, the symptoms become more obvious as an interview proceeds.

2. *Confusion or Subdelirium*

The patient is obviously disorientated and out of touch with his surroundings. As disorientation for time can occur in full consciousness, it is disorientation for place and person that is the essential feature. Only the simplest questions can be comprehended and then the answers are extremely brief. Left to themselves, patients fall asleep.

3. *Delirium*

All the above features are present, but in addition abnormal experiences, such as hallucinations, often visual, may occur. The patient easily becomes frightened and may try to run away. As co-ordinated activity is not possible, he may be merely restless or may fall or try to climb out of bed. If the patient is restrained, he may struggle fiercely against what he conceives as attacks.

4. *Coma*

As the patient's condition deteriorates, activity diminishes to a feeble restlessness and picking at the bed-clothes. Speech is reduced to a faint incomprehensible muttering. The patient finally sinks to a state where there is little or no response to any stimuli and only the basic respiratory and cardiac reflexes are present.

Twilight States

Consciousness is restricted and dominated by a few ideas, delusions or visual hallucinations. General behaviour is fairly well ordered, but the patient may become very excited. Recovery may occur suddenly and the patient has an almost complete amnesia for the episode. Typically, these attacks follow on an epileptic fit, but they may also end with a fit.

Fugues

These are wandering states with some degree of loss of memory. Consciousness is disordered by brain disease or, which is more common, by anxious preoccupation. There is no sharp distinction from twilight stages. Fugues occur in acute coarse brain disease, in hysteria and in suicidal depressives.

Sleep Disorders

Hypersomnia

This is an increase in the amount of sleeping. It occurs in diseases of the hypothalamus, in hysteria and in psychopathic personalities in trouble.

Narcolepsy

The patient suddenly falls asleep. Attacks are often provoked by emotion and it occurs in lesions of the hypothalamus.

Insomnia

It is never easy to be sure if a complaint of insomnia is true or hypochondriacal. Anxious patients have difficulty in getting to sleep. Depressive patients are liable to have difficulty in staying asleep, which usually consists of waking at 2 or 3 a.m. and having difficulty in getting back to sleep. Some of these patients may wake two or three hours before their usual time and lie awake until it is time to rise. Some depressives have broken sleep, waking and drowsing throughout the night. Anxious depressives have difficulty in getting to sleep and in staying asleep.

Some patients claim that they do not sleep at all. Usually this is either hypochondriacal or hysterical exaggeration.

Inversion of Sleep Rhythm

The subject sleeps through the day and is awake and restless at night. This is produced by hypothalamic lesions.

Sleep Deprivation

Deprivation of sleep for 36 hours or more can produce hallucinations and paranoid attitudes. Such deprivation may occur during prolonged first stage of labour, in anxious mothers with restless infants, and also in those addicted to amphetamine.

DISORDERS OF EMOTION AND FEELING
Definitions
1. *Feeling and Emotion*

It is usual to distinguish between feeling and emotion. Arnold (1961) gives the following definitions:

FEELING
'A positive or negative reaction to some experience.'

EMOTION
'The felt tendency toward anything intuitively appraised as good (beneficial), or away from anything intuitively appraised as bad (harmful). This attraction or aversion is accompanied by a pattern of physiological changes organized towards approach or withdrawal. The patterns differ for different emotions.'

2. *Affect*

The term 'affectivity' includes the whole of the emotional side of life, but an 'affect' is a sudden accentuation of emotion of short duration and marked intensity, often reactive.

3. *Mood*

This is an emotional state, usually of some duration, in which the total experience of the subject is completely coloured by the prevailing emotion.

Mood Changes

Mood changes and affective swings in the mentally ill are sometimes a normal response to an abnormal experience. Thus many schizophrenics become very frightened when they first hear voices.

Abnormal mood states can be divided into: (1) elation; (2) depression; (3) anxiety; and (4) irritability. It is often assumed that elation and depression are necessarily qualitative exaggerations of the cheerfulness and unhappiness which are a natural part of everyday life, but the mood changes in manic-depressive illnesses often seem to be qualitatively different from normal.

1. *Elation*

This is a state of marked cheerfulness associated with infectious gaiety. It occurs in mania, but is occasionally seen in patients with lesions affecting the hypothalamus.

Euphoria is a state of mild unwarranted cheerfulness. This is often associated with a sense of bodily well-being called 'eutonia'.

2. *Depression*

This is a feeling of dejection which colours all thought and activity. The same word is used to signify normal reactive unhappiness and also the morbid unpleasant mood which occurs in constitutional depressive illnesses. The term 'autonomous dysthymia' has been proposed for the latter but has not been generally accepted. 'Depression' is also used as a shorthand term for depressive illness.

3. *Anxiety*

This term is a translation of the German word *Angst* which means 'a fear without an object or a dread', since the word *Furcht* meaning 'fear' must always have an object. Unfortunately, the word 'anxious' in everyday speech is used for being worried about something.

As a psychiatric term anxiety is 'an unpleasant affective state with the expectation, but not the certainty, of something happening' (Lewis). Quite often, however, in psychoanalytic and psychodynamic discussions the word 'anxiety' is used in the sense of fear.

TENSION
Patients are usually aware of the increased muscular tension which accompanies anxiety.

PANIC
Occurs when severe anxiety or fear leads to chaotic motor behaviour.

PHOBIA
Is an anxiety or fear restricted to one situation, object, or idea. Phobias can be due to different causes:

Conditioned or learned phobias: the child learns to be frightened of something such as a mouse or frog, either because a parent or parent substitute is frightened by these things, or because of some traumatic experience associated with such events or animals.

Obsessional phobias (*see* p. 45): The patient is frightened that something might happen. He is compelled to think about it although he realizes it is ridiculous or at least that it persists in his mind without cause.

4. *Irritability. Ill-humoured Mood States*
Some patients have states of ill-humoured mood, in which they are unhappy, miserable, angry, resentful and irritable. These states most commonly occur in epilepsy, but can be seen in depressive states, in abnormal individuals, in paranoid mania and in compensation neurosis.

Abnormalities of Emotional Expressions
Emotional Indifference
Here the patient shows complete indifference to one situation, or, to put it in another way, all emotion associated with a given event is dissociated. It is often seen in children and adolescents who, being unable to tolerate the emotional complications of their interpersonal relationships, say that they do not care and act as if they did not.

Belle indifférence
Here the patient shows a bland indifference to some severe hysterical symptom.

Emotional Lability and Emotional Incontinence
Many normal people are easily moved to tears and in some cultures weeping is acceptable in both sexes. In Britain men are expected not to weep, so that tears in a British man are usually the sign of a serious upset. Many depressives are easily moved to tears.

Emotional incontinence occurs when the subject bursts into tears or laughter for little or no reason. Usually it is weeping and this occurs in coarse brain disease, especially in arteriosclerotic dementia. A few patients with brain disease have attacks of forced laughing or crying.

Inadequate Expression of Affect

The patient shows insufficient or inappropriate affect in relation to the situation. This occurs in schizophrenia and when well marked it is diagnostic. It should be remembered that some anxious patients smile foolishly when talking about serious topics, as do deaf people when they have not heard all that has been said to them. Some middle-aged depressives may smile when talking about their deficiencies and make wry jokes about themselves, a sort of 'gallows humour'.

Depersonalization

The subject has the feeling that he has no feeling. He finds that the normal swing of emotion when he sees his friends and loved ones is absent and if depressed he may reproach himself bitterly for this apparent callousness. This is often associated with derealization in which the environment is changed so that it appears strange, distant or even unreal. The patient may say the world looks flat or 'made of cardboard'.

Depersonalization may occur in depression, schizophrenia, hysteria and normal subjects.

Perplexity

The patient is puzzled and bewildered. This may occasionally be due to anxiety or depression produced by situational difficulties. In the early stages of schizophrenia the apophanous experiences may produce bewilderment.

Ambivalence

This is the presence in the mind of the opposite attitudes towards a person, idea, or action. All of us have contradictory attitudes towards certain ideas, but one of the two attitudes is dominant. In schizophrenia these two opposed emotional attitudes and ideas may be more or less present at the same time or alternate rapidly in the conscious mind.

Ambivalence towards an act, or ambitendency, is a disorder of motor behaviour in which the subject stops and starts a voluntary act several times before completing the act, or failing to do so. This is especially well seen in some catatonic patients.

DISORDERS OF INTELLIGENCE

Definition of Intelligence

Wechsler defines intelligence as: 'The aggregate or global capacity of the individual to act purposefully, to think rationally, and to deal effectively with his environment.'

Dementia

This is a permanent loss of intelligence due to coarse brain disease. The term should not be used for reversible intellectual impairment due to acute coarse brain disease, or for personality deterioration in schizophrenia.

Deterioration

Schizophrenia was originally called 'dementia praecox' and chronic patients were said to be 'demented'. Such patients have no coarse brain disease and are therefore 'deteriorated'.

Amentia

This was used in English to mean a lack of intelligence obvious at an early stage. In German it is used to designate subacute delirious states.

MOTOR BEHAVIOUR

Subjective Experience of Behaviour

Obsessions and compulsions can be regarded as disorders of behaviour of this kind, since the normally subjective experience of the progress of thought and action is disturbed.

The most outstanding abnormalities of this kind are the feelings of passivity, when the patient has the experience that his thoughts, feelings and actions are not his own and that he is made to do these things by outside influences. This may be attributed to rays, radio waves, atomic rays, television, witchcraft and so on. These 'made' experiences are diagnostic of schizophrenia.

Classification of Objective Motor Disorders in Mental Illness

Motor disorders can be classified into:
1. Disorders of adaptive movements
    a. Expressive movements.
    b. Reactive movements.
    c. Goal-directed movements.
2. Non-adaptive movements
    a. Spontaneous movements.
    b. Induced movements.
3. Disorders of posture
    a. Distorted normal postures. Manneristic postures.
    b. Abnormal postures. Stereotyped postures.
4. Abnormal behaviour patterns
    a. Non-goal-directed patterns of behaviour.
    b. Goal-directed abnormal patterns of behaviour.

Disorders of Adaptive Movements

Expressive Movements

In manic-depressive disease there is an excess of expressive movement in mania and a lack of it in depression. The manic shows a wide range of expressive movements and tends to use his hands and upper trunk to express his feelings, so that large expansive movements are made. In contrast the depressive shows poverty of facial expression and what there is is sad and provoked by morbid topics. These patients, rather like actors, may smile with their lips but not with their eyes. Depressed retarded patients often have an angulation of the inner end of the fold of skin in the upper eyelid (Veraguth's sign).

In schizophrenia expressive movements may be severely affected. Thus in catatonia the face is usually flat and expressionless, or at least facial movement is stiff, although the eyes may show some liveliness. Other catatonics have excessive grimacing and facial contortions. Sometimes they show *Schnauzkrampf* in which the nose is wrinkled and the lips are excessively pouted, giving the appearance of an animal's snout.

In post-encephalitics the face is usually flat and expressionless and very greasy-looking—'the ointment face'.

Reactive Movements

These are the immediate adjustments to stimuli which are carried out automatically. In catatonia and motility psychoses these movements may be lost before voluntary movements are affected. This gives a general stiffness of movements which is difficult to describe.

In anxiety reactive movements tend to be rapid and excessive. In retarded depression they are diminished.

Goal-directed Movements

These are usually carried out effortlessly and smoothly. In depression movements may be slow and tired, but in anxiety they are quick and tremulous. In catatonia they are often awkward and lacking in grace. Voluntary movements reflect the personality and mood state, so that the movements always show some individuality. If this individuality is excessive, then we can speak of a mannerism which is an unusual variation in the execution of a goal-directed movement or normal posture. Mannerisms occur in abnormal personalities and in some schizophrenics.

Non-adaptive Movements

Spontaneous Movements

The commonest spontaneous movement is tremor, which occurs in anxiety. The various organic tremors will not be considered here, but it must be pointed out that organic tremors can vary in severity and are made worse by anxiety so that such variations are not indicative of the psychogenic origin of a tremor.

Tics are short, jerking movements of the face, neck and upper trunk. They are often provoked by anxiety, but they cannot be regarded as hysterical conversion symptoms.

Spasmodic torticollis consists of spasms of twisting of the head. This is made worse by psychological stress, but is determined by an abnormality in the nervous system.

Choreiform movements are short, jerking movements affecting the whole body, looking like half-formed purposive movements. In Sydenham's chorea they are fine movements and affect the periphery more than the trunk. In Huntington's chorea they are coarser and effect the face, upper trunk and arms. Grunting and snorting noises also occur in chorea.

Stereotypy consists of the repeated performance of a non-goal-directed action in a uniform way. Sometimes it is possible to discern the remnants of some purposive movement. This leads psychoanalysts to interpret these movements as representing some symbolic act. Stereotypies occur in catatonia and in organic states.

Some catatonics show parakinesia, in which there is a continuous irregular activity of the whole musculature, including the face, and resembling the movements of Sydenham's chorea.

Abnormally induced Movements
These can be regarded as the result of undue compliance on the part of the patient:

a. AUTOMATIC OBEDIENCE
The patient carries out all instructions. This is sometimes called 'command automatism', but this term has also been used for the syndromes of waxy flexibility, echolalia and echopraxia.

b. ECHOPRAXIA
The subject imitates all the actions of the examiner. Echolalia is present when he repeats what is said to him. Echolalia and echopraxia occur in schizophrenia and dementia.

c. PERSEVERATION
This is the repeated useless repetition of a goal-directed act. This may occur in speaking, so that the patient repeats his reply to a question several times. Perseveration is most commonly seen in the dementias, but can occur in catatonia. Palilalia and logoclonia are special varieties of perseveration affecting speech.

d. FORCED GRASPING AND GROPING

In forced grasping the subject takes the examiner's hand every time it is offered *despite instruction to the contrary*. This is different from the grasp reflex, in which the patient grasps everything which touches his palm. The grasp reflex occurs bilaterally in widespread cortical lesions, but may occur unilaterally in tumours of the frontal lobe. A few patients will grope after the examiner's finger if he repeatedly touches the palm of the subject's hand while slowly moving the finger away. This is the so-called 'magnet reaction'. Forced grasping may occur in catatonia and in coarse brain disease.

e. COOPERATION OR MITMACHEN

The patient allows his body to be moved without the slightest resistance and when the doctor stops the body slowly reverts to its rest position. *Mitgehen* is an extreme form. These movements are found in some catatonics and can occur in frontal lobe lesions.

f. OPPOSITION

The patient resists all passive movements to the same degree as the force being applied by the examiner. If movements are carried out very gently then the patient often does not resist them, but as soon as abrupt forceful movements are attempted opposition occurs.

Disorders of Posture

Manneristic postures are odd, stilted postures which are not rigidly maintained, while stereotyped postures are abnormal postures which are rigidly maintained. This distinction is not always easy to make. One stereotyped posture which is seen in both catatonics and dements is the 'psychological pillow'. The patient lies for hours with his head two or three inches off the pillow.

Flexibilitas cerea or waxy flexibility occurs in patients with catatonia and in those with lesions affecting the brain-stem. The patient allows his body to be placed in awkward positions and there is a feeling of plastic resistance as the examiner moves the body. The position is maintained for more than one minute. Preservation of posture or catalepsy occurs when the patient maintains a position in which the examiner puts him, but there is no sense of plastic resistance.

Abnormal Behaviour Patterns

1. *Non-goal-directed Behaviour: Stupor and Excitements*

a. STUPOR

This can occur in depression, catatonia, hysteria and coarse brain disease. The patient lies or sits motionless and does not reply to questions, or if he does he gives muttered monosyllabic replies. In depressive illness psychomotor retardation occurs in which all thought and motor activity are slowed down. When this becomes extreme, stupor occurs, but usually the face looks depressed and is not entirely expressionless as in catatonic stupor and there is some emotional response to affect-laden questions. Incontinence of urine and faeces frequently occurs in catatonic and organic stupor, but hardly ever in depressive or hysterical stupor. In organic and catatonic stupor disorders of posture such as flexibilitas cerea may be present. In catatonia the stupor may pass into an excitement or be briefly interrupted by an impulsive act.

Some catatonics show very little spontaneous activity but will eat when food is put before them and micturate and defecate when placed on the toilet. As they can, therefore, unlike the stuporose patient, be pushed into activity, this state can be called 'akinesia'.

b. EXCITEMENTS
These occur in mania, in severely agitated depressives, in catatonia, in paranoid schizophrenia, in delirium, in psychogenic reactions in mental defectives and unsophisticated individuals, in psychopathic personalities, in hysterical females, in epilepsy (epileptic furore) and in other organic states. The gay, infectious mood in the absence of hallucinations usually makes the diagnosis of manic excitement fairly easy. The other conditions are not easy to differentiate from one another.

c. NEGATIVISM
This is an active striving against all external attempts to influence behaviour. The more the examiner insists on examining the patient the greater the resistance, so that excitement may occur.

2. Goal-directed Abnormal Behaviour
This covers the whole of mental illness, so that only the following outstanding behavioural patterns sometimes seen in severe mental illness can be discussed:

a. SILLY BEHAVIOUR
Some hebephrenics smile foolishly and behave in a childish, silly way.

b. UNPLEASANT TRICKS
Some abnormal personalities and manics get much enjoyment out of practical jokes. Some hebephrenics play unpleasant pranks on their fellow patients.

c. BRUTALITY
Such behaviour is common in aggressive psychopaths, but some emotionally devastated chronic schizophrenics behave in a brutal, inconsiderate way.

d. MANNERISTIC BEHAVIOUR

Some abnormal personalities carry out complicated patterns of behaviour in a manneristic way. This is also seen in some chronic schizophrenics.

e. IMMORAL BEHAVIOUR

This *per se* is no indication of mental illness, but immoral behaviour may be released by coarse brain disease, schizophrenia, or mania. Thus in so-called simple schizophrenia one of the outstanding features is the ethical and moral deterioration.

f. MURDER

Despite the popular press and novelists this is not a common feature of mental illness (*see* p. 245). In Britain most murders are committed by distressed, unhappy people, and not by the insane.

SPEECH AND WRITING

General Disorders of Speech

Some schizophrenics show abnormal attitudes towards the questioner. They may always turn to the speaker or turn away when spoken to. The former (adient) patients may always speak when spoken to or merely stare fixedly at the examiner. If they speak it may be drivel, i.e. it is grammatically well-formed, but the content is nonsense; or there may be verbigerations consisting of the repetition of the same senseless syllables.

Mutism occurs in stuporose states due to all causes, but is also seen in some catatonics in whom it appears to be a mannerism. Such patients may write, although they refuse to speak. Mutism can occur as an isolated symptom in hysteria, but is not as common as hysterical aphonia.

Perseveration (*see* p. 61) occurs almost exclusively in coarse brain disease. In some dementias, such as Alzheimers' disease, palilalia occurs. This is the repetition of a phrase with increasing speed. Logoclonia, the rapid repetition of the last syllable of what has just been said, e.g. 'I am all right-ite-ite-ite-ite-ite', also occurs in the same conditions.

Writing in the Mental Disorders

Schizophrenic patients show mannerisms and stereotypies in their writing. Letters may be distorted or embellished and the lines of script may be arranged in a design. Some schizophrenics show much more thought disorder in written than in spoken productions, but the reverse also applies. Handwriting may become large and bold in mania and small and cramped in depression.

NOTE ON NEUROLOGICAL DISORDERS OF SPEECH AND ALLIED TOPICS

Since some schizophrenics show features like aphasic disorders and some dements have aphasia, a short account of aphasia and related subjects will now be given.

Aphasia

The incoming sensations are recognized as percepts in the cortical area in which they terminate, but these areas must be connected to the other sensory areas and to a central co-ordinating area on the left side in the right-handed, comprising the posterior part of the first temporal convolution and the adjacent parts of the parietal and occipital lobes. In this area preliminary schemata for words are elaborated and impulses pass forward to the posterior part of the first frontal convolution to evoke the motor schemata for speech, giving rise to impulses which pass the lower end of the precentral convolution, which gives rise to impulses which pass to the speech musculature via the appropriate motor nuclei. Lesions interrupting the appropriate motor paths will affect the production of speech, but dysarthria so produced is not, strictly speaking, a disorder of speech function.

Aphasias can be classified according to whether the disorder is predominantly receptive, intermediate, or expressive.

1. *Receptive Aphasia*

a. PURE WORD DEAFNESS
Words are heard, but not understood. The lesion is in the first temporal convolution near the first transverse temporal gyrus.

b. AGNOSIC ALEXIA
Words are seen but not recognized, although the patient can write spontaneously and to dictation. The lesion is one which interrupts the connection between the visual cortex on both sides and the left angular gyrus in the right-handed.

2. *Intermediate Aphasia*

a. NOMINAL APHASIA (AMNESTIC APHASIA)
The names of objects cannot be evoked. The lesion is in the left temporoparietal region in the right-handed.

b. CENTRAL APHASIA
There is a defective comprehension of written and spoken words and also of grammatical relationships, together with grammatical and syntactical errors and the misuse of words in spontaneous speech. The lesion is in the posterior part of the left temporal convolution.

3. *Expressive Aphasia*

a. VERBAL OR CORTICAL MOTOR APHASIA

There is difficulty in the use of words, so that in severe cases speech is almost entirely absent. Words are often distorted and the patient knows what he wants to say, but cannot find the right words. There is a greater facility of impulsive utterances. The lesion is in the posterior two-thirds of the first frontal convolution.

b. PURE WORD DUMBNESS

All spoken speech is lost, but inner speech and writing are preserved. This disorder occurs in lesions affecting different parts of the anterior portions of the brain.

Apraxia

This is an inability to perform or carry out a volitional action in the absence of any motor or sensory loss or disorder of co-ordination.

Limb-kinetic Apraxia

There is an inability to appreciate the constituent elements of a movement. Some neurologists claim that this is due to a slight damage to the pyramidal tract.

Ideomotor Apraxia

The subject can imagine the act which he wants to perform, but he is unable to do it. A lesion in the dominant parietal lobe produces this disorder bilaterally, but a lesion in the corpus callosum may cause this apraxia on the opposite non-dominant side.

Ideational Apraxia

The patient is unable to carry out a complex series of acts, although he may be able to imitate simple movements. The lesion is in the dominant parietal lobe.

Constructional Apraxia

Individual movements can be carried out accurately but actions cannot be properly ordered in space. This is due to a failure in the integration of kinaesthetic and visual elements in spatial perception.

Apraxia for Dressing

The patient is not able to relate his body to his clothes, so that this is partly due to apraxia and partly to a disorder of the body image. It occurs in lesions of the parieto-occipital region in the non-dominant hemisphere.

The Agnosias

In agnosia the subject experiences the sensations in the given sense modality, but cannot recognize objects in this modality, while he is able to do so in other modalities. Agnosias are due to an interruption of the connections between the specific cortical area and the rest of the brain. When these disorders occur in isolation they can be mistaken for hysterical complaints. Thus a patient with visual object agnosia said he was blind and this was interpreted by the examining doctor as hysterial, since the patient could obviously see.

Chapter 5

Abnormal and psychopathic personalities

Personality can be defined as the whole system of relatively permanent tendencies, physical and mental, which are distinctive of a given individual organism, tendencies which determine its adjustment to its psychological, social and material environment. The scientific study of personality approaches it either by way of surface characteristics, i.e. traits, or by underlying tendencies, which may be described in terms of drives, needs, constructs, unconscious mechanisms, etc. A trait may be defined as a generalized predisposition to consistencies of behaviour. The existence of a vast number of trait names testifies to a folk tradition which, despite all the work carried out on other approaches, remains the most popular and comprehensible way of describing personality.

In any one person, traits of personality do not cover the whole field of behaviour, e.g. a person may be friendly, honest, tidy, careful, etc. in some situations and not in others. Traits tend to be associated into groups, giving rise to types of personality. Because of the limited field of particular traits in any one person, it is therefore possible for individuals of the same type to behave very differently in similar situations.

Traits vary in intensity and when sufficiently strong can be regarded as abnormal in the statistical sense, i.e. on the general principle that extreme forms are less common than the average. However, at a sufficient level, they can then interfere with the individual's relations with other people. When they pass beyond the bounds of what is socially tolerable, they will be regarded as abnormal in the sense of being morbid. Sociologists believe that abnormality of behaviour is merely that which is beyond the bounds set (arbitrarily) by society. Mental illness is therefore different from the normal only quantitatively, not qualitatively. This theory is most applicable to abnormal personality.

From their clinical experience, psychiatrists have described types of abnormal personality based on the dominant trait (though mixed varieties are acknowledged). Schneider (1958) has described ten types which are generally accepted by German-speaking psychiatrists although modifications have been suggested by Leonhard and Petrilowitsch. When the traits are not quite outside normal limits, Leonhard has called these subjects 'accentuated personalities'.

LEONHARD'S CLASSIFICATION OF ABNORMAL PERSONALITIES

The Epileptoid Personality

This has nothing to do with epilepsy and is called by others the 'explosive' personality. When something does not suit these persons, they flare up and react impulsively. When they are frustrated or in a bad mood severe excitement may occur. They change their job frequently and tend to drink to excess. The *uncontrolled personality* is the milder form.

The Anankastic Personality

In Britain this is commonly called the *obsessional personality* and in the USA the *compulsive personality*. Within normal limits it is the overprecise personality. The anankast is a rigid inflexible person who loves order and discipline because he cannot bear to live outside a known framework. His pedantic and self-righteous attitude towards others, which arises from his inability to understand a different viewpoint, may give rise to difficulties. He is the perfect subordinate but in a position of leadership cannot make decisions. He is usually a highly respectable person and a living example of moral rectitude. Such persons usually have a low sexual drive, but occasionally this may be accompanied by vivid sexual fantasies, which may lead to perverse or promiscuous behaviour. Although some anankasts have minor obsessional symptoms, such as counting, checking and rechecking, there is little connection between this type of personality and obsessional states (neurosis).

The Hysterical Personality

Jaspers pointed out that the essential feature of this type of personality was an excessive need for appreciation. If they do not get this, they overact or behave in a way which increases the concern of others for them. They are described as egoistic, vain and self-centred, exhibitionistic, emotionally capricious and volatile, histrionic, emotionally shallow and mendacious, though typically they convince themselves more than they do others. Although coquettish in behaviour, they tend to be frigid.

Traditionally, hysterical personality has been associated with hysterical symptoms, although nowadays most patients with hysteria do not have a hysterical personality. As this diagnosis used to be regarded as applicable only to women, and as the descriptions were made by men, the result is that, as pointed out by Chodoff and Lyons (1958), the hysterical personality 'is a picture of women in the words of men and. . . amounts to a caricature of femininity'. Most psychiatrists tend to be somewhat anankastic in type and therefore dislike the hysterical personality. In consequence, their descriptions of this type of person emphasize the unpleasant aspects and ignore the great emotional sympathy and empathic qualities which make these people so sensitive to the feelings and mood of others. When they also have talent, they may become great performers in the world of the arts.

Paranoid Personalities

This type has a need to be recognized for what he considers to be his true worth. He tends to overvalue his abilities and readily attributes his failures to the ill will of others. There is an excessive sensitivity to supposed or actual injuries or slights. Leonhard believes that there is an abnormal persistence of the effects of emotionally loaded experiences, which tend to accumulate and bias thought. The name comes from the fact that delusion-like ideas may develop in these persons, who come to believe that they are the victims of intrigues against them. They are ambitious, striving and very sensitive to criticism. They are easily offended and may be inclined to fight for the rights of others. In mild form, these persons may be described as *overpersistent.*

The Reactive-labile Personality

The reactive-labile personality is emotionally sensitive and reacts to emotionally charged situations, whether they be happy or sad. These persons are much more likely to develop 'reactive depressions' than the average. Milder forms are known as *emotive personalities.* It is difficult to decide if they feel more deeply than others or if they merely have an increased emotional responsiveness.

The Cyclothymic Personality

The cyclothymic personality is abnormally sensitive to external influences, but is not reactive to the same degree. External events act as releasing agents rather than causes of mood change, which arises from an internal lability. The mood tends to continue for some time and may outlast the immediate emotional upset. Sometimes the variations in mood are entirely the result of internal events so that the cyclothymic may become depressed or elated for hours, days or weeks for no obvious reason. Some of these persons are liable to affective disorders, but not all.

When the variations are extreme, ranging from rapture to utter despair, Leonhard considers them to be reminiscent of anxiety-elation psychosis. Mild forms are called *mood-labile personality.*

Subdepressive, Hypomanic and Anxious Personalities

These three types may be regarded as attenuated forms of the corresponding disorders.

Mixed Types

Leonhard believes that combinations of abnormal or accentuated personality traits can occur and the traits can sometimes modify each other. For example, he suggests that anankastic and hysterical traits appear to compensate each other.

OTHER PERSONALITY TYPES

Some personality types described by Schneider are not accepted by Leonhard. These are the sensitive, fanatical, affectionless, weak-willed and asthenic personalities. Clearly, there is scarcely any limit to the number of types which can be described, but that is of greater interest to literature than to psychiatry.

The International Classification of Diseases lists nine types of personality disorder: paranoid, affective, schizoid, explosive, anankastic, hysterical, asthenic, sociopathic and others. Sexual deviations, alcohol and drug dependence are listed separately.

Attempts have been made to classify abnormal personalities by psychometric methods, using data derived from questionnaires or observer ratings. The usual methods are factor analysis, which groups the personality traits, or cluster analysis, which groups together individuals, according to their resemblance. For example, Blackburn (1975) examined 79 non-psychotic male offenders admitted to Broadmoor Hospital, using 12 scales from the Minnesota Multiphasic Personality Inventory, and found four profile types covering 80 per cent of his subjects. Type 1 were undersocialized, impulsive, aggressive, extrapunitive and relatively lacking in anxiety and other subjective disturbances. Type 2 had high levels of anxiety, depression, social avoidance, but were more hostile, aggressive, impulsive and undersocialized than Type 1. Type 3 denied psychological problems and had a high degree of control. Type 4 showed social shyness, introversion and depression; they were moderately hostile. Tyrer and Alexander (1979) used a structured interview schedule, from which factor analysis gave four factors. Cluster analysis gave six types: Explosive, Asthenic, Paranoid aggressive, Histrionic, Anankastic and Schizoid. The first and third differed chiefly on severity as did also the second and fourth. When these pairs were combined, the four clusters closely resembled those obtained from the factor analysis.

PSYCHOANALYTIC THEORY: THE CHARACTER NEUROSES

In neurosis the repressed material breaks through into consciousness in a form which is foreign to the ego, but in character disorders the form is not alien to the ego. Character traits are of two types: sublimation of instinctual drives, and a part of a countercathectic measure which keeps certain instinctual drives in check. The first type is not pathological, but those in the second type can distort social relations severely.

It is possible to classify character types according to the stage of libidinal development which had the most effect on the character. Thus there is the oral type which may be frustrated or gratified. The gratified oral type is optimistic, self-assured, and generous, while the frustrated variety is pessimistic, impatient, irritable, selfish and demanding. Marked exaggerations of these oral types are found among antisocial personalities. The anal character is orderly, obstinate and stingy, while the urethral traits are impatience and ambition.

PSYCHOPATHIC PERSONALITIES

Most German-speaking psychiatrists have followed Kurt Schneider and regarded psychopathic personalities as abnormal personalities who suffer, or cause society to suffer, from their abnormality. However, even among German-speaking psychiatrists, the term 'psychopathic personality' has acquired a pejorative meaning. Both Petrilowitsch and Leonhard have pointed out that the negative aspects of the psychopathic personality have been overstressed and that the same psychopath who is a burden to society can, given the right circumstances, be a worthwhile member of society. Leonhard and Petrilowitsch do not use the terms 'psychopathic personality' or 'psychopath', but use the term 'abnormal personality' instead.

Characteristics
1. Signs and symptoms of mental illness are not essential.
2. The disturbance is of action and in social behaviour.
3. They live predominantly in short term values.
4. Their conflicts are acted out in social life, not in personal symptoms.
5. Inability to learn by experience.

These points are open to criticism. Although psychopaths are not mentally ill in the usual sense, many of them experience much anxiety and depression and may react with severe symptoms to the stresses they experience. To say that short term values dominate their lives does not distinguish them from so many others who are not psychopathic. The inability to learn by experience merely signifies that the punishments inflicted on them by society for their misdeeds have little effect on their patterns of behaviour, but a style of life is not easily changed.

Classification
1. Aggressive—uncontrolled explosive outbursts.
2. Sociopathic—antisocial behaviour, when due to the personality (constitution) of subject, and is not secondary.
3. Persistently abnormal character.

Aetiology

Heredity—history in parents and family, including other types of illness. Adoption studies have provided good evidence for hereditary factors.

Environment—poverty, broken homes, parental alcoholism, illegitimacy.

Organic factors—encephalitis, chorea, brain injury, sometimes epilepsy.

1. Aggressive

These subjects experience outbursts of violent conduct, in the form of episodes usually precipitated by environmental factors. The outbursts described usually are homicidal attacks, but can include alcohol and drug addiction (in bouts), because of similarity in types of personality (dipsomania).

There is usually a long history of wayward, impulsive, violent behaviour. The high intensity and fierceness of episodes are accompanied by great hate and frustration. The personality often shows coldness, hardness and indifference to others' feelings.

2. Sociopathic

(*a*) The petty delinquent, involved in thieving, lying and swindling. They are impulsive, lacking in foresight, egocentric, irresponsible and show little or no compunction towards others. They are at war with all others and society.

(*b*) Pathological liars, who lie habitually and without need, chiefly wishful fantasies, and sometimes with real falsification of memory. Usually light-hearted, irresponsible, plausible, complacent and self-confident, they are full of information which is superficial and unreliable. This type shades into the pathological swindler. It includes those who show the Münchausen syndrome, a repeated simulation of disease for which they gain admission to hospital and undergo treatment, including surgical operations.

(*c*) Inadequate—weak-willed, tired, drifters, tramps, beggars, etc.

3. Persistently Abnormal Character

This covers a wide variety of types which are difficult to classify. The distinction between normal and abnormal is even more difficult to make here than with other types.

(*a*) Paraphilia—homosexuality, sadism and masochism, paedophilia, fetishism, exhibitionism and bestiality (*see* Chapter 13).

(*b*) Arsonism, kleptomania. The latter group can be distinguished from 'shop-lifters' because they steal only one object, which sometimes they succeed in accumulating in enormous quantities.

(c) Alcoholism (see Chapter 8).
(d) Drug addictions.
(e) Eccentrics.

Many of these conditions are mixed together and within one group there are different varieties with different aetiologies, e.g. alcoholism. Many eccentrics and tramps are suffering from schizophrenia.

Discussion

Possible Organic Basis

Young post-encephalitics may behave just like aggressive psychopaths, which suggests a possible physical basis for psychopathy. Williams (1969) found non-specific abnormalities of the EEG in 57 per cent in those showing persistent aggressive behaviour, compared with 24 per cent in offenders with a solitary violent crime, and 12 per cent in the population at large.

Immaturity

Much of the abnormal behaviour of aggressive psychopaths can be understood as due to immaturity, and this fits in with the EEG findings. Maddocks (1970) found that after a mean of 5·6 years of follow-up, 10 out of 59 (17 per cent) seen in outpatients had settled down, 39 (66 per cent) had not, 3 (5 per cent) had died and 7 (12 per cent) could not be found.

The Criminal

Some criminals are produced by a criminal subculture although they may conform to the criteria of psychopathy. It is not justifiable to regard these criminals as being mentally abnormal. Antisocial behaviour is a poor criterion for classification, because all varieties of personality can be found among criminals. It is not difficult to find anankastic, paranoid and hysterical personalities in prison. The anankast, for example, can be a trustworthy upright member of society or he can be a highly skilled and meticulous safe-breaker. It is preferable not to use the terms 'psychopathic personality' and 'psychopath', but to use the term 'antisocial personality' and then go on to specify the variety of abnormal personality.

THE TREATMENT OF PSYCHOPATHIC PERSONALITIES

Psychotherapy

On the whole these patients do not respond well to individual psychotherapy, because they 'act out' in the treatment situation. In the case of the 'episodic psychopath' supportive psychotherapy and environmental adjustment are necessary during a crisis. However, it is important that the psychiatrist should not allow the psychopath to use psychiatric illness to escape the natural consequences of his actions.

Group therapy appears to be a more rational treatment of the psychopath, because his unusual behaviour is much more obvious in the group situation and he can learn to cope with it in the social environment of the group. On the whole, the results of treatment are disappointing. Counselling of 'pre-delinquents' showed little benefit, when compared with a control group (Mannheim, 1955) and Cornish and Clarke (1975) found that residential treatment for deliquency did not improve the reconviction rate.

Criminal Psychopathic Institutions

These are special penological institutions in which individual and group therapy can be carried out. In some countries the courts, on psychiatric advice, can commit a criminal psychopath to a special institution for a period not greater than a normal prison sentence. The prisoner can then be discharged by a review board only after a prolonged period of trial leave.

Guardianship

Many countries have legal provisions for guardianship designed to prevent unstable or mentally ill individuals from exposing themselves and their families to social distress. English law allows a court to place a psychopath under guardianship after he has been convicted of an offence. It is possible that this may be done in some cases of psychopathy in order to supervise the patient and prevent him from getting himself into difficulties.

Chapter 6

Psychogenic reactions, personality developments and neuroses

In this chapter we consider a number of syndromes which can best be thought of as reactions of types of personality to stress, and also two others which have certain features in common with the rest but are difficult to classify.

The normal, accentuated and abnormal personalities respond to psychological trauma in many different ways. The symptoms and the severity of the psychiatric disturbance depend on the previous personality and the nature and extent of the psychological trauma. Sometimes the response is an acute reaction which dies away in a few days or weeks. This may be referred to as a psychogenic reaction. In other cases the disorder may run a chronic course and last for months or years. Sometimes the abnormal response begins slowly and fluctuates in severity, but over a period it steadily becomes worse. This is a personality development, i.e. the result of a chronic interaction between an abnormal personality and the environment. The distinction between a personality development and a psychogenic reaction is not always a sharp one because a patient may have what appears to be an acute psychogenic reaction but it may continue as a personality development as a result of an unfavourable environment.

Psychogenic reactions and personality developments can be classified as follows:
1. Anxiety reactions.
2. Goal-directed or hysterical reactions and developments.
3. Depressive reactions.
4. Hypochondriacal developments.
5. Paranoid reactions and developments.

ANXIETY REACTIONS
The Classification of Anxiety States
Classification is somewhat arbitrary, as the different forms shade one into another.

1. *Acute Anxiety States*
    a. Fright reactions.
    b. Acute traumatic and reactive anxiety states.
    c. Acute exacerbations of chronic anxiety states.

76

2. *Chronic Anxiety States*
   a. Chronic reactive anxiety state.
   b. Phobic-anxiety state.

1. Acute Anxiety States

a. Fright Reactions

These reactions follow a catastrophic experience, such as an earthquake, an explosion, or a traffic accident. The symptoms are very variable. Sometimes there is stupor with mutism. Sometimes there is panic-striken behaviour which may put the subject into greater danger. There may be a euphoric mood with pressure of speech and overactivity, or a twilight state with marked restriction to consciousness. The fright reaction lasts for a short time, but can pass over into a hysterical reaction. Immediate treatment is effective and consists of a dose of hypnotic adequate to give prolonged sleep of up to a day.

b. Acute Traumatic and Reactive Anxiety State

The subject undergoes some terrifying experience which threatens his life. He becomes tense, anxious and tremulous. He is easily startled and his sleep is broken by anxious dreams concerned with the traumatic event. Treatment by abreaction became popular during World War II. Recovery occurs so long as there is no marked secondary gain.

Less acutely, the patient suddenly experiences some disruption of normal personal or social relationships. Most individuals become anxious when their usual adaptation is disturbed. The severity of the anxiety depends on the severity of the stress and the resilience of the personality. Such patients should be reassured that they are not ill, but as having a normal reaction to difficulties. Sedation should be given to tide the patient over the crisis, but should not be continued for long, to avoid habituation. Patients should be encouraged to cope with their problems and given such help as may be necessary.

c. Acute Exacerbations of Chronic Anxiety States

Chronically anxious patients are liable to react acutely to stresses. They need to be tided over the acute phase and treatment is then directed to their chronic condition.

2. Chronic Anxiety States

a. Chronic Reactive Anxiety States

These can be regarded from two viewpoints. On the one hand they can be considered as the characteristics of a person with an abnormally anxious disposition. This may have a genetic background or may have arisen as the result of experiences in early life. These people have a low threshold for the arousal of anxiety, which once it has developed, fades away slowly. Given sufficient stress, the symptoms may reach disturbing and disabling levels, and the fading away may be indefinitely prolonged. From this point of view, a chronic anxiety state is a personality development. This is the traditional viewpoint. On the other hand, the symptoms may appear in a person who may or may not be obviously anxious, but having once appeared, perhaps precipitated by stress, they persist and can thus be regarded as an affective disorder, i.e. a disorder in which the central feature is a disturbance of mood. Evidence is accumulating for this latter viewpoint, and for this reason, the symptoms, treatment, etc. of chronic anxiety states are dealt with in Chapter 9.

b. Phobic Anxiety State

Many patients experience specific phobias against a background of more or less anxiety. These are usually grouped into three types, specific animal phobias (e.g. dogs, moths), situational phobias (e.g. darkness, thunderstorms) and social anxieties (e.g. eating in public). The first two usually date from childhood, having been brought on by some traumatic experience. The last tends to have developed later in life. On the whole, these phobias repond well to behaviour therapy.

Distinct from these is the anxiety-phobic-depersonalization syndrome. Most of these patients are women and the symptoms often appear in the second and third decade. The previous personality is characterised by insecurity, dependence and sometimes hysterical traits. The characteristic symptom is a fear of going out of doors alone (agoraphobia) and of being in crowded places. The patient is afraid that she will experience an attack of panic or dizziness and will faint or collapse. An attack of panic or dizziness and faintness occurring against a background of chronic anxiety may have precipitated the syndrome. Some of these attacks have been shown to be associated with mitral valve prolapse. In about two-thirds, patients experience bouts of depersonalization. The response to treatment is unsatisfactory.

GOAL-DIRECTED OR HYSTERICAL REACTIONS
Definition

The presence of mental or physical symptoms for the sake of some advantage although the patient is not fully aware of their nature.

The term 'hysterical' is used in at least three senses. It may be used to designate a goal-directed reaction or what is called a 'hysterical illness' in the English-speaking world. The term may also be used to designate a type of personality (see Chapter 5) or it may be used for importunate attention-seeking behaviour.

In the USA the term conversion reaction is used for hysterical reactions in which physical symptoms occur, while the term dissociative reaction is used for those hysterical reactions in which psychological symptoms are present. Although the two terms are convenient, they imply a theory about the nature of the mechanisms producing symptoms which not everybody accepts. Janet used the concept of dissociation to explain all hysterical symptoms.

Aetiology

Intelligence, Education and General Background

Dull and unsophisticated persons are likely to have well-marked hysterical symptoms when in conflict. In more intelligent individuals and in cultures in which 'neurosis' is respectable, hysterical symptoms may take the form of anxiety and phobias.

Physical Illness

This may suggest to the patient the idea that illness is a solution to his problem, leading to a hysterical exaggeration and prolongation of the disability originally produced by a physical disease.

Sometimes a diagnosis of hysteria has to be changed eventually to one of organic cerebral disease. This suggests that the hysteria may be adopted as a solution to life's difficulties because of lowered functional capacity of the brain. Hysterical symptoms are more common with temporal lobe lesions.

Psychological Theories

Janet's Theory of Dissociation

Fatigue, puberty, physical disease, and emotion can all lower psychological tension. This lowering of tension in hysteria affects only one function which disappears from consciousness, i.e. it is dissociated.

The subject has a conflict which produces anxiety, allowing dissociation to occur. A mental representation of a bodily or mental function is split from consciousness. Physical or mental illness is then accepted as the cause of the distress produced by the mental conflict, so that the anxiety is replaced by *belle indifférence.*

Freud's Theory

The fixation point is at the genital stage of libidinal development, so that when introversion occurs due to loss of a loved object (*see* p. 27) the freed libido regresses to reactivate the unsolved conflicts in the Oedipal situation.

The incestuous love object is symbolized by the symptoms, or the subject identifies with it, so that there is a somatic dramatization of an unconscious fantasy.

The hysterical symptom may symbolize the Oedipal conflict or the current conflict, or may be based on some mild organic defect. The hysterical phobia symbolizes the current conflict and the Oedipal conflict.

PRIMARY GAIN

The symbolic solution of the current conflict leads to a relief from anxiety. This is the primary gain.

SECONDARY GAIN

The symptom itself may produce fortuitous environmental changes which are advantageous to the patient. This is the secondary gain and may be so great as to provide an unconscious motive for continuation of the hysterical symptom after the current conflict has been resolved.

Any symptom due to mental or physical illness can be used unconsciously for secondary gain.

ANXIETY HYSTERIA

A term used by Freudians to describe hysteria in which anxiety is also present; it also covers phobic states and sometimes obsessional states. It is a term which is better avoided.

Sociological Theory

This is derived from the notion of 'role taking'. The 'sick role' carries with it many privileges and exemption from many social obligations, including working for a living. Other people are under the obligation to be sympathetic, kind and helpful. The adoption of the 'sick role' may therefore be a way of getting out of a difficult situation which appears to be impossible to deal with. This can also happen with a patient who feels ill in a way he finds difficult to explain. Hysterical symptoms then provide, in the words of W. S. Gilbert, 'corroborative details to give an appearance of verisimilitude to an otherwise bald and unconvincing narrative'. The disadvantages of the sick role may be more than counterbalanced by its benefits, e.g. in compensation 'neurosis'. The theory does not distinguish adequately between hysteria and malingering. However, it could be said that every hysteric is a bit of malingerer and every malingerer is a bit of a hysteric.

Symptoms

General Points

Any physical or mental disorders which can be imagined by a normal person can be hysterical symptoms.

Negative physical findings are not diagnostic of hysteria, since it can be some time before unequivocal indications of physical disease appear. Hysteria is a positive diagnosis, so that the psychiatrist must be able to show that the symptom is related to the patient's situation. Until he can do this he should not assume that the illness is hysterical merely because a general physician cannot find any positive signs. Symptoms can be sensory, motor, or mental.

Sensory Symptoms
These consist of blindness, deafness, anaesthesia and pain. They tend to occur under great stress and among the unsophisticated. Hysterical abdominal pain may have led in the past to multiple partial eviscerations by uncritical surgeons.

Motor Symptoms
These take the form of paralysis, spasms and tremor. When the patient tries to move his 'paralysed limb' the antagonists contract as well as the appropriate muscle groups, and associated movements occur in the paralysed limb when the normal one is moved. Hysterical fits occur when there is an audience and consist of a thrashing about of the limbs with the eyes firmly shut, quite unlike the tonic and clonic contractions of the epileptic. Mild blackouts may be difficult to diagnose and it must be remembered that a single negative EEG does not exclude epilepsy.

Mental Symptoms
1. AMNESIA, FUGUES, TWILIGHT STATES AND MULTIPLE PERSONALITIES
Loss of memory may only be partial when it affects some memory which is very painful or it may affect all knowledge of the past and the personal identity. This total lack of memory is in striking contrast to the preservation of the ability to deal reasonably with the immediate environment, whereas a dement with the same degree of memory loss cannot fend for himself.

The hysterical memory loss is usually associated with wandering. This is a hysterical fugue or wandering state. During such states the subject sometimes re-enacts traumatic events in a very dramatic way.

The boundary line between hysteria and malingering in these states is impossible to define. Multiple personalities are artefacts created by hysterics with the assistance of gullible psychiatrists.

2. HYSTERICAL PSEUDODEMENTIA AND GANSER STATES
Ganser described a twilight state in prisoners, in which there was clouding of consciousness and approximate answers. Other psychiatrists claimed that true clouding of consciousness did not occur in this condition. In hysterical pseudodementia the patient gives approximate answers in the absence of any change in consciousness. Care has to be taken to distinguish between approximate answers (*Vorbeireden*) and paraphasic speech disorder which may occur in generalized brain damage when it is associated with clouding of consciousness. It is questionable whether the Ganser state and hysterical pseudodementia should be regarded as hysterical conditions. It seems much more logical to consider them to be varieties of malingering.

3. STUPOR
This usually occurs under severe stress. There is no incontinence and the patient will often eat when not observed.

4. HYSTERICAL EXCITEMENTS (HYSTERICAL 'PSYCHOSES')
These may be shortlived outbursts of violence in hysterical psychopaths or excited states with aggression and self-mutilation lasting for several months. These latter patients are usually adolescent or young adult females who have had a very disturbed childhood. They have vivid visual hallucinations and slash their wrists and forearms repeatedly. Despite the severe excitement it is easy to make rapport with them.

5. HYSTERICAL ANXIETY AND DEPRESSIVE STATES
Here the patient reacts to unpleasant situations with anxiety and/or depression. The symptoms solve the situation to some degree so that they are continued because of the secondary gain, or they subside and remain as a symptom pattern which can be used hysterically in the future.

Special Varieties of Hysterical Reactions
Compensation Neurosis
The desire for compensation and the anxiety associated with the legal proceedings are responsible for the illness. Other factors, such as unspoken fear of dangerous jobs (e.g. a face worker in a coal mine), and increasing difficulty in heavy manual work with age may be brought to the patient's attention by the accident and act as unconscious motives for the neurosis, so that cure is impossible. A pension rather than a lump sum is likely to continue the disability.

The symptoms are usually gross conversion hysteria mixed with anxiety and depression. Anger and resentment are only just below the surface. If there are no complicating factors recovery occurs after the compensation is settled but not always.

Engagement Neurosis
This is a neurosis or psychogenic reaction which occurs in either sex when firm plans have been made for marriage.

The personality is usually obsessional and often there is undue dependence on an overprotective mother.

Depression and anxiety are common symptoms, but gross hysterical symptoms may occur. The intended spouse is told: 'I am ill, darling; it would be unfair to marry you.' He or she replies: 'You are ill, darling; you need me all the more. I will look after you.' There is thus no escape from the prospect of marriage.

These patients dissociate their engagement from their illness, so that the illness can be called hysterical, although in the absence of gross conversion symptoms it can be regarded as a psychogenic reaction.

Treatment

This depends on the relative importance of the situation and the personality in determining the illness. Psychotherapy (see p. 218) should be directed towards the discovery of the basic conflict and patients should then be encouraged to make a rational solution of their conflicts. Situational adjustment must be made where possible. If this can be done, then almost any face-saving treatment is effective. In engagement neurosis both marriage and termination of the engagement lead to a disappearance of the symptoms.

Prognosis of Hysteria

This depends on:

1. THE CURRENT CONFLICT
If this is mild, then there is a vulnerable personality, so that further illnesses are likely. If the conflict is insoluble then the outlook is poor.

2. SECONDARY GAIN
If this is great, recovery will be less likely.

3. COMPENSATION
Psychotherapy will be useless until compensation is settled.

4. PREVIOUS PERSONALITY
Recurrence is likely in hysterical personalities who have suffered from previous illnesses.

5. INTELLIGENCE
'Deep' psychotherapy is useless in the dull and backward, but suggestive therapy may be effective if the illness is no longer useful. If the IQ is low and readaptation impossible then the outlook is hopeless.

6. AGE
Recurrence is likely if the patient has experienced repeated hysterical illnesses until well on into middle life.

7. DURATION OF ILLNESS
The longer the illness has lasted the less the likelihood of cure. By this time secondary gain is very great and loss of skill increases employment problems.

8. PRESENCE OF PHYSICAL ILLNESS
A physical defect enhances the patient's belief in the physical basis for all his disability. Many chronic invalids are persons with slight physical illnesses with a marked hysterical overlay.

DEPRESSIVE REACTIONS

Reactive unhappiness is a normal event, but some personalities, particularly the reactive-labile, subdepressive and cyclothymic types, easily become depressed and the depression lasts an undue length of time. Severe prolonged reactive unhappiness is often called 'reactive depression' although it is quite different from a depressive illness. The reactive depressive is often angry and resentful and blames others for his condition, while the patient with a depressive illness usually blames himself. Delusions or overvalued ideas of ill health, self-reproach, persecution and poverty do not occur in reactive depression. This disorder is also known as a 'neurotic depression', but if one applies the criterion of insight, mild depressive illnesses without delusions can be called neurotic depressions. As a depressive illness can be provoked by psychological trauma it is not always easy to decide if a mild depression is a depressive illness or a reactive depression (*see* p. 117).

HYPOCHONDRIACAL DEVELOPMENTS

These are more likely to occur in anankastic, overprecise, overpersistent and asthenic personalities. The patient develops the fear or the overvalued idea that he has a physical illness. Sometimes the disorder begins after a transient autonomic disturbance, such as a burst of extrasystoles. In other cases it follows some event which makes the patient become more observant of his bodily functions. A friend may die from cardiac infarction and this may make the patient worry about slight aches and pains in the chest. In other cases the hypochondriasis begins after extramarital sexual intercourse, when the patient is frightened that he has been infected with venereal disease. The fears of disease give rise to anxiety which causes autonomic symptoms which reinforce the patient's fear.

Some hypochondriacal patients are frightened that they may have a physical illness, while others appear to experience unpleasant sensations which give rise to hypochondriasis. Leonhard has called the first type 'ideohypochondriacal' and the second 'sensohypochondriacal'. The sensations which the sensohypochondriacal patient complains of are plastic descriptions of pain and abnormal sensations which on the whole are incomprehensible to the ordinary healthy person. The treatment of these patients with psychotherapy is not very easy, as they are unable to get away from their fears of, or beliefs in, physical illness.

PARANOID REACTIONS AND DEVELOPMENTS

These can also be called delusion-like reactions and developments, because the delusions which occur are understandable results of the interaction of the personality and the environment. They are more likely to occur in paranoid and overpersistent personalities and also in patients with deformities and deafness.

Ideas of persecution may develop in a paranoid or overpersistent personality when subjected to constant bullying by a harsh insensitive superior. The ideas of persecution naturally die away when the patient is removed from the stressful situation. Sensitive personalities may develop paranoid reactions when their weaknesses are exposed by some key experience. For example, a sensitive personality may be worried about his illegitimacy and when this fact accidentally becomes public knowledge, he may develop a paranoid reaction. Some paranoid and overpersistent personalities have hypomanic traits and tend to become querulous. They are always fighting for their rights and for the rights of others. They may get themselves involved in law suits, which they carry on interminably.

Morbid jealousy is a common paranoid development, in which the patient has delusions that the spouse is unfaithful. It can occur in either sex, but appears to be more common in men, so that it is sometimes known as the 'jealous husband' or the 'Othello' syndrome. Usually the patient comes from a broken home or a social background in which marital infidelity is not uncommon. Accusations of infidelity are at first intermittent, but later they become almost continuous, although they fluctuate in intensity. The wife may be beaten or cajoled into a false confession. These patients may be extremely violent and can severely injure or even murder their wives. Often the patient gives a detailed account of an episode of suspicious behaviour on the part of the wife and claims that he knew after this event that his wife was unfaithful to him. For example, a patient said that while he was lying in bed during the day he saw his wife and son-in-law misbehaving in a mirror which hung on the wall of the corridor opposite his bedroom. He could not explain why he did not get out of bed and tax his wife with her immoral behaviour. Accounts of this kind are always produced long after the patient has begun to accuse his wife of infidelity and are of the nature of retrospective falsifications. These patients often produce ridiculous evidence that their wives are unfaithful. They claim that there are seminal stains on the wife's underwear, that the vagina is moister than usual, and that she looks debauched.

Erotomania is a rare psychogenic reaction or personality development in which the patient, usually a woman, believes that someone of the opposite sex is in love with her although the alleged lover has given no substantial indication of his love. The patient knows that she is loved because of the way in which the lover looks at her or the way he shakes her hand and so on. Often the patient has only seen the lover at a distance and has not spoken to him. Erotomania can be a transient disorder in adolescence or a personality development in middle life, but schizophrenia may begin as erotomania and clear schizophrenic symptoms may only become obvious after many months.

OBSESSIONAL OR ANANKASTIC REACTIONS

Aetiology

The illness sometimes begins in adolescence and childhood. There is a family history of obsessional illness in about 30 per cent. The population prevalence is about 0·05 per cent.

Psychoanalytic Theory

The regression activates conflicts at the anal sadistic stage of libidinal development. Some displacement occurs, but the main mechanisms used are 'undoing' and isolation. In undoing, the material representing aggressive fantasies appears in consciousness followed by its opposite which cancels out the effect of the preceding anxiety-laden material. In isolation, different aspects of an ambivalent attitude are separated in time and place.

The Clinical Picture

Obsessive Compulsive Behaviour

The patient may have obsessional ideas or images, in which case a phrase or vivid memory image dominates his mind, or he may be troubled by obsessional impulses or compulsions. He may be obliged to touch things or count things. Sometimes the impulse is one of carrying out some antisocial act. In other patients the obsession takes the form of a phobia and the individual is frightened that something might happen, although his common sense tells him that it is ridiculous. This often takes the form of fear of infection and contamination, which leads to washing rituals and complicated patterns of behaviour designed to avoid dirt and disease. Over half the patients are obsessed with causing harm to themselves or others. Sometimes the obsessions are complicated ruminations about one particular thing or idea or very complicated trains of thought which have to be thought through before the patient can be satisfied.

Often the rituals or ruminations have to be repeated until the patient is satisfied that they have been carried out correctly. In mild cases this may be two or three times, but in severe ones the repetitions may be much more numerous.

If the patient is prevented from carrying out his obsession he becomes very tense. Some patients with very abnormal personalities may become very angry and even violent when they are prevented from performing a ritual or compulsion.

Anxiety and Depression

When the obsessions are very marked the patient is usually very anxious and depressed, because of the torturing nature of the symptoms. In some patients the mood change seems to be partly or wholly independent of the obsessional symptoms and is associated with the typical features of depression.

A few patients have manic-depressive illnesses and their obsessions are much worse during the depressive phases and hardly noticeable in the manic phases.

General Behaviour

Some patients suffer from their symptoms, while others involve their friends and relatives in their obsessional rituals and may do this by threats as well as endearments.

Usually obsessions do not lead to criminal behaviour. However, obsessional thoughts of suicide or of murdering the children, which may occur in some depressives, may be carried out, and such patients should always be admitted to hospital for treatment.

The Course of the Illness

It tends to fluctuate in severity, but improves as the years go by. About half eventually make a complete recovery. Sometimes the symptoms stop suddenly and start again just as suddenly some time later. Patients who come for treatment for the first time in middle life sometimes describe a mild bout, lasting only a few months, occurring during adolescence.

Differential Diagnosis

Depression

Some depressed patients have obsessions, but usually single obsessions. Very rarely some female depressives are obsessed by a short four-lettered word. They are terribly ashamed, intensely depressed, and usually suicidal.

Early morning waking, diurnal variation of mood, well-marked guilt and self-reproach, and hypochondriasis suggest the depressive bias of an obsessional state.

Schizophrenia

In the author's experience obsessions rarely occur at the onset of schizophrenia. If they do occur other indications of schizophrenia can usually be found.

Many obsessional neurotics are very peculiar people, so that if they suffer from a depression or a psychogenic reaction they may present with very strange symptoms. Atypical illness of this kind may be mistaken for schizophrenia.

Organic States

Some post-encephalitic patients have forced thinking during oculogyric crises. The features of post-encephalitic Parkinsonism are usually clearly present. Other organic states are rarely complicated by obsessions.

Treatment

Psychoanalysis

These is no clear evidence that obsessional neurotics are cured by psychoanalysis. All psychoanalysts agree that it is a difficult illness to treat.

Supportive Psychotherapy and General Measures

The therapist and the patient discuss the symptoms. This often helps the patient because his symptoms seem so bizarre to him that he cannot talk about them with friends and relatives. Behaviour therapy has been shown to be effective in some patients.

The individual must be kept fully occupied. In severe exacerbations inpatient care is recommended with a full programme of occupation.

Drugs

The benzodiazepines and phenothiazines may be useful when the patient is very tense. Controlled trials have shown (Insel et al., 1983) that tricyclic antidepressant drugs, especially clomipramine, can be very effective and this is not related to their antidepressant effect.

Leucotomy

It has been suggested that a modified leucotomy is indicated in the patient with severe obsessions associated with marked tension, but with a good previous personality, who has made great efforts to carry on with his life with the help of supportive psychotherapy for several years and who is severely crippled by his symptoms.

A grossly abnormal personality, onset in childhood and atypical symptoms are contraindications.

ANOREXIA NERVOSA

Incidence

This is an uncommon disorder, but all the evidence indicates that the incidence is increasing. Estimates vary widely, from 0·8 to 10·8 per 100000 among women aged 15–34. One inquiry found that among women university students, 2 per cent had a history of this disorder. Among patients, less than one-tenth are men.

Aetiology

A high incidence of affective disorder has been found in the relatives. Winokur et al. (1980) found that 22 per cent of the relatives had histories of primary affective disorder, compared to 10 per cent among the controls. Hudson et al. (1983) found that the risk of affective disorder among the relatives was 27 per cent compared with 12 per cent in relatives of bipolar affective disorder.

The typical patient is a quiet, anxious, sensitive and unsocial person. She is hard working and has little interest in boys. It is said that great feelings of inadequacy and a striving for self-control and perfection dominate her psychological attitudes. The commonest age of onset, between 13 and 17 years, indicates that it is related to the onset of puberty and the problems of adolescence. In a considerable proportion, the disorder appears in the twenties, indicating the importance of other factors.

It is accepted that sufferers come from families with disturbed interrelationships, but how much this is the result of the situation created by the disorder is uncertain. At one time much emphasis was placed on the effect on a submissive girl of a dominant mother and a passive father, but with the increasing incidence, this particular family constellation has become relatively uncommon. One theory regards the condition as being essentially based on a rejection of the adult feminine role and a desire to return to childhood, but this does not fit well those cases where the disorder appears in a married woman with children. The psychoanalytic theory, that the disorder comes from fantasies of oral impregnation, fatness being regarded unconsciously as equivalent to pregnancy, has been largely abandoned.

Physiological theories concerning hypothalamic dysfunction derive their significance from the fact that in a quarter of cases the cessation of menstruation appears well before loss of weight. Endocrine abnormalities have been found, e.g. low levels of luteinizing hormone, follicular stimulating hormone and oestrogens, which are not related to the starvation.

Sociologists point out that the increased incidence of this disorder has occurred during a period of increasing emphasis on feminine slimness. Books on slimming have reached extraordinarily high sales and are regular among the 'best sellers'. All women's magazines have articles regularly on slimming, and there are even magazines devoted entirely to that subject.

Clinical Features

Nearly half the patients are overweight at the beginning. The patient develops a morbid fear of fatness and starts to diet. Gradually her consumption of food diminishes until it reaches surprisingly low levels and the patient becomes emaciated. Despite this she continues to be busy and active and insists that there is nothing wrong with her. When the family tries to persuade her to eat more normally, she complains that the food chokes her and she has no appetite. In fact, the appetite is normal ('anorexia' is a misnomer) and the patient is intensely preoccupied with food and even dreams about it. It has been shown that these patients' perception of their body image is distorted in the direction of fatness.

Menstruation ceases soon, if it has not already done so. In men, the equivalent is loss of libido and impotence. The limbs are cold and cyanotic. There is no abnormality on physical examination other than an increase of lanugo, especially on the back.

Bulimia nervosa is a closely related disorder, or perhaps a variation. The patients are liable to attacks of gorging, sometimes to the point of being painfully bloated with food, after which they induce vomiting. They feel very guilty and self-contemptuous about this behaviour. Abuse of laxatives is common. The vomiting may lead to alkalosis, with low potassium blood-levels, tetany and even epileptiform fits. Menstruation is not disturbed.

These patients are usually older and sexually more experienced than anorexics. The syndromes may occur together. There is evidence that bulimic behaviour of a mild type is not uncommon. Halmi et al. (1981) found it in 19 per cent of female and 5 per cent of male college students.

Diagnosis

The triad of symptoms: emaciation, much physical activity and denial of symptoms, is characteristic of the disorder. The possibility of malabsorbtion syndrome or cerebral tumour should be borne in mind, but in the presence of typical symptoms there is no need to engage in elaborate investigations for other possibilities. Food faddists may become very thin, but they are not actively seeking thinness. In mild or late onset cases, the features of the illness may be atypical. In doubtful cases, it is helpful to admit the patient and keep a careful watch on the amount of food she eats.

Prognosis

In the past, patients often died of inanition, pulmonary tuberculosis or other intercurrent infection. Modern treatment can prevent this but patients often lose weight again after discharge from hospital and have to be readmitted, often within the next 2 years. Even after 5 years, about 5 per cent are still severely anorexic. Nearly half eventually recover completely, but patients are known who have continued to show symptoms even in late life. Late onset cases are more chronic. The mortality is about 5 per cent.

Treatment

A weight of less than 60 per cent of the average requires intervention. If it is below 50 per cent it is life threatening. It may be necessary to go through a confrontation before the patient will accept treatment.

Mild cases can sometimes be treated as outpatients, but the majority of patients are better admitted into hospital. The patient should be kept in bed at first and put on a diet of 1500 kcal daily increasing to 4000 kcal daily. It is easier to control intake if the diet is liquid at first. A crisis may occur when the weight first starts to increase but feeding difficulties diminish as the weight increases. Chlorpromazine or thioridazine in doses of 300 mg daily has been recommended but is not necessary. The nursing staff should take care that the patient does not dispose of her meals in various ways while pretending to eat them. As the weight comes back to normal the patient is allowed to get up a little and obtains more and more privileges as the weight improves. Behaviour therapists carry out this procedure using a carefully planned progressive regime. Family therapy is the best form of psychotherapy but patients are generally reluctant to co-operate. Sometimes they are trying to get away from the family! Some form of psychological support will be required for a long time.

A recent controlled trial has shown that imipramine (and probably a wide range of anti-depressants) is an effective treatment for bulimia.

Chapter 7

Psychosomatic disorders

DEFINITIONS AND GENERAL PRINCIPLES
Definition

The term 'psychosomatic' has been used in two ways. In a broad sense it has been applied to that approach by the physician which takes into account the social and psychological factors as well as the physical ones relating to the development, course and treatment of illness. For example, it has been shown (Rahe and Arthur, 1978) that more illnesses are experienced soon after a stressful experience than at other times, although the relationship is weak. 'Psychosomatic' has now been replaced by the more fashionable 'holistic medicine'. This is the correct practice of medicine and should not need a special designation. In a narrow sense, 'psychosomatic' has been applied to disorders which are not neuroses or psychoses, but in which psychological factors appear to play an important part. Even in the narrower sense, it has been claimed that the term is redundant, because it can be said that psychological and social factors are important in all illnesses. Be that as it may, it is a covenient description and can be defined as follows.

Freudian Views

Freud distinguished between neurotic symptoms which were symbolic of a conflict, i.e. conversion symptoms, and those neurotic symptoms due to a neurotic misuse of a given function. His followers have called this second variety 'organ neurotic'.

Despite the non-symbolic nature of organ neurotic symptoms many psychoanalysts give 'dynamic' explanations of psychosomatic diseases.

Personality Theories

At one time it was said that various psychosomatic disorders appeared in specific types of personality. This opinion has now been generally abandoned, but in coronary artery disease there is some evidence that infarction is more likely to occur in a particular type of personality.

RESPIRATORY DISORDERS
Bronchial Asthma

The basic disorder in bronchial asthma is the narrowing of the lumen of the smaller bronchi as a result of the contraction of the circular muscle of the bronchus and/or swelling of the bronchial mucosa. Three factors play a part in bronchial asthma: (1) allergy, (2) infection and (3) emotional disturbance.

In any given case one, two or all three of these factors may play a part. There appears to be an inherited predisposition to asthma, because there is an excess of bronchial asthma and infantile eczema in the families of asthmatics. Asthma begins in childhood and often produces a vicious circle of anxiety. The mother worries about the child and transmits her anxiety to him and this may cause further asthmatic attacks. What would otherwise have been a normal mother–child relationship is distorted by the natural anxiety produced by the illness. Another factor is that the attacks of asthma give the child a special status in the family and he may use his illness to gain attention or to get his own way.

There is very clear evidence that asthma can be caused by emotional disturbance or by suggestion. Thus Herxheimer found that when asthmatics were placed in situations in which they had previously been exposed to allergens they had attacks of asthma, although they were not exposed to an allergen. The situation became a conditioned stimulus for an asthmatic attack. Many different investigators have shown that allergic reactions can be accentuated by stress. The relation between allergy and emotion in asthma is very well illustrated by the story about the famous physician Trousseau, who suffered from asthma and was allergic to oats. Normally when he went into his stables he had a mild wheezing, but not a severe attack of asthma. One day he went into his stables and discovered that his coachman had been swindling him. He became very angry and had the worst attack of asthma he had ever had in his life.

Various types of personality have been described as typical of patients with asthma, but these claims have not been substantiated. Objective studies with the Maudsley Personality Inventory and the Cornell Medical Inventory by Rees have shown that the asthmatic tends to have a score midway between normals and neurotics. Rees (1956) found a higher prevalence of psychological factors in asthmatics who developed asthma for the first time after the age of 45.

Vasomotor Rhinitis

This consists of attacks of rhinorrhoea, with sneezing and difficulty in breathing through the nose. The immediate cause of the symptoms is an excessive secretion of the nasal mucosa with swelling and increased vascularity. Allergy, infection and emotional disturbances may all play a part in producing attacks (Rees, 1964).

Hay Fever

This is an allergic condition, in which the nasal mucosa is allergic to pollen. In 36 per cent of allergic patients Rees (1959) found a close temporal association between emotional tension and the precipitation of signs and symptoms of hay fever, such as rhinorrhoea and sneezing. Such patients had a higher incidence of instability of personality, timidity and over-anxiety than the others. Compared with a control group, the patients were significantly more anxious, obsessional and ambitious.

GASTROINTESTINAL DISORDERS

Peptic Ulcer

This term will be used for ulcers affecting the prepyloric portion of the stomach and the duodenum. These ulcers are quite different from gastric ulcers affecting the body of the stomach, and in the following discussion gastric ulcers will not be considered.

Experimental Evidence

It has been known for many years that damage to the hypothalamus produces gastric and duodenal ulceration. Lesions of the brain following cerebral thrombosis in human beings have been known to cause gastric ulceration.

Personality Types

Various types of personality have been alleged to be associated with duodenal ulceration. Fry (1964) found that patients with duodenal ulcer were three times more liable to neurosis than expected. The notion of a specific type of personality has been largely abandoned, but there is no doubt about the highly anxious disposition.

Response to Treatment

Often when intractable duodenal ulcers are treated with gastrectomy some new nervous symptoms appear. Browning and Houseworth (1953) compared the results of surgical and medical treatment in two groups of patients with intractable ulcer symptoms. In the surgical cases 43 per cent still had ulcer symptoms after operation, but the incidence of other psychosomatic symptoms increased from 13 per cent before operation to 37 per cent after operation and neurotic symptoms increased from 50 per cent to 100 per cent. Other interesting findings are that the suicide rate is higher after gastrectomy for peptic ulcer and that alcohol addiction is also more common.

The Irritable Colon Syndrome

This has also been called the spastic colon and mucous colitis. It is characterized by alternating diarrhoea and constipation, abdominal pain, flatulence and at times excessive quantities of mucus in the stools. It seems that patients with this complaint have colons which react more readily to parasympathetic stimulation than the normal.

ENDOCRINE DISORDERS

Endocrine Psychosomatic Relationships

In the past there has been a tendency to look upon hormones as the primary cause of emotional and behavioural patterns. In fact hormones release, potentiate, or inhibit patterns which are laid down in the nervous system and are, therefore, only partial causes of patterns of behaviour. The endocrine glands are directly or indirectly under the control of the nervous system. Thus there are areas in the hypothalamus which directly or indirectly control the release of pituitary hormones. The final result of the activity of these centres is fed back to them, so that their activity is controlled. The hormones which are produced by the peripheral endocrine glands may in turn have an effect on other hypothalamic centres producing change in behaviour patterns. Thus the gonadotrophic hormone of the pituitary stimulates the ovaries to produce oestrogen which has an effect on the female genitalia, but this hormone also affects the hypothalamic centres making the female animal sexually receptive.

Hyperthyroidism (Graves' Disease)

There is no doubt that psychological factors play a part in the illness.

Psychological Trauma

In some cases the illness appears to follow a severe emotional trauma. For example, a farmer came home to find his house on fire and despite all his efforts his wife and children were burnt to death before his eyes. Shortly after this he developed severe thyrotoxicosis. In other cases bereavement or prolonged emotional tension appears to have precipitated the illness.

Any explanation of the cause of thyrotoxicosis must account for the fact that this illness is much more common in women. As in other psychosomatic disorders it seems necessary to postulate an inborn mechanism which is the essential cause of the illness.

Diabetes Mellitus

This has been regarded as a psychosomatic disorder, but the accepted view is that it is an acquired or inherited organic disorder. Cases have been reported in which the onset of the disease was preceded by severe emotional stress, but these may be chance findings. It has, however, been shown that stressful situations in the established diabetic may produce marked changes in the insulin requirements. Situations which cause feelings of frustration, loneliness, or dejection are often followed by glycosuria and an increase in the insulin requirements, while satisfactory solution of psychological conflicts which leads to greater security may lead to a decrease in insulin requirements and hypoglycaemia.

Menstrual Disorders

Amenorrhoea

This may result from psychological trauma. For example, 73 women of a series of 732, who had been sexually assaulted, had amenorrhoea which was not due to pregnancy. Out of a total of 450 women who were interned in the Hong Kong Japanese internment camp 234 developed amenorrhoea following internment, although the diet was adequate at the time. Some depressed patients have amenorrhoea and a few chronic female schizophrenics do not menstruate, though this is rare.

Menorrhagia

This can occur in women under stress and sometimes occurs in depressive illnesses.

Dysmenorrhoea

It has been claimed that this is due to a faulty attitude towards sex and that the woman with dysmenorrhoea is rejecting the female role. Dysmenorrhoea is very common, and Coppen and Kessel (1963) in an unselected sample of women of menstrual age found that 12 per cent had severe pain and 33 per cent had moderate pain at the onset of a period. Dysmenorrhoea was not affected by marriage, but declined with parity. The same investigators administered the Maudsley Personality Inventory to a sample of 500 women and found that dysmenorrhoea was not associated with high scores on neuroticism or extraversion, which would be expected if the disorder was hysterical. On the other hand, they found that women with premenstrual tension had high neuroticism scores. The finding that dysmenorrhoea does not appear to be a neurotic condition is confirmed by an investigation of 800 female students, in which it was found that there was no greater incidence of psychological disorders in those students with dysmenorrhoea.

Premenstrual Tension

In this condition physical and mental symptoms occur in the second half of the menstrual cycle. The patient becomes anxious, tense and irritable and there may be depression, bloated feelings, fatigue, nausea, painful swelling of the breasts, headaches, dizziness and palpitations. Less often there is increased sexual desire, excessive thirst, increased appetite and hypersomnia. The symptoms begin 7–14 days before the period and pass off when menstruation begins. It has been claimed that this syndrome is the result of faulty luteinization, so that the action of the oestrogen produced by the ovary is not antagonized. The physical symptoms may be sometimes relieved by giving diuretics or substances with progestin activity, such as dimenthisterone and norethisterone. Benedek-Jaszmann and Hearn-Sturtevant (1976) obtained good results with bromocriptine, which suggested to them that the symptoms may be related to excess prolactin.

CARDIOVASCULAR DISORDERS

Essential Hypertension

In Britain many physicians do not accept that this is a psychosomatic disorder. Pickering, who has made a life-time study of the illness, paid no attention to the possible psychological causation of hypertension.

Nevertheless, there is much evidence that there is some relation between stress and raised blood pressure. For example, Heine, Sainsbury and Chynoweth (1969) found that in patients with a long history of depression with agitation, blood pressure correlated with ratings of anxiety and agitation. Cobb and Rose (1973) found that hypertension was four times more frequent in air-traffic controllers than in second-class airmen.

Coronary Artery Disease

Various groups of investigators have claimed that stress will disturb the coronary artery circulation. The most popular theory of the aetiology of coronary artery disease is that it is due to hypercholesterinaemia caused by diet and constitutional predisposition.

Personality Theories

A typical coronary personality (Type A) has been described as a compulsive man who drives himself too hard and, because of a chronic sense of time urgency, strives to accomplish more and more in less and less time (Friedman and Rosenman, 1959). This is much like the alleged psychosomatic personality of other disorders, but the evidence of a personality abnormality in this illness is a little more convincing.

Epidemiological Studies

Most epidemiological work suggests that restricted physical activity plays a part in the causation of coronary thrombosis. Thus Morris showed that sedentary workers had coronary thrombosis more often and more seriously than physically energetic workers. Some other findings contradict this to a degree. On the whole, epidemiological studies tend to discount the role of personality in coronary thrombosis and to incriminate physical inactivity, diet, smoking, and certain occupations. An important exception is the study of Rahe, Romo, Bennett and Siltanen (1974) which showed a clear increase in life-changes in the 6 months preceding myocardial infarction and death from coronary disease.

Paroxysmal Tachycardia

In an unselected series of patients with paroxysmal tachycardia, Fish found that the majority were suffering from a reactive anxiety state or a depressive illness. Stokvis trained a patient to think himself into an attack of paroxysmal tachycardia in order to prevent his deportation from Holland to a German concentration camp. There is little doubt that this condition has a neurophysiological basis, but nevertheless psychological factors appear to bring the patients to the cardiologists.

RHEUMATOID ARTHRITIS

Aetiology

The most popular aetiological theory is that rheumatoid arthritis is an auto-immune disease. As with other illness where the aetiology is obscure rheumatoid arthritis has been supposed to be a psychosomatic disease. Baker and Brewerton (1981) found that women with rheumatoid arthritis of recent onset had had significantly more stresses in the preceding months than a matched control group.

SKIN DISORDERS

The fact that psychological factors play a part in skin diseases has been recognized by dermatologists for years and anxiolytics have often been prescribed for the skin patient.

Psoriasis

It is well known that this condition may be provoked by psychological trauma, but it may also follow infectious illnesses and skin trauma. It is probably the result of an inherited predisposition of the skin to react in a special way.

Urticaria

It has been claimed that personality disorder is common in chronic urticaria, while emotional stress is often found in acute urticaria. The relation between urticaria and emotional stress is well shown in the case of the patient who always had an attack of urticaria when he was annoyed. He was admitted to hospital for investigation and the nursing staff were persuaded by the investigators to accuse the patient falsely of some minor infringement of the hospital rules. This made him angry and within a few minutes he developed an urticarial rash. Perhaps the most interesting patient is the woman who was dining with her lover and eating lobster when her husband surprised her and she immediately developed generalized urticaria. Previously she had not been allergic to lobster, but after this episode she always had urticaria whenever she ate it.

SUMMARY

Since many people with the same psychological difficulties which are allegedly specific causes of psychosomatic disorders suffer from neuroses and may even pass for normal, it is difficult to regard the psychological factors in psychosomatic disorders as more than contributory. There must be some, as yet undiscovered, disorder of the nervous system in each variety of psychosomatic disorder.

Chapter 8

Drug Dependence

Drug Dependence

The Expert Committee of the World Health Organization (1969) defined drug dependence as 'a state, psychic and sometimes also physical, resulting from the interaction between a living organism and a drug, characterized by behavioural and other responses that always include a compulsion to take the drug on a continuous or periodic basis in order to experience its psychic effects and sometimes to avoid the discomfort of its absence. Tolerance may or may not be present. A person may be dependent on more than one drug.' Six types were defined in terms of the typical drug: morphine, barbiturate or alcohol, amphetamine, cocaine, cannabis and hallucinogens.

ALCOHOLISM

This term is used rather loosely to designate heavy drinkers of all kinds. It is better to use the following terms:

1. Habitual Drinkers

These may have a high consumption but can control it if they wish.

2. Psychological Dependence

The drinking problem is related not so much to the quantity as to the reasons for drinking. There is psychological dependence if the person: (a) drinks to cope with difficulties; (b) engages in surreptitious drinking; (c) takes steps to ensure that drink is always available.

CLINICAL FEATURES

The drinker will experience 'blackouts' (anterograde amnesia, palimpsest memory) in which even after a moderate intake of alcohol he behaves normally but has no memory of what he has done. In addition, he will suffer from loss of appetite and indigestion. Anxiety and depression are common.

The drinking gives rise to difficulties with the spouse. Impotence or refusal of sexual intercourse will add to these. At work, the drinker may arrive late (especially on Mondays) or absent himself frequently. The excessive amount of money spent on drink may lead to financial difficulties. There may be outbursts of aggressive behaviour. Despite this, the drinker will deny he has a problem or blame others for all his difficulties.

3. *Physical Dependence*
In this state the subject has no complete power to make decisions about drinking: whether to refrain or to stop before becoming drunk. This is often called 'loss of control', but the loss is a gradual process.

CLINICAL FEATURES
The previous symptoms and difficulties become worse. In addition, drinking may occur at unusual times, e.g. in the morning, before an important interview. The person will experience a craving for drink, brought on by anxiety, depression or by surroundings conducive to drink. Tolerance gradually develops. Withdrawal symptoms begin to appear: 'morning shakes' (hand tremor), sweating, malaise, nausea and retching.

Aetiology
Social Factors
Some people become alcoholics because they live in an environment where heavy drinking is the rule, for example, business men, publicans and barmen. Anything which leads to the rapid drinking of hard liquor will lead to dependence, for example, inappropriate licensing laws and poor drinking conditions.

Psychiatric Illnesses
On the whole, the major psychoses are not associated with alcohol dependence in Britain. Chronic anxiety states may lead to drinking when the patient finds that alcohol calms him down.

Personality Abnormalities
Some psychopathic personalities are *inter alia* alcohol dependent. Gloomy, anxious, inadequate people may drink for relief and become dependent. Periodic drinkers are psychopathic personalities with periodic crises in which they drink to seek oblivion.

Genetic Factors
Studies of family histories, twins and adopted children of alcoholics have shown that in some cases there is a hereditary tendency to alcohol dependence. This may explain why heavy drinkers do not always become dependent.

Treatment
This is mainly by psychotherapy, but some physical methods may be helpful adjuncts.

Psychotherapy: The Basic Rules

1. The patient must agree that he is an alcohol addict and that he must not drink alcohol for the rest of his life. About 5 per cent of addicts can return to 'social drinking', but to hold out the hope of this to the patient is to lay a trap for the other 95 per cent.
2. No pledges or promises should be extracted from the patient.
3. The patient must be frank with the therapist and contact him as soon as possible in the event of a relapse.
4. The patient must be treated as an adult by the therapist and the relatives. He must make his own decisions and be responsible for his actions.
5. Threats of physical, mental, or social ruin are worse than useless and may produce an 'I don't care if I do die' attitude.

POINTS ABOUT PSYCHOTHERAPY

The problem is to help the patient find something worthwhile which will fill up the gap in his life left by giving up alcohol. Religious activities or some kind of help for others may fill this gap. Alcoholics Anonymous (A.A.) is an organization of ex-alcoholics who help alcoholics to give up drinking. This is really a variety of group therapy with the additional advantage that the patient is able to live a life with some meaning, i.e. he helps himself by helping others. When patients are admitted to hospital, preparations should be started immediately for providing food, shelter and work on discharge.

Physical Treatment

DISULFIRAM (ANTABUSE, CRONETAL)

This substance inhibits the enzyme responsible for the breakdown of acetaldehyde, an intermediate metabolite in the utilization of alcohol. If the patient drinks while taking the drug he is upset by the acetaldehyde, which causes flushing, tachycardia, dyspnoea, nausea and vomiting. A dose of 0·5 g of the drug is given daily for a week, and then reduced to 0·25 g daily. Towards the end of the first week a test dose of 50–100 ml of spirits in 150–250 ml of water is taken. This produces a reaction so that the patient knows what to expect. This drug is a useful prop in a reasonable patient who is likely to have drink forced upon him. It should not be given to patients with severe chest, heart, or liver disease.

Citrated calcium carbimide (Abstem) has been introduced as a milder substitute for disulfiram. It produces no toxic reactions or side-effects. Sensitivity to alcohol appears within a few hours, but the reaction to a test dose of alcohol is usually much milder than with disulfiram.

AVERSION THERAPY
This consists of attempting to condition the patient against alcohol by making him vomit with apomorphine when he drinks. The value of this treatment is extremely doubtful.

Prognosis
The best results are obtained in those patients who have become alcohol dependent due to social pressures. On the whole, the prognosis is not good. When alcoholism is associated with depressive illness, it has been shown by Merry et al. (1976) that prophylactic lithium therapy can be of great help in reducing incapacity.

PSYCHOLOGICAL DISORDERS ASSOCIATED WITH ALCOHOL
Pathological Intoxication
After taking a small quantity of alcohol some individuals develop a mild clouding of consciousness and very violent behaviour. The normal signs of drunkenness are absent. On recovery there is usually no memory of the episode. Many of these patients have abnormal EEG records. The illness is an organic twilight state produced in a susceptible subject by excessive fluid intake and alcohol.

Delirium Tremens
Aetiology
Delirium tremens develops after many years of misuse of alcohol, so that it usually occurs in the fifth and sixth decades. Infection or injury may initiate the illness. Abstinence from alcohol is probably the most important causative factor, so that the disorder can be regarded as a withdrawal phenomenon.

The Prodromal Period
This may come on a few days or a week before the onset. The patient is anxious, tremulous (most obvious in the hands) and restless, with hypersensitivity to noise and light. Nausea is common, especially in the mornings, together with anorexia. Isolated visual hallucinations occur, especially in the dark and when the patient is alone, in about a quarter of cases. The symptoms increase in severity until disorientation and delirium are produced. Epileptic fits in about 10 per cent of cases occur in the prodromal period and may mark the onset of the delirium.

The Delirium
The general appearance is characteristic. The face is red, there is marked sweating, with high pulse rate and dilated pupils and a severe tremor affecting the hands, the speech and the upper part of the body. Visual

hallucinations are outstanding. Small animals, such as beetles, mice and snakes, are seen, usually accompanied by severe anxiety or intense terror. Occasionally Lilliputian hallucinations occur, associated with marked pleasure. Scenes and pictures are sometimes hallucinated. Hallucinations can be suggested and the patient may be persuaded to read from a plain piece of paper. Hallucinatory voices are rare, but noises, isolated words and music may be heard. Hallucinations of touch, muscle senses and equilibrium are very common.

Consciousness is changed in a dream-like way. Disorientation for time and place is complete, but there is no disorientation for person. Attention can be obtained for short periods, especially if the examiner speaks loudly, slowly and clearly. In these circumstances the patient will answer questions and accept reassurance.

There is marked restlessness with pressure of activity. Sometimes the patient carries out the actions of his trade (occupational delirium). The mood swings between euphoria and anxiety.

There is absolute insomnia and the illness often ends with a so-called critical sleep lasting 24–48 hours, at the end of which the patient wakes recovered or with a Korsakoff state.

Course and Prognosis

Usually it lasts from 2 to 6 days, but abortive cases lasting 1–2 days occur. Mortality varies from 1 to 15 per cent in different series and depends on age and presence of complicating illnesses and injuries.

Treatment

This consists of sedation with phenothiazines, but diazepam may be used if necessary. Antibiotics are given for complicating illnesses. It has been claimed that large doses of vitamin B complex (Parentrovite) are curative, but the evidence is contradictory.

Alcoholic Hallucinosis

This occurs in heavy drinkers. Hallucinatory voices become suddenly apparent in a state of clear consciousness, or a mild, transient, delirious state lasting a day or so ushers in the hallucinosis, which continues in clear consciousness. The voices seem to come from above the patient's head; they talk about him in the third person, abuse him and call him a homosexual. Because of the voices the patient believes that he is being persecuted.

Illusions and delusional misinterpretations of sensory stimuli and occasionally visual hallucinations occur at night, so that a mixture of delirium tremens and alcoholic hallucinosis is sometimes present.

The hallucinosis lasts longer than in delirium tremens, but half the patients recover within a month. Patients who do not recover within 6 months remain chronic and have intellectual impairment.

Treatment is the same as that recommended for delirium tremens.

The Alcoholic Korsakoff State

Korsakoff described a syndrome characterized by failure of immediate memory and associated with polyneuritis. It was later realized that it was due to alcohol, but that the same sort of memory defect occurred in subacute brain disease produced by many different diseases. The clinical picture with loss of registration as its main feature is called the 'Korsakoff state' or 'amnestic syndrome', but when there is also a polyneuritis it can be called 'Korsakoff's psychosis'.

The Clinical Picture

Disorientation for time and place is complete, but orientation for person is preserved. Despite the gross disorientation the patient can usually find his way about the ward and his behaviour is in keeping with the environment.

Memory for knowledge acquired earlier in life is well preserved, but often there is a retrograde amnesia for events immediately preceding the illness, which sometimes stretches back to a point many years before. It is often said that impressibility (registration) is disordered, but although one of the major disorders is that of 'minute memory' (*see* p. 150), experiments involving recognition and relearning show that new memories can be acquired with difficulty but cannot be evoked or recalled. Confabulation usually occurs, but may not be spontaneous. In such cases the patient can usually be persuaded to confabulate. The confabulation covers up the gaps in the memory.

Thinking is disordered in that there is difficulty in changing the direction of thought, so that all incoming sensations are distorted in terms of the current train of thought, which only changes direction when disturbed by some intense stimulus from without or within. The mood is usually one of euphoria. There is no insight into the disorders of memory and orientation. The general attitude is one of passivity, and often these patients are extremely suggestible. Polyneuritis is usually, but not invariably, present.

Treatment

It is customary to give large doses of vitamin B complex.

Prognosis

This is poor, since some degree of dementia is often the final result.

Wernicke's Encephalopathy

The direct cause is a deficiency of thiamine (aneurin). This can be produced by poor diet, excessive vomiting, or secondary dietary deficiency due to alcoholism.

Pathology

Acute haemorrhagic lesions are found in the periaqueductal grey matter in all cases, in the mamillary bodies in most, and in the dorsomedial nucleus of the thalamus in over 50 per cent of cases. This is more or less the same as the distribution of gliosis in alcoholic Korsakoff states. It is probable that both disorders are due to thiamine deficiency and the difference between them is merely in the tempo of the morbid processes.

Clinical Picture

Eye signs are characteristic. There is lateral nystagmus and ophthalmoplegia, most frequently a lateral rectus palsy. Ataxia is well marked and the patient walks on a wide base and tends to reel.

Spontaneous speech is minimal and there is a strange aversion. The patient answers questions in a perfunctory manner and cannot focus his attention on any topic. He may turn over and go to sleep during a conversation. The typical memory and thought disorder of the Korsakoff state is often present. There is, in fact, no sharp boundary between Wernicke's encephalopathy and the Korsakoff state.

Treatment

Large doses of vitamin B complex are given. The administration of thiamine alone might unmask other vitamin deficiencies.

Outcome

Death often occurs. In some series 50 per cent died. As a rule, when the acute signs die away a Korsakoff state is left behind.

Alcoholic Dementia

This may come on insidiously or may follow delirium tremens, alcoholic hallucinosis, the Korsakoff state, or Wernicke's encephalopathy. CAT scans have shown that cerebral atrophy is much more common in heavy drinkers than had been realized.

Alcoholic Delusions of Jealousy (Alcoholic Paranoia)

The alcohol addict may develop delusions of jealousy, which may at first only occur during drunkenness. The condition is often attributed to the alcoholic's diminished potency, his increased desire when drunk, and the wife's refusal to have sexual intercourse because of his lack of consideration and general unpleasant behaviour when drunk. The wife's refusal is misinterpreted.

There are probably three different types of jealous alcoholics: (1) jealous husbands (*see* p. 144); (2) inadequate insecure persons who become jealous when drunk—this stops when the patient gives up drinking; and (3) schizophrenics who are also heavy drinkers.

DRUG DEPENDENCE
Drugs Involved
There are three main groups depending on pharmacological effects.
1. *Opiates.* Morphine, heroin, pethidine and other synthetic drugs.
2. *Euphoriants.* Cocain, marijuana, the sympathomimetic amines and the hallucinogenic drugs.
3. *Hypnotics.* The barbiturates, benzodiazepines and other anxiolytics.

Opiate Dependence
All the analgesic drugs cause tolerance, physical dependence, and emotional dependence. Liability to dependence ranges continuously from those whose life is quite unaffected by regular consumption of the drug, to those whose life revolves around it, with nothing left for work, career or friends. Dependence on morphine will be used as a paradigm.

The Administration of the Drug
Initially it is taken subcutaneously and in some subjects this may cause nausea, vomiting and malaise at first, but after repeated injections the side-effects decrease in intensity. The subject drifts off into a light sleep and then wakes and nods off repeatedly. During the drowsiness, dreams related to the usual fantasies occur.

Intravenous morphine ('mainline') produces dizziness, flushing, itching and rumbling in the stomach. A sensation occurs in the abdomen like an orgasm, but it does not affect the genitals.

Symptoms during Addiction
The pupils are constricted, constipation is always present and libido declines. Women usually stop menstruating and rarely become pregnant. As long as the addict gets an adequate supply of the drug he can carry on with his job and is in fairly good health. Emaciation is secondary to the use of available cash to buy drugs instead of food.

The Abstinence Syndrome
The clinical features of this condition are shown in *Table 1.*

This syndrome is due to a physiological change in the whole of the nervous system. An adequate dose of morphine or an equivalent drug will reverse the abstinence symptoms completely within a few minutes. The abstinence syndrome is best treated with methadone linctus (2 mg in 5 ml). In Stage 1, 10 mg methadone should be given and 20 mg can be given 1 hour later if the symptoms do not subside. If Stage 2 has been reached 20 mg methadone should be given and repeated in 2 hours. When withdrawal symptoms appear in the course of treatment, it has been found that propanolol can alleviate them considerably (Hage and Jensen, 1975).

Table 1. THE ABSTINENCE SYNDROME

PERIOD OF ABSTENTION SYMPTOMS

Stage 1	14–18 hours	Yawning, perspiration, rhinorrhoea, mild lacrimation
Stage 2	18–24 hours	Absolute insomnia, worsening of above symptoms Muscular twitchings, aching in legs and back. Hot and cold flushes Patient curls up and covers himself with blankets
Stage 3	36–48 hours	Extreme restlessness. Patient gets in and out of bed Retching and vomiting. All other symptoms increase in severity Rapid weight-loss. Extreme misery Temperature rises by about 1°C Blood pressure rises by 15–30 mmHg Increase of respiration rate
Stage 4	48–60 hours	Peak intensity of all symptoms—may then decline
Stage 5	7–10 days	Objective signs absent Insomnia, weakness, jitteriness, aches and pains persist for weeks

Other Opiates and Morphine Substitutes

In general, if a drug is as effective an analgesic as morphine it is likely to have the same addiction-producing property.

Addiction to the synthetic analgesics is roughly the same as morphine addiction, but the intensity of the abstinence syndrome is somewhat less. This is especially the case with methadone (Physeptone). Heroin, which is diamorphine, has slight side-effects, but the abstinence syndrome is as bad as that of morphine.

Meperidine (Pethidine) taken subcutaneously produces severe dizziness and elation. As the duration of its action is brief the addict takes it at 2–3 hour intervals throughout the 24 hours. The drug is irritant, so that indurated patches occur in the skin and muscles and large skin ulcers may occur. Tolerance is marked and daily doses of 1000–4000 mg may be reached. Unlike morphine, tolerance is not complete and the drug has a toxic effect. Tremors, confusion, visual hallucinations and fits may occur. The EEG shows paroxysms of high-voltage slow waves and spike and wave discharges.

Abstinence symptoms are like those of morphine but occur in 3–4 hours and are maximal after 8–12 hours.

The Diagnosis of Drug Addiction

Isolation will produce abstinence symptoms; a morphine antagonist will produce abstinence symptoms. Naloxone given intravenously will produce discernible withdrawal symptoms in a dose of 0·1 mg. Larger doses, up to 0·8 mg in 2 ml given slowly i.v., will detect minimal dependence. The effect of the injection lasts 20–30 minutes.

When a teenager starts on heroin, it may be recognized by such changes as loss of appetite, loss of interest in his appearance, staying secluded in his room, unexpected absences from home (to obtain supplies), sleeping out and giving up organized activities (Rathod et al., 1967).

Treatment

The first step is to withdraw the drug. This must be done in an institution and the patient's physical health should be good. Methadone given orally is substituted for the opiate (1 mg methadone = 4 mg morphine = 2 mg heroin = 20–30 mg meperidine). Once substitution has been made the methadone is withdrawn over 3–10 days, depending on the response. If the patient is in poor physical health it may be withdrawn more slowly.

When the patient has been detoxified and shows no dependence (as demonstrated by a test with nalorphine), he can be put on naltrexone, which prevents the euphoriant effect of narcotics. The drug is taken by mouth in liquid form, starting with a small dose increased to 50 mg in 3 days. This dose is effective for 24 hours, 100 mg for 2 days, and 150 mg for 3 days. Maintenance is by 100 mg on Mondays and Wednesdays and 150 mg on Fridays.

Physical treatments must be regarded as only a first step in treatment and rehabilitation. Individual psychotherapy appears to be of little value, but group therapy can be helpful. Experience in the USA has shown that the 'Synanon' communes can be very effective in the rehabilitation of some drug addicts.

The outcome of heroin dependence is poor, even if not quite as bad as was once thought. In one series, after 10 years, 40 per cent had become abstinent, 40 per cent continued, and 15 per cent had died. The rest were lost to the follow-up.

Euphoriants

These drugs are all different in chemical structure but all produce euphoria and there is no complete tolerance to them.

Cocaine

The drug is taken as snuff, or intravenously, usually in conjunction with heroin or morphine. It produces an ecstatic sensation of extreme mental and physical power, with the abolition of all sensations of fatigue and hunger. The effects wear off quickly in several minutes and the doses have to be repeated every time the effect disappears. This causes toxic symptoms such as tachycardia, rise in blood pressure, severe sweating, tremors, twitching, muscular spasms and occasionally convulsions.

If the drug is taken for some time a paranoid psychosis develops: the patient believes that he is being watched by detectives, and may assault innocent bystanders. Formication, the feeling of insects crawling on the skin, occurs. This is known as the 'cocaine bug'.

The Sympathomimetic Amines

Dextroamphetamine sulphate and methylamphetamine hydrochloride are the drugs of this group which are most commonly taken. Often barbiturates and/or alcohol are taken as well. Some tolerance occurs, but toxic effects always occur in high doses. An intake of 2000 mg a day has been recorded. A paranoid psychosis indistinguishable from schizophrenia often results from high doses.

Marijuana

Hashish or marijuana is usually smoked, mixed with tobacco, in the 'reefer' cigarette. It produces elation and a distortion of space and time. The conjunctivae are injected and pseudoptosis occurs. There is no tolerance and dependence on it is very similar to that on alcohol.

Hallucinogenic Drugs

Officially, according to the Poisons Regulations (Hallucinogenic Drugs), 1967, the following drugs are included in this designation: dimethyltryptamine, lysergic acid diethylamide (LSD), mescaline, psilocybin and psilocin. The latest fashion for 'street drugs' now includes phencyclidine. Severe panic, chaotic behaviour and suicide may occur during the psychosis induced by these drugs. Permanent schizophrenic psychoses have been reported, but experimenting with LSD occurs in the age groups in which schizophrenia is not uncommon. Physical dependence on LSD probably does not occur, but psychological dependence does. It has been found that LSD can cause chromosomal damage.

Barbiturates and Benzodiazepines

Barbiturate dependence was once common in the UK, but has ceased to be a problem (except for abuse with 'street drugs') now that the prescribing of barbiturates as anxiolytics has been largely abandoned. Barbiturates have been replaced by the benzodiazepines not only because they are much safer in overdosage, but also because they are much more effective in relieving anxiety and have fewer and less severe side-effects.

Rebound effects can be seen in the EEG after as short a period of use as 1–2 weeks. Dependence can occur with therapeutic levels of dosage after 4 months. Dependence can be either of the type associated with increasing dosage, or with a steady dosage at therapeutic levels.

Abstinence Symptoms

The commonest withdrawal symptoms (in descending order of frequency) are: anxiety and tension, disturbed sleep, loss of appetite, metallic taste, paraesthesia, sore eyes and photophobia, headache, incoordination and vertigo, muscle aches and twitchings, tremor, nausea and retching. Convulsions (unlike with the barbiturates) are rare.

Treatment of Dependence

This is best carried out in hospital. The drugs consumption is reduced to zero over a period of 4 or, at the most, 8 weeks. No advantage is gained from a longer period.

Dependence on Other Hypnotics

Dependence on paraldehyde, chloral hydrate and meprobamate can occur. The symptoms are like barbiturate dependence and the effects of withdrawal are about the same. Chloral addicts tend to have red puffy eyes. Any drug as effective as a quick-acting barbiturate in relieving anxiety will probably be just as prone to produce dependence.

Psychological Theories of Addiction

General Psychiatric Views

Some addicts are normal personalities who become addicted due to the injudicious use of analgesics. Others are neurotics, psychopaths, or people with both psychopathic and neurotic traits.

*Personality Types**

There are five personality types of addicts:

1. Normal individuals in whom addiction is due to unwise use of analgesics by doctors.

2. Neurotic individuals who take drugs to relieve anxiety.

3. Psychopathic individuals who take drugs to produce elation or a 'lift' of some kind.

4. Individuals with both neurotic and psychopathic characteristics.

5. Psychotic individuals who take the drug to relieve depression.

Wikler's Pharmacodynamic Interpretation

Wikler suggests that the specific pharmacological effect of the drug may help the subject with his psychological problems. Thus, since opiates reduce primary drives such as hunger, pain and sex, and also decrease aggression, the addict will be someone whose main sources of anxiety are associated with these drives. The effect of the drug is useful to the addict. When physical dependence occurs a new need for the drug is

*The terms 'psychopath' and 'neurotic' are used here in the standard Anglo-American sense.

created, so that addiction is partly maintained by this secondary factor. The immediate relief of withdrawal symptoms by the drug leads the addict to treasure it, and he then uses the drug for any discomfort. Any unusual situation requires an injection, so that the addict is 'conditioned'.

General Social Factors

Social factors determine the availability and the use of drugs in a given community. In Britain where control of the import of drugs has been strict, addiction for a long time occurred only among those with access to dangerous drugs, such as doctors, nurses, and so on. In 1959 there were very few heroin addicts in Britain under the age of 35 years, but by 1965 there were 100 known addicts under the age of 20. The epidemic of heroin addiction that followed was partly controlled by stricter regulations on the prescribing of heroin, but at the end of 1974 there were 1980 registered narcotic addicts in Britain, and the numbers are still growing. The control of dangerous drugs in Britain is by the Misuse of Drugs Act 1971 and the Regulations of 1973. Such Regulations are brought up to date by the Home Office on the advice of the Advisory Council on Misuse of Drugs.

Chapter 9

Affective psychoses and manic-depressive illness

GENERAL PRINCIPLES

Manic-depressive Disease

Kraepelin isolated manic-depressive insanity as a group of illnesses which were usually recurrent, in which recovery usually occurred, and in which disorder of emotion determined all the symptoms. These illnesses occurred in individuals who showed some mood abnormality even when apparently well, particularly 'cyclothymia', which means swings of mood in opposite directions. Thus manic-depressive insanity consisted of mania, depression, or both, in an individual with an inherited predisposition to mood disorders. The following types of illness could be observed: (1) a single depressive attack; (2) a single manic attack; (3) recurrent depression; (4) recurrent mania; (5) circular psychosis, i.e. attacks of mania and depression at different times; (6) mixed affective states; (7) constitutional excitement (hyperthymia); (8) cyclothymia, i.e. an alternation of mild manic and depressive moods.

Are All Affective Psychoses Manic-depressive?

Kleist regarded manic-depressive illness as a bipolar illness, because either features of the opposite condition could be seen in any given clinical picture, or attacks of mania and depression occurred at different times in the patient's life. Leonhard, following Kleist, has distinguished pure melancholia, pure mania, five varieties of pure depression and five types of pure euphoria from manic-depressive disease.

There seems to be little point in making such fine subdivisions and the introduction of effective treatment has shown that they are irrelevant. What has been increasingly recognized as important is that many patients have recurrent attacks of depression without ever experiencing any mania.

It is always possible for such patients to have an attack of mania, and Perris (1966) has shown that the probability of such an occurrence drops to low levels after three to four attacks of depression. Genetic studies suggest that pure recurrent depressions (unipolar depressions) have a genetic background different from the depressions with mania (bipolar depressions). If then it is accepted that not all depressions are manic-depressive, then it is necessary to subsume the manic-depresive disorders under the broader grouping of affective disorders. This does not require any alteration of the definition that the primary disturbance is a change of mood, but immediately raises the question of the place of the anxiety states. Logically, they should be included with the affective disorders and, fortunately, clinical evidence provides support for such a classification.

There are then three main groups of affective disorders:

1. Mania.
2. Depressions.
3. Anxiety states.

The manias have often been subclassified into (a) mania, (b) hypomania and (c) chronic mania.

The depressions are clearly a very mixed group and classifying them seems to be a favourite preoccupation of some psychiatrists. It is convenient to distinguish between the following types:

a. Bipolar disorder, in which recurrent bouts of depression are interspersed with attacks of mania. A common form is when the mania precedes the depression.

b. Unipolar depressions.

c. Single depressions.

Another method of classification, and one which is of practical value, is based on the pattern of symptoms. One can distinguish between two extremes (a) retarded and (b) anxious (or agitated) depressions. There is much controversy nowadays as to whether this distinction merely refers to the differences between the extremes of a distribution, in which intermediate types are common, or whether it refers to two types which are distinct, implying that intermediate forms are relatively uncommon.

Other classifications distinguish between 'psychotic' and 'neurotic' depressions, about which sufficient has already been said (see p. 201); or between 'reactive' depressions, where the illness is precipitated by psychological stress, and 'endogenous' depressions where it is not. These distinctions are sometimes confused, as in the phrase 'an endogenous depression precipitated by psychological stress', or muddled, e.g. endogenous versus neurotic depressions. This is analogous to classifying races as African versus Redheads.

INCIDENCE

The average incidence of affective disorder demanding psychiatric treatment is 3–4 per 1000 of the population. Depressive illnesses of the milder sort are extremely common. The peak incidence of hospital admissions is between 55 and 65 years.

AETIOLOGY

Heredity

The tendency to mood disorder rather than this illness as such is inherited. The incidence of manic-depressive illness among the parents of patients is 10·2 per cent and among children is 12·8 per cent (Slater, 1938). Studies of twins have shown that 68 per cent of monozygotic twins are concordant for affective disorder, whereas for same-sexed dizygotic twins the concordance rate is only 23 per cent. Perris (1966) found that the risk of affective illness in the first-degree relatives of patients suffering from bipolar illness was 10·1 per cent for bipolar illness, but only 0·5 per cent for unipolar illness. Correspondingly, in relatives of patients with unipolar illness, the risk for unipolar illness was 5·0 per cent, but only 0·3 per cent for bipolar illness. It seems almost certain that manic-depressive psychoses are heterogenous genetically.

The Basic Personality

Four varieties of personality are found in association with manic-depressive disorder. They are as follows:

1. *The Depressive Personality (Dysthymic)*
Gloomy, conscience-stricken individuals, embittered by fears and cares.

2. *The Manic Personality (Hyperthymic)*
Cheerful, happy, bustling, self-confident 'go-getter'.

3. *The Irritable Personality*
Querulous, quarrelsome, embittered and easily upset.

4. *The Cyclothymic Personality*
All three of the previous types may swing into the opposite mood state for a short time, whereas the cyclothymic has mood changes of depression or elation which last for days or weeks and are never in equilibrium.

The Physical Constitution

The pyknic body build, as described by Kretschmer, is common in manic-depressive disorder. This is a stocky build, with a broad, rounded face with no sharp features, a short, massive neck and rotund abdomen, large visceral cavities, tendency to fat on the trunk, slender extremities, tapering to small hands and feet. On the whole, all one can say about body build and mental disorder is that the thick-set are more often found among manic-depressives and the thin and ill-thriven among schizophrenics; but there is a marked overlap. Other physical factors are:

Race
Bipolar disorder is said to be more common among Jews.

Sex
Admission rates for affective disorders usually show a proportion of at least 3 females to 2 males.

Physical Disease
Affective psychoses, especially depressions, may be released by brain disease: for example, general paralysis of the insane, cerebral arteriosclerosis, etc.

Endocrines
Depression and tension occur in the premenstrual period. Adrenal hormones may cause affective disorders in the predisposed. Affective disorders are common after childbirth and at the menopause.

The Diencephalon
Foerster and Gagel (1933) pressed on the intact hypothalamus during an operation under local anaesthesia and elation and flight of ideas occurred. Manic clinical pictures may occur in disorders affecting the hypothalamus.

Perris (1966) found that 17 per cent of 148 depressed patients had 'immature' EEGs. More recently (Perris, 1975) he showed that some variables in the EEG correlated with severity of depression.

Reserpine
This drug has been used as a 'tranquillizer' and also for the treatment of hypertension. It has been shown that even one single dose will deplete the cerebral stores of serotonin and these do not return to normal for at least a month. It can produce severe depressive illness in some patients receiving this drug, presumably those who have a predisposition to affective disorder. This condition is not relieved by withdrawal of the drug and must be treated in the same way as a primary depressive illness.

Biochemical Abnormalities
There is evidence that depressives have some deficiency of serotonin in the brain and possibly of catecholamines. The mono-amine oxidase inhibitors and the tricyclic antidepressants increase the amount of free amines in the brain, the former by decreasing their metabolism and the latter by inhibiting their re-uptake. Tryptophan is a precursor of serotonin and it has been shown that it is probably an effective antidepressant, especially when combined with MAO inhibitors.

Other biochemical disturbances in the affective disorders are related to water and electrolyte balance. It has been shown that residual sodium (cell sodium and a small amount in bone) is increased in the affective disorders by as much as 50 per cent in depression and as much as 200 per cent in mania. The administration of lithium lowers the residual sodium. Lithium seems to have a specific effect on manic symptoms, whereas neuroleptics give rise to a drug-induced quietude. There is a loss of extracellular fluid at the onset of a depressive illness and this is regained as the patient improves clinically. These changes are accompanied by corresponding changes in the weight of the patient, and can occur even when the dietary intake is stabilized.

Reactive Factors

Most illnesses are due to the reaction between constitutional and external factors. The latter can range from obvious stress to none at all and the illness will therefore range between 'reactive' and 'endogenous'. In assessing the role of external stress, it is possible to make errors either way. Everybody has troubles of some sort and therefore it is very easy to blame an illness on to them. Patients are prone to account for their illness in this way but sometimes a careful history will show that symptoms began before the apparent precipitating stress. Errors can occur in the opposite direction: to state that no precipitating stress occurred can mean only that none has been found. Even then the significance of a traumatic event must be considered from the patient's point of view. What may appear trivial to the observer may be a threat to all that the patient holds most dear.

Psychoanalytic Theory

The Fixation Point in Depression

This is at the oral stage of libidinal development. Fixation at this stage produces an individual who is unduly dependent on supplies of affection from others.

Development of the Depression

An experience causes loss of self-esteem or narcissistic supplies, i.e. supplies of affection which bolster up the self-esteem. The patient reacts to his loss of the love object by introjecting, so that he has the fantasy that he has devoured the ambivalently loved object. The sadistic nature of the mechanism of introjection gives rise to guilt.

Mourning and Melancholia

When a loved person dies the lover is still linked to the lost love one by a large number of memories. These ties have to be broken and this is a difficult and painful process. The mourner incorporates an image of the lost loved one and the normal person finds it easier to loosen the ties with an introject than with an external object.

The reaction to bereavement will be more intense when: (1) the object has not been loved on a mature level, but has been used as a source of narcissistic supplies; (2) the relationship with the lost object was ambivalent; or (3) there is oral fixation with unconscious longings for sexualized eating. These characteristics are found in people predisposed to depression.

Mania

The same conflicts occur in mania as in depression, but the patient uses the defence mechanisms of denial and overcompensation. This idea of the denial of depression in mania is sometimes expressed in the phrase 'manic defence'.

CLINICAL STATES

General Symptomatology

The symptoms are commonly described as occurring in one of three main spheres. These are: (1) psychomotor activity, (2) emotion and (3) volition.

If the activity in these three spheres is increased then there is a manic illness; if diminished, a depressive illness. If activity is increased in one sphere and diminished in another then there is a mixed affective state. We can now consider: (1) mania, (2) depression, (3) mixed affective states and (4) anxiety states.

1. MANIA

In contrast to the depressions, mania is an uncommon disorder. It has been said that it is becoming less common, but clear evidence is wanting.

Mood and General Behaviour

The mood ranges from exuberant cheerfulness and pleasant overhelpfulness to wild, unruly high spirits. All inhibitions have disappeared. The patient is domineering and rejects control. He may suddenly become very irritable or very sad and even weepy for a minute or so. He is full of jokes and witty comments, but easily steps beyond normal bounds when he notices the vanities and conceits of others and makes fun of them. His remarks can then hurt and are not easily tolerated. In chronic cases, the mood becomes more and more tinged with angry excitement with marked ideas of persecution, such as unjust detention or legal committal, etc. Sexual activity is often increased. The patient feels superbly well and denies that anything is wrong with him.

Pressure of Activity

Patients are overactive; they undertake a multitude of things which they cannot carry through. If the illness is severe there may be ceaseless activities; they shout until they are hoarse, and smash things without reason. They often play tricks and practical jokes.

Pressure of Speech

Speech ranges from over-talkativeness to a never-ending chatter. The puns, allusions and 'clang' associations become more and more based on chance and environmental influences until it becomes impossible to follow the connection between one thought and the next, the typical 'flight of ideas'.

Delusional Ideas

Grandiose ideas and a general superior attitude are evident. As they upset other people they may resent the natural results of their own offensive behaviour and believe that others are against them. They may have erotic ideas about strangers. Hypochondriacal ideas may occur, but do not have the sense of urgency which they have in depression.

Hallucinations

Misinterpretations and illusions are common, but true hallucinations are rare.

Bodily Changes

Loss of weight and early morning wakening are common, but unlike the depressive the patient has a good appetite and looks well, with a fresh, youthful appearance and quick, forceful movements. If the mania is severe then exhaustion may occur.

Severity of Symptoms

In hypomania there are mild overactivity and cheerfulness which may pass as normal to lay persons. In mania overactivity may be very severe and in acute mania life may be threatened from exhaustion and intercurrent diseases.

Differential Diagnosis

When the typical symptoms are present, the diagnosis is easy, but typical symptoms are not all that common. Manic patients often experience brief periods of depression, sometimes even shedding a few tears. The inexperienced psychiatrist may confuse this with the emotional lability of dementia.

In acute mania, the speech may become so disturbed that it is impossible to follow the connection of ideas. Euphoria may be difficult to distinguish from excitement and the clinical picture comes to resemble that of schizophrenia. In chronic patients, euphoria tends to fade away and the patient becomes more and more frustrated by the refusal of others to accept his wonderful ideas and ingenious schemes. Thus his attitude and speech become increasingly paranoid.

The Treatment of Mania

1. Phenothiazines

In marked excitement chlorpromazine should be given 50 (occasionally 100) mg 4- to 6-hourly by intramuscular injection. At the same time the drug should be given orally, 25 mg three times a day on the first day, 50 mg three times on the second, and 75 mg four times a day on the third. The intramuscular administration of the drug can be stopped as soon as the patient is no longer excited, and occasional doses may be given later if the excitement worsens. Usually it is not necessary to continue the intramuscular chlorpromazine longer than 48 hours. The oral dose of chlorpromazine may have to be increased to 400–500 mg a day or in rare cases to 1000 mg a day. Since chlorpromazine has been known to cause severe jaundice, another phenothiazine may be preferred. A dose of 25 mg of chlorpromazine is roughly equivalent to 25 mg of thioridazine, 2 mg of perphenazine, and 2·5 mg of trifluoperazine. It may be necessary to give antiparkinsonian drugs in addition, such as orphenadrine hydrochloride 50 mg three or four times a day, or benztropine methanesulphonate 1 mg three times a day.

2. Haloperidol

This is a butyrophenone. In acute excitements 5 mg of this drug can be given intramuscularly 6-hourly and once the excitement is under control 1·5–3 mg can be given orally three times a day. Doses of up to 7·5 mg a day can be given without any complications apart from Parkinsonism and torsion dystonia, which can be controlled with antiparkinsonian drugs. Torsion dystonia in which the neck is twisted and the patient is unpleasantly excited also occurs during the administration of perphenazine and trifluoperazine.

3. Lithium

This can be given as lithium carbonate 600 mg, or lithium citrate 1200 mg three times a day. This controls manic excitement, but the therapeutic dose is quite close to the toxic dose, and it is essential to maintain a normal salt intake and to monitor the blood level to between 0·8 and 1·2 mmol/l.

4. Electroconvulsive Therapy

Repeated ECT, such as three treatments a day for the first day, two a day for the next two days, and one daily when necessary, will control mania, but there is a risk of cerebral damage. This treatment was useful in severe mania before the introduction of phenothiazines, but should rarely be necessary nowadays.

2. DEPRESSION

The depressive illnesses are among the commonest of mental disorders. The majority of individuals suffering from a depressive illness do not go to a doctor, and of those who do a large proportion complain of somatic symptoms, or loss of energy or 'feeling run-down', and are not therefore diagnosed. Fortunately, most of these patients recover within a few weeks or a few months at most.

Mood

Although the change in mood is regarded as central, patients may not complain of this symptom and if they do admit to feeling depressed, they regard it as secondary to their other misfortunes and disabilities. Some patients may be able to distinguish their mood from a state of being miserable or unhappy. The patients with wrinkled brows, look depressed, tired and self-concerned. Everything appears gloomy and hopeless to them. They feel inadequate and helpless. They burst into tears easily and sometimes find themselves weeping for no reason at all. Any expression of sympathy with their condition brings tears to their eyes. In milder states they feel better after an outburst of weeping, but this relief disappears as the depression increases. A point is reached where they would like to weep but cannot; they are 'beyond tears'.

When mild, the depression can be concealed with an effort, and will even disappear in the presence of congenial company. When more severe, this is not possible and patients try to avoid mixing with other people. Classically, the mood undergoes diurnal variation, being worse in the mornings and improving as the day goes on. Some patients say that they feel at their best in the mornings. Diurnal variation is often absent.

Most patients are also anxious as well as depressed and the amount of anxiety may range from minimal to a level at which it obscures the depressed mood completely. When such patients are given sedatives to diminish their anxiety, the depressed mood becomes more obvious.

Anxiety is accompanied by difficulty in concentration as the patients are preoccupied with unpleasant possibilities and various fears. They then complain of poor memory and forgetfulness.

Guilt

This is a very typical symptom though not always apparent. Patients may be preoccupied with vague feelings of inadequacy and may blame themselves for having fallen into their present state. They may also become preoccupied with trivial delinquencies in their past. They may say that they have been bad husbands or wives and even give evidence about this; but then cannot explain why they should suddenly feel guilty about a long-standing pattern of behaviour. In severe cases, they may say they have committed unutterable sins or dreadful crimes, but do not know what they are. Very rarely delusions and even hallucinations of guilt may be present.

Motor Activity: Retardation

In retarded depression all psychomotor activity is inhibited. There is poverty of movement, the gait is dragging and the patient walks as if bowed down by a weight on the shoulders. The patient sits with a peculiar stillness and, if left alone, seems not to be fully aware of his surroundings. When spoken to there is often a delay in replying and the speech is quiet and monotonous. The facies is lacking in expressive mobility. Retardation may progress to stupor but is rarely severe and almost never with incontinence of urine and faeces, which is common in catatonic stupor.

Motor Activity: Agitation

This is the motor expression of anxiety, but retarded patients can be anxious, so there is no simple relation between the subjective feeling of anxiety and agitated behaviour. Mild degrees of agitation can co-exist with mild degrees of retardation.

Agitation ranges from mild fidgeting to ceaseless movement, with hand wringing, skin picking and continuous pacing. Patients may talk incessantly about their preoccupations, thus showing pressure of speech. They may fasten on to doctors and nurses, continually demanding reassurance and help. In severe cases, they may moan continually and inarticulately. Severe agitation is now very rarely seen as it is particularly responsive to treatment with ECT.

Agitation is more common and more marked in depressions occurring in middle life and old age.

Depersonalization

The patients feel changed and lacking in proper emotions. They feel cut off from normal human contacts. This symptom is closely related to derealization, in which patients complain that the world seems changed, distant and far away, lacking in vividness and even unreal. Both these symptoms are uncommon.

Obsessions

Obsessional thoughts and ruminations may occur but they are very uncommon nowadays.

Hypochondriasis

Some individuals have a hypochondriacal personality and this may range from mild health fads to a way of life in which the dominant theme is the maintenance and protection of health. Hypochondriasis may appear for the first time in relation to the onset of a depressive illness. It may range from an excessive emphasis on bodily symptoms, through vague feelings that there must be some bodily disease present, to moderate convictions that the patient is suffering from cancer, tuberculosis, etc. The patient repeatedly asks for reassurance and may demand investigations. At the best these produce only temporary reassurance and the patient soon returns with other complaints. Classically, older depressives complain that their bowels are 'blocked'.

Delusions

The symptoms of guilt and hypochondriasis may progress to delusional intensity. In the former case patients may confess to imaginary wicked sins and crimes and say that they are going to be punished, arrested and killed for them. In the latter they may say that their brains have rotted, their bowels have been blocked for months, etc. Delusions of poverty occur rarely.

Mild ideas of reference are common, but occasionally they may become well marked, though not clear persecutory delusions. Such delusions should not be confused with delusions of guilt, in which the patient believes that, because of his wickedness, he is going to be punished, tortured or executed.

Hallucinations

These are rare. They are usually reproaching voices calling out odd words or phrases such as 'Rotter', 'Kill yourself', etc. The 'voices of conscience' may be heard. Continuous auditory hallucinosis suggests schizophrenia or organic psychosis. Some patients believe that they smell and it is difficult to decide if this is hallucinatory or delusional.

Intelligence and Memory

Anxiety or retardation may hinder concentration and lead to poor intellectual performance and memory.

Suicide

This may be the first and last symptom of depression. It occurs when retardation is slight and anxiety not too great. The retarded depressive cannot begin the attempt and the very anxious cannot think it out or carry it through successfully. Depressives may kill loved ones; the depressed mother may kill her child. Attempted suicide or successful homicide may have a cathartic effect and the patient may feel much better. The possibility of suicide should always be considered, however mild a depressive illness may be.

Bodily Symptoms
These are as follows:

1. *Anorexia*

Loss of appetite with marked loss of weight are common. Constipation is supposed to be associated with these symptoms but is uncommon. Very rarely there is excessive appetite, usually in the milder depressions and accompanying anxiety.

2. *Fatiguability*

The patient complains of loss of energy and being easily tired. Sometimes this is a severe and intractable symptom.

3. *Sleep*

In classic sleep disorder the patient gets to sleep but wakes at 2–4 a.m. and lies awake for hours. Other forms of insomnia are: (*a*) waking and falling asleep again repeatedly through the night; (*b*) possible difficulty in getting to sleep.

Note on Involutional Melancholia
This disorder was described as occurring during the involution in rigid obsessional personalities with little interest outside the family and home, for example, in a 'house-proud housewife'. When full-blown there is marked hypochondriasis, especially connected with the bowels, severe agitation, and paranoid ideas. Nihilistic delusions, such as that the patient is dead, everything is destroyed, etc., may also occur. There is little point in distinguishing this syndrome from other forms of depression.

Differential Diagnosis
1. *Depressive Reaction*

This is the natural unhappiness which occurs in a normal person who has a severe disappointment or in an inadequate personality reacting to mild stress. The classical symptoms of depressive illness are absent. Usually resentment and anger are not far from the surface. There is a tendency to blame others and no self-reproach or ideas of guilt.

2. *Anxiety States*

Anxiety states may usher in depression or anxiety symptoms in depression may lead to neglect of depressive symptoms. If a previously well-adapted adult suddenly develops an anxiety state one should look for an affective or organic illness.

3. *Schizophrenia*

Depression in an abnormal personality may be very atypical. Some depersonalized depressives have difficulty in explaining their strange apparent lack of emotion and the peculiar change in their perception of the world which occurs in derealization. In some patients delusions of persecution are very marked, but no other non-understandable symptoms are present (*see* p. 135).

4. Symptomatic Depression

Cerebral arteriosclerosis frequently causes depression. General paralysis of the insane, encephalitis lethargica and paralysis agitans may be associated with depression. The organic illness is usually obvious on physical examination, but it is advisable to carry out a Wassermann reaction in all cases of severe depression. Depression can precede obvious signs of arteriosclerosis.

Management of Patients on Drug Treatments for Depression

The first step in the proper treatment of depressives is the making of a correct diagnosis. It is therefore necessary to distinguish between those patients who are suffering from a primary depressive illness and those who are manifesting an excessive depressive reaction to stress, the sort of reaction that occurs in some kinds of emotional personality. The correct treatment for such patients is to refrain from giving them drugs and to give them reassurance and comfort, to rally round the family to support them and to help them with their problems. Patients suffering from depressive illness require the same help from their physicians as the previous group but in addition they need more specific treatment. When the diagnosis is in doubt, the patient should be seen frequently and treated as a psychogenic reaction. If there is no improvement within a reasonable length of time, the patient should then be given antidepressive drugs. The pattern of symptoms shown by these patients is of little relevance to the distinction being made, despite traditional beliefs.

If the illness is very severe or it is considered that the patient is actively suicidal, then the correct treatment is a course of ECT. If there is doubt, then the patient should be admitted to hospital and put on drugs. If the patient's condition then worsens or if there is no sign of response in 4 weeks then the patient should be given a course of ECT.

Most antidepressive drugs produce their side-effects almost immediately, but their therapeutic action takes 2–3 weeks to develop. Because of this delay, it is advisable to see the patient weekly or fortnightly for the first 4 weeks or till signs of improvement appear. As side-effects tend to diminish with time, the patient should start with a half dose and build up to the full dose in about a week to 10 days. The action of these drugs is slow and cumulative, so it is quite unnecessary to adhere to the tradition of giving a dose three times a day; the full daily dose can be given at night, but in appropriate circumstances (*see below*) it can be divided into morning and evening doses.

It is of the greatest importance to explain to the patient that the side-effects appear early and the therapeutic effect appears late. Without this, it appears to the patient that the burden of side-effects is added to the burden of illness but without relief. Proper examination and reassurance prevent the patient becoming frightened by the appearance of side-effects. Such explanations do not alarm the patient and do not add to the symptoms; depressive patients are not suggestible. When the physician gives such explanations he should check that the patient understands them and also the regime of treatment. Explanation and reassurance are like any other treatment, they should be given in adequate doses and repeated as often as is necessary.
adequate doses and repeated as often as is necessary.

The physician should check that the patients are taking their drugs properly. Various methods have been proposed for detecting whether patients do so, but this is always an unsatisfactory approach to the problem. If patients trust their physician and understand what is expected of them, they will take their drugs; if they do not, and they discover that they are being 'spied upon', then they will find ways of evading detection.

If there is a good response to the drug, then continuous improvement can be expected for at least 4 months. The patient should be kept on the drug for at least 6 and preferably 8 months. It is then possible to test the effect of reducing the dosage slowly at monthly intervals and if symptoms start to recur, to go back one or two steps. During this period it is important to keep reminding the patient to adhere to the regime of treatment and not to change it without seeking advice first. General experience has shown that a maintenance dosage of drug is at about the level of half the therapeutic dose.

The following minor points can be important in clinical practice. Elderly patients should be started on comparatively small doses which should be increased only slowly. Postural hypotension is not uncommon as a side-effect in these patients although it is rare in others. For this reason, it is advisable not to give them their dosage at night only, but to split it into morning and evening doses. Such patients often have to get up at night to empty their bladders, and if they fall down there may be nobody near at hand to help them. The physician should avoid yielding to his importunate patients and falling into the trap of giving treatment for symptoms. Patients are much disturbed by their loss of energy, fatiguability, loss of appetite and, above all, by insomnia. The physician should always emphasize that these are symptoms of the illness and as the patient responds to treatment they will go. In consequence, there is no need to do anything for particular symptoms.

Drugs (Symptomatic Treatment)

Treatment of symptoms should be avoided as much as possible. In the long run it does not help the patient, it demoralizes the physician and leads easily into habits which militate against correct diagnosis and proper treatment. However, symptomatic treatment is useful during temporary exacerbations.

1. *Hypnotics*

It should be made clear to the patient that hypnotics will be prescribed for a short period only. These drugs are of limited use in the treatment of depressive illness. Although a sufficient dose will 'knock out' a patient who has difficulty in falling asleep, the drugs have very little effect in delayed insomnia and the patients still wake in the early hours of the morning. Increasing the dose does not prevent them from waking but ensures that they are thoroughly 'groggy' for the morning and much of the rest of the day.

Barbiturates should not be prescribed as it is too easy to commit suicide with them. Benzodiazepines are safer and the current favourites are nitrazepam and flurazepam. The dose given should be the minimum that will relieve the patients from the worst effects of lack of sleep, rather than that which will give them a 'night's sound sleep'.

2. *Day-time Sedation*

Diazepam and lorazepam are the current favourites but any of the benzodiazepines with which the prescriber is familiar will do. Prolonged use will lead to dependence so they should be given only for a short limited period when anxiety is intense. Agitation is only moderately diminished by them.

3. *Euphoriants*

Amphetamine and its derivatives should not be prescribed, partly because their effect wears off within a few weeks, but chiefly because they are so addictive. They should be regarded by psychiatrists as obsolete. Other euphoriants such as methyl phenidate and, the most recent introduction, pemoline may have some use in the treatment of depressive illness but their value has not yet been determined.

Antidepressive Drugs

1. *Tricyclic Antidepressants*

The first of these drugs to be introduced was imipramine and it still tends to be regarded as the standard against which others are measured. Many derivatives and allied compounds have since been introduced, of which the most popular now is amitriptyline. Dothiepin, iprindole, opipramol and dibenzapine are similar compounds but not closely related to the others. Although clinical trials have shown there are differences between the effects of these drugs, they do not come to much in clinical practice. The chief value of a wide choice of drugs is that some patients may show particular intolerance or an idiosyncratic reaction to one and may therefore have to be switched over to another. With most of them the effective range of dosage is between 75 and 150 mg daily. If patients do not respond to 200 mg daily then they are unlikely to respond to higher dosages. Because postural hypotension is more common and more dangerous in old and frail patients, the starting dose should be 20 mg and should not be increased more rapidly than twice a week. For these patients, the dose should be divided into a morning and evening dose. These drugs usually take 10–20 days to affect the depression, although protriptyline is said to come into effect in about half that time.

About 30 per cent of outpatients show no improvement on these drugs, but for those who do improve treatment should be continued for at least 6 months. It is then possible to reduce the dosage slowly to about half of the previous level. There is good evidence that maintaining the patients on the drug for at least a year does diminish the possibility of recurrence of depressive illness. Nevertheless, it is advisable at 3–4 months' intervals to attempt to reduce the dosage or stop the drug altogether. If symptoms return, the dosage should be increased to the full effective level for another 3 months.

These drugs have anticholinergic properties which give rise to side-effects. The most common is dryness of the mouth, followed by palpitations, sweating, dizziness and loss of accommodation. Postural hypotension and vomiting also occur.* It has been shown that many of these drugs produce mild changes in the ECG but these are of little significance except in patients. with heart disease. Patients should be warned of these side-effects and encouraged to continue with the medication despite them, as they diminish with time. In general, the newer introductions do have less side effects.

2. Tetracyclic Antidepressants

Maprotiline is the first of this new class of drugs. It is of interest that it inhibits the uptake of noradrenaline only and not of serotonin. Nevertheless, it is as effective as imipramine and amitriptyline and appears to have less side-effects. Mianserin is a more recent introduction and has received favourable reports.

3. Other Classes

New antidepressive drugs continue to be developed and some of them are completely different in chemical structure from those already described. An example is viloxazine, which is a bicyclic compound. The few clinical trials on them which have been reported indicate that they are about as effective as the older classes of drugs and that the indications for their use are much the same. Some clinical trials in the

*The risk of effects on glaucoma is small, but it is always useful to check on a history of glaucoma in the patient or family, or pain in the eyes accompanied by halos seen around lights. Pupil size can also be checked easily (Reid et al., 1976).

USA have shown that the phenothiazines and the thiothixenes, generally regarded as neuroleptics of value in the treatment of schizophrenia, also have some antidepressive effects. There seems very little point in using them for this purpose though they are sometimes combined with antidepressive drugs in the hope that they will diminish anxiety.

Tryptophan, an amino acid normally found in food, has been shown to have a mild antidepressive action. It also potentiates the effects of monoamine oxidase inhibitors and clomipramine. It is given in doses of 1000–1500 mg per day.

Lithium appears to have no effect as a treatment of depressive illness, but it is of great value in the prophylaxis of recurrences of unipolar and especially of bipolar disorders. It should be given in doses which will maintain a serum level of 0·8–1·2 mmol/l.

4. Mono-amine Oxidase Inhibitors (MAOI)

The varieties available have now dwindled very much and for practical purposes the field is dominated by two: phenelzine, which is a hydrazine derivative, and tranylcypromine which is a non-hydrazine compound. Dosages of the former run from 15 to 90 mg per day and of the latter from 10 to 50 mg per day. The use of these drugs has declined because of the fears of the danger of 'hypertensive crises'. The evidence suggests that these fears have been exaggerated. The difficulty with these drugs is their erratic action; some patients respond very well to them and a large number do not respond at all. Distinguishing between potential responders and non-responders is not yet possible, despite many popular beliefs about it.

Side-effects are increased pulse-rate, hypertension, drowsiness, dizziness, constipation and dry mouth. Hypertensive crises have already been mentioned. The crisis consists of severe headache, tachycardia, nausea, vomiting and even subarachnoid haemorrhage. It may occur after eating certain foods, such as cheese or yeast, which contain a high content of tyramine; also after drugs such as procaine and morphine analgesics, adrenaline, its analogues and derivatives, and methyldopa. It has been claimed that when MAOI drugs are given with tricyclics, then severe crises may occur but there is evidence to show that this is probably a very rare complication.

Electroconvulsive Therapy

This treatment is indicated when the patient is actively suicidal or so severely ill that it would be inhumane to wait for the drugs to take effect. It should never be administered without being preceded by an intravenous anaesthetic and a short-acting muscle relaxant. The treatment should be given twice a week but if the patient shows a very rapid response, the frequency should be decreased to once a week. It is a clinical tradition that longer intervals between treatments decrease the possibility of impairment of memory. The minimum course is six treatments and the maximum is 12. Minor transient complications are memory defect and confusion, which occur more quickly in elderly subjects. The chief risks of this treatment come from the anaesthetic and muscle relaxant. There are no absolute contraindications for this treatment but if the patient's occupation requires a good memory, every effort should be made to avoid the use of straight ECT either by giving drugs or administering unilateral ECT. Clinical experience and sound judgement are required when this treatment is considered for patients suffering from heart failure, recent coronary thrombosis or hypertension.

Psychotherapy

The nature of the illness must be explained to the patient and relatives. Firm and repeated assurance with simple explanations of symptoms should be given. Help should be given with the patient's personal and social problems, but when he improves he is generally capable of dealing with his difficulties without assistance. The patient should be discouraged from making important changes in his life-style while he is ill.

Prognosis

General

Prognosis for individual attacks is good, but recurrence is common. Mental hospital admission figures suggest that less than 20 per cent of depressive illnesses are single attacks. Mania probably very rarely occurs as a single attack. The intervals between attacks of bipolar disorder decline from a median of 4·3 years between the first and second attacks to 1·7 years between the fourth and fifth attacks. Depressive attacks tend to occur as the patient grows older and tend to become longer and more severe with each repetition, whereas manic attacks remain the same length or even become shorter with each repetition.

Clinical Features

Clear-cut classical manic or depressive illness in a previously good personality has the best prognosis and if there have been previous mental illnesses then they have been typical affective psychoses. If the previous personality was inadequate and showed neurotic traits the prognosis is bad. Gross hypochondriasis and severe depersonalization have been alleged to be poor prognostic signs. If these symptoms occur in a typical depressive illness this is not so.

3. MIXED STATES

Kraepelin (1921) described six mixed affective states of which only one, agitated depression, is at all common. Many of the others are doubtful varieties, and if they occur, they do so when the patient is passing from depression to mania or vice versa. Some patients may quickly pass from one mood to the other and while in transition show a mixture of symptoms. Some patients may have a manic illness, but depressive elements such as hypochondriasis and self-reproach frequently emerge, making the diagnosis difficult.

4. ANXIETY STATES

With the exception of hysteria, the anxiety states are generally regarded as the most psychogenic of all mental disorders and the most responsive to psychotherapy. The evidence for the former is by no means satisfactory. Anxiety is very responsive to stress and persons who in common parlance have an anxious disposition, i.e. have a low threshold for the development of anxiety under stress, can find 'psychological precipitants' all too easily. As for the latter, such patients respond quickly to comfort and reassurance, and the belief that extensive psychotherapy is more effective has little basis. In recent years there has been great activity in the development of new treatments by behavioural methods, even in the USA, and this at least indicates that traditional psychotherapy is not as effective as has been claimed.

Anxiety States as Affective Disorders

1. There is a strong genetic component in the constitution which predisposes to anxiety states, as illustrated by twin studies. Slater and Shields (1969) reported that in monozygotic twins 13 out of 20 pairs (65 per cent) were concordant for marked anxiety symptoms, whereas in same-sexed dizygotic twins only 5 out of 40 pairs (13 per cent) were concordant.

2. A large proportion of patients show considerable improvement and even recovery by 2 years from the onset of symptoms. Recurrent cycles are not by any means as clear as in manic-depressive disorder but are recognized (Snaith, 1968).

3. Depressive illnesses with typical symptoms sometimes occur as an acute flare-up of symptoms in patients who have been considered to be suffering from typical anxiety states, even for years.

4. The boundary between depressive illness with marked anxiety (anxious depressions, 'neurotic' depressions) and anxiety states is not at all clear.

5. Some patients with 'anxiety states' respond very well to treatment with mono-amine oxidase inhibitors. Panic attacks, which may be the basis for agoraphobia, may respond to treatment with tricyclic anti-depressants. Although this does not actually prove anything, it does suggest that there is a common element between depressive and anxious illnesses.

Symptoms of Anxiety

Anxiety occurs in many different psychiatric disorders. It is important to recognize anxiety symptoms, because the anxious patient often complains of the physical accompaniments of anxiety and not of anxiety as such. The presenting physical symptoms of anxiety are determined by the patient's previous experience of disease and his constitutional predisposition to different patterns of autonomic overactivity.

Cardiovascular Symptoms

Palpitation is the most common symptom of this kind and is a sensation of forceful beating in the praecordial region. In severe anxiety the sensation may spread into the neck and upper abdomen. Patients often complain of headache, sometimes experienced as a band round the forehead or as a pain below the occiput.

Respiratory Symptoms

Breathlessness is common in anxiety and usually manifests itself as a difficulty in filling the chest with air. It is therefore often accompanied by sighing respiration. Attacks of breathlessness may occur when the patient is at rest. Sometimes patients may develop a hyperventilation syndrome. In this case the prolonged deep breathing leads to a loss of carbon dioxide and a respiratory alkalosis, so that the patient feels weak and dizzy and has paraesthesiae in the hands and feet. Some chronically anxious patients have the syndrome of left inframammary pain; when they complain of aching and soreness in the lower part of the breast.

Gastrointestinal Symptoms

Dryness of the mouth is often caused by anxiety and can give rise to mild difficulty in swallowing. The commonest abdominal symptom of anxiety is an unpleasant churning sensation in the epigastrium. A patient may also complain of eructation and a burning sensation in the epigastrium, which may lead him to believe that he has 'indigestion'. In severe anxiety, spasm of the pylorus and reversed peristalsis may give rise to vomiting. In less severe anxiety the patient may feel continuously nauseated. Anxiety sometimes leads to a loss of appetite, but a few anxious women overeat and find that eating allays anxiety to some degree. Some anxious patients have an increased motility of the gastrointestinal tract and may complain of abdominal distension after meals and frequent soft stools.

Genitourinary Symptoms

Increased frequency of micturition may result from anxiety. Sexual drive may be diminished. A few patients have an increase in sexual drive and some anxious males have erections when their anxiety becomes severe.

Motor Symptoms

Anxiety may cause a general increase in the tone of voluntary muscles, which is experienced by the patient as a feeling of tension. Tense patients often complain of being weak and exhausted. Tension in the frontal and temporal muscles may cause a tension headache which is experienced as a tight band across the forehead. Typically the patient with an anxiety state complains of frontal headache, while the patient with a depressive illness tends to complain of occipital headache. Anxiety often produces tremor, which is usually most marked in the hands and which increases during voluntary movements or when attention is drawn to it.

Psychological Symptoms

Anxiety causes increased distractibility, so that the patient is unable to think clearly or to concentrate on an intellectual task. Difficulty in concentration leads to a poor memory, because the patient is unable to attend to what is going on around him. Poor memory and difficulty with intellectual tasks may lead the intelligent introspective patient to think that he is going out of his mind. Some anxious patients feel bewildered and perplexed, while others complain of a 'muzziness' or feeling of fullness in the head. Dizziness or a sense of unsteadiness may be the presenting complaint of an anxious patient. The physiological basis of this symptom is not clear, but in some cases it appears to be an accentuation of normal postural dizziness which occurs when the subject rises from a sitting position.

Sleep

Anxious patients have difficulty in falling asleep. When anxiety is severe the patient may have frightening dreams from which he awakes in terror.

The Diagnosis of Anxiety States

Many acutely depressed patients have severe anxiety which may overshadow the depressive symptoms. Acute anxiety states in the absence of some severe traumatic event or unpleasant life situation should be investigated carefully for depressive mood, diurnal variation and the typical sleep disorder.

Treatment

The establishment of good rapport with the patient is fundamental to the treatment and management of the anxiety states. On this basis, explanation and reassurance will generally produce a considerable amelioration of symptoms. Drugs and psychotherapy (*see* Chapter 14) are the foundations of treatment, but sedatives and tranquillizers should be kept at a minimum. If patients are liable to attacks of panic and especially if these occur in specific situations they can be given a capsule of sodium amytal 50 mg or lorazepam 1 mg to take in anticipation. Quite often, the possession of the capsule is sufficient to tide them over the emergency. Some patients who suffer from 'anxiety-phobic' states respond well to treatment with MAO inhibitors. Marked autonomic symptoms show a good response to beta-blockers.

Chapter 10

Schizophrenia and paranoid states

THE CONCEPT OF SCHIZOPHRENIA

Schizophrenia was originally isolated as an illness which always caused a deterioration of the personality (*see* p. 14). Then it was realized that some patients with typical schizophrenic illnesses recovered completely. Thus Kraepelin (1919) found that 2·6 per cent of his patients with dementia praecox made complete and lasting recoveries. If the course of the illness is not used to separate this psychosis from others then the only alternative is to use some psychological symptomatological criterion. The most suitable one is that of 'understandability', i.e. a symptom is schizophrenic if it cannot be understood as arising emotionally or rationally from the personality and the affective state of the patient. This approach gives the following definition of schizophrenia:

'A group of mental disorders in which there is no coarse brain disease and in which many different clinical pictures can occur. The form and content of some of the symptoms cannot be understood as arising emotionally or rationally from the affective state, the previous personality, or the current situation, with the proviso that if paranoid delusions are present the diagnosis cannot be made in the absence of other "non-understandable" symptoms.'

AETIOLOGY

Heredity

The general risk is 0·8 per cent. If both parents are schizophrenic, then 41 per cent of their offspring will be schizophrenic. If one parent is schizophrenic then 12 per cent of the children will be schizophrenic and 33 per cent will be schizoid personalities even if adopted and brought up in a non-schizophrenic family. Of the grandchildren 3 per cent will be schizophrenic. The risk of a sibling of a schizophrenic is 8 per cent if the parents are free from schizophrenia, and 14 per cent if they are not.

There is good evidence that schizophrenia is genetically based, but other genes and psychological and physical factors play an important part in determining the onset of the disorder. In the main, the concordance figures for schizophrenia are found to lie between 35 and 65 per cent in monozygotic twins and between 9 and 26 per cent in same-sexed dizygotic twins, according to whether the concordance rates are based on cases found in mental hospitals or population studies, and whether strict or wide concepts of schizophrenia are employed.

Personality

An abnormal premorbid personality is often found, for example, the so-called schizoid personality. Persons of this type are shy, quiet, shut-in, sensitive individuals who show little emotion and are unsociable. Some patients (30–50 per cent) show no mental abnormality before onset. There is a tendency to be wise after the event, but schizoid personalities are more common in relatives of schizophrenics.

Development

Alanen (1968) has described families of schizophrenics as tending to be either chaotic or rigid. In the former the atmosphere was incoherent and irrational, dominated by one parent's disturbed thought and behaviour. In the latter there was excessive rigidity of roles, emotional impoverishment with unbending attitudes and expectations. Singer and Wynne (1965) concluded that the parents of schizophrenics were unable to focus attention selectively on shared percepts or feelings. Communication was of such a style that it ended up with lack of understanding. This emphasis on the form of communication is the opposite of the theories of Bateson (Bateson et al., 1956) who emphasizes the content of parent—child communication in which verbal and non-verbal communications are contradictory and lead to the 'double-bind' relationship. These ideas have been further developed by Laing and Cooper. These findings are contradicted by investigations of the children of schizophrenics who have been adopted at an early age. It has been found that they are just as liable to develop schizophrenia as are the children of schizophrenics brought up by their biological parents, as compared with the adoptive siblings who do not shown an increased tendency to develop schizophrenia (Rosenthal and Kety, 1968).

Social Isolation

Goldberg and Morrison (1963) and Dunham (1965) have shown that although the proportion of schizophrenics coming from social class V and from socially isolated areas of cities was excessive, this was largely due to the downward drift in social level of such patients.

Disorders of the Nervous System

Schizophrenia occurs more frequently in association with epilepsy than would be expected by chance, and this is particularly so in relation to temporal lobe epilepsy (Slater et al., 1963).

Birth complications and neonatal asphyxia tend to damage the mesial temporal lobe and evidence of such damage is common in patients suffering from temporal lobe epilepsy. The offspring of schizophrenic mothers who subsequently themselves become schizophrenic have a much higher incidence of birth complications than those children who do not become schizophrenic. In the case of monozygotic twins discordant for schizophrenia, the same applies to the proband twin.

Neurotransmitters have now been shown to play an important part in the development of the symptoms of schizophrenia. The drug L-dopa, which stimulates dopaminergic neurones, has been known to produce schizophrenic symptoms and all neuroleptics blockade such neurones. Chronic intoxication with amphetamine (which is a potent releaser of dopamine) can produce symptoms indistinguishable from schizophrenia. There is some evidence that viral infection of the CNS may be a factor in the development of schizophrenia.

Metabolism

Metabolic activity of schizophrenics varies between much wider limits than in normals but no definite pattern is discernible. Gjessing found disturbance of nitrogen balance in certain periodic catatonics.

Precipitation

Physical Illness

Occasionally infectious illness or childbirth precipitates schizophrenia. However, the superimposition of the symptoms of organic psychosis on an affective disorder may make the diagnosis of puerperal psychosis difficult.

Psychological Stress

The onset of schizophrenia is occasionally associated with severe psychological stress. This does not occur in the majority of cases.

Psychoanalytic Theory

Regression extends back as far as the early narcissistic stage. There is therefore a loss of object relations. Symptom formation thus consists of the reactivation of archaic functions and the conflict is solved by the denial of reality. Fantasies of world destruction, bodily hallucinations, feelings of grandeur, schizophrenic formal thought disorder and some catatonic symptoms are due to regression. However, the patient tries to restore his object relations, so that some symptoms are attempts to do this. These are world reconstruction fantasies, hallucinatory voices and some catatonic symptoms.

Paranoid Delusions

Freud believed that paranoid delusions were ways in which the patient could deny his wish for a homosexual relationship.

Neo-Freudian Views

Some Freudians, such as Federn, have suggested that the ego is not entirely dependent on the id for its energies. Federn sees schizophrenia as a breakdown of ego boundaries.

Klein regarded schizophrenia as a regression to the paranoid schizoid position, where there is a tendency for the ego to fragment.

SYMPTOMATOLOGY

1. Thought Disorder (see p.43)

a. *Disorder of the Stream of Thought*
Blocking, in which the train of thought suddenly stops and a completely new one begins, is diagnostic of schizophrenia. Inhibition of thought, pressure of thought, or flight of ideas may occur, but is not characteristic.

b. *Formal Thought Disorder* (see p.48)
This is a gross disorder of conceptual thinking in the presence of evidence that at some time in his life the patient had an adequate intellectual performance. In the absence of coarse brain disease this disorder is diagnostic of schizophrenia. In the early stages it appears as poverty of ideas and associations, obscurity of expression, vagueness and a stilted and pontifical woolliness.

c. *Alienation of Thought* (see p. 45)
Thought deprivation, insertion and broadcasting are diagnostic of schizophrenia.

d. *Disorder of Thought Content—Delusions*
i. PRIMARY DELUSIONAL EXPERIENCES; APOPHANY (see p.45)
Apophanous experiences occur in the acute stages of the illness. However, they are soon woven into secondary delusions based on mood and hallucinations, so that they cannot be recognized in the later stages of the disease.

ii. DELUSIONS OF PERSECUTION
These are based on primary delusional experiences, feelings of bodily change, hallucinations of all kinds, and on misinterpretations based on mood and ideas. The natural reactions of other people to the patient's illness are also misinterpreted. Delusions of persecution by Jews, Freemasons, etc., have been replaced by more topical persecutors.

iii. DELUSIONS OF GRANDEUR
These consist in beliefs of omnipotence, e.g. being Jesus, God, and so on. They may occur early in the illness or later on. They cannot be explained as justification of persecution.

iv. HYPOCHONDRIACAL DELUSIONS
These are based on bodily hallucinations, but may at times be due to thought disorder. Sometimes they are a presenting symptom.

2. Sense Deceptions (*see* p. 36)

a. *Auditory Hallucinations*

i. VOICES

Hallucinatory voices in a clear state of consciousness are very common in schizophrenia. They may be clear or unclear. Voices may talk to the patient or talk about him in the third person. Running commentary voices may occur and are diagnostic. The voices may be abusive and hostile or reassuring. They may give orders which the patient may or may not carry out. The patient may hear his own thoughts spoken aloud, so-called *Gedankenlautwerden*. This is diagnostic. The voices may be attributed to real or imaginary people or to machines, such as radio and television.

The voices may be intermittent or virtually continuous, and the patient then hallucinates during conversation. Frequently the voices cease when the patient is occupied in work or conversation. Continuous auditory hallucinations in the absence of organic disease are mostly likely to be due to schizophrenia.

ii. ELEMENTARY HALLUCINATIONS

Buzzing, whistling, etc., may occur and be used to support paranoid delusions about machines and so on.

b. *Visual Hallucinations*

Visions occur but usually are distinguished from reality. Visual hallucinations are rare.

c. *Bodily Hallucinations*

Sensations of heat, cold, pain and electric shock may be felt. Sexual sensations and orgasms may be complained of. These experiences are felt as foreign and are diagnostic of schizophrenia.

d. *Hallucinations of Smell and Taste*

These occur in the acute stage, but are not characteristic.

3. Emotional Disorders

a. *General Disorders of Mood*

Mood elevation, depression, anxiety and perplexity may occur, but are not characteristic. Acute illness often begins with depression, anxiety, or both.

b. *Abnormalities of Emotional Expression*

Loss of finer feelings for relatives and unaccountable rages are often an early sign. Characteristic disorders are: (1) flattening of affect; (2) incongruity of affect; and (3) stiffness of affect.

Mild degrees of flattening and incongruity are difficult to assess and must be used cautiously in diagnosis, since the range of emotional expression in abnormal personalities is very wide. Failure of rapport may be diagnostic or may be due to a failure on the part of the examiner.

4. Motor and Behaviour Disorders (Catatonic Disorders)

a. *Subjective Feelings of Passivity*

The patient feels that his thoughts, feelings, speech and actions are not his own, and that he is made to carry out these activities by outside influences. This may be interpreted in a delusional way. These feelings are diagnostic of schizophrenia.

b. *Excitements*

Senseless excitements occur. The mood is not cheerful and destruction of clothes, fittings, and furniture occurs. Violent senseless assaults may be made on nurses and fellow patients. Excitements may be short-lived or may alternate with stupor. Mild excited states may continue for long periods and take the form of tearing, restless wandering, or senseless moaning. These states usually respond to phenothiazines and are not seen very often today.

c. *Akinesis and Obstruction*

The patient is motionless but can be pushed into action. Movements may begin and then stop suddenly.

d. *Stupor*

Patients sit or lie motionless with or without increased muscle tension. They do not reply to questions or react to stimuli and the facies is expressionless. Emotional changes may be seen, such as a transient incongruous smile, and the eyes may be lively. A 'psychological pillow' is common. Saliva dribbles from the mouth, and there is incontinence of urine and faeces. Stupor may be interrupted by excitement or a sudden impulsive act.

e. *Other Catatonic Symptoms*

Negativism, stereotypies, mannerisms, waxy flexibility, echolalia, echopraxia, *Mitgehen, Mitmachen* (co-operation) and parakinesia (*see* pp. 60–62) may occur.

f. *Speech*

Some patients are mute, while others reply to every question with drivel or with incoherent nonsense. Verbigeration may occur. Some patients talk past the point (*Vorbeireden*).

g. *Autism*

This is a detachment from reality with a relative or absolute predominance of inner life. It is often used in a vague way to indicate that the patient is withdrawn or has difficulty in making personal contacts.

5. Disorders of Consciousness

During acute shifts the patient may be preoccupied with vivid hallucinations and appear disorientated—the so-called oneiroid state. In chronic patients delusions, talking past the point, autism and general disinterest may give rise to apparent disorientation.

6. Disorders of Memory

No disorders of memory can be found on formal testing.

a. *Delusional Memories*

A delusion may acquire the characteristic of a memory image, or a delusion may be back-dated.

b. *Misidentification*

This may be positive or negative. That is, strangers may be claimed as acquaintances, or vice versa.

c. *Confabulation*

Some chronic schizophrenics produce fantastic confabulations.

d. *Apophanous Memories*

An abnormal significance may be attached to a memory image.

CLASSIFICATION OF SCHIZOPHRENIA

Many different classifications of schizophrenia have been put forward, but Bleuler's modification of Kraepelin's original grouping is as good as any other. The dividing lines are not hard and fast, and patients may begin with one form of the disease which may then develop into another.

1. The Paranoid Form

Hallucinations and delusions are continuously in the foreground in this form of the illness.

2. The Catatonic Form

Motor symptoms predominate in this variety.

3. The Hebephrenic Form

In this type there is general deterioration, in which thought and affectivity are affected without paranoid or motor symptoms being prominent, although they occur.

4. The Simple Form

Thought disorder and affective disorder are present, but paranoid and motor symptoms are absent throughout the course of the illness.

SPECIAL FORMS OF SCHIZOPHRENIA

Schizo-affective Illnesses or Mixed Psychoses

The Problem

Some patients have illnesses in which there is a marked affective component, usually depressive, but there are some symptoms which are non-understandable and cannot be derived from the affective symptoms. These illnesses are probably one of the following: (1) depressive illness with undetected organic complications; (2) depressive illness in abnormal personalities; (3) psychogenic reactions in abnormal personalities; (4) a special illness separate from schizophrenia and manic-depressive disease; (5) schizophrenia with marked depressive features.

Cycloid Psychoses

Leonhard has described three cycloid psychoses which are not manic-depressive or schizophrenic. These psychoses are bipolar, i.e. they may show clinical pictures at either end of a continuum. The clinical pictures are not hard and fast, so that features of one cycloid psychosis may be found in another.

ANXIETY–ELATION PSYCHOSIS

The patient has a mood disorder either of anxiety or ecstasy. In anxiety there are ideas of reference and sometimes hallucinatory voices and illusions. Often there are complaints of bodily sensations. In ecstasy the patient wants to help others and may have hallucinations of hearing and vision.

CONFUSION PSYCHOSIS

Here thinking is primarily affected. In the excited state there is incoherent pressure of speech, with ideas of reference and auditory hallucinations. In the inhibited state poverty of speech, even amounting to mutism, perplexity, ideas of significance, illusions and hallucinations occur.

MOTILITY PSYCHOSIS

Psychomotor activity is mainly affected. In the excited phase there is hyperkinesia, consisting mainly of expressive and reactive movements. In the akinetic state all movements are restricted. Reactive and expressive movements are affected earlier than voluntary ones, so that in mild cases reactive movements are absent and posture and mimicry are rigid, although voluntary movements are carried out.

Oneirophrenia

In some acute schizophrenics there seems to be a dream-like change in consciousness, which Mayer-Gross called the *oneiroid experience*. He considered that it was due to intense delusional experiences and hallucinations which occupied the patient's entire attention. Meduna and McCulloch (1945) called schizophrenia with clouding of consciousness 'oneirophrenia', and claimed that these patients had an anti-insulin factor in the blood. This has not been confirmed.

Pseudoneurotic Schizophrenia

This variety of schizophrenia resembles a neurosis, but anxiety affects all aspects of the psychic life and many different neurotic symptoms may be present at the same time. Short-lived psychotic episodes occur in which ideas of reference, depersonalization and hypochondriacal ideas are present. This is probably neurotic pseudoschizophrenia, as these patients seem to be psychopathic personalities in Schneider's sense, who are reacting badly to stress.

Pfropf or Grafted Schizophrenia

Some high-grade mental defectives develop schizophrenia, so that it is grafted on the defect. However, some defectives are really childhood schizophrenics, so that schizophrenia in a defective can in some cases be a shift in a long-standing schizophrenic illness. Further diagnostic difficulties are created by the occurrence of depressive illnesses in mental defectives. Such conditions may be atypical because the patient cannot explain his symptoms.

Periodic Catatonia

Gjessing found that a few catatonic patients showed phases of excitement or stupor in association with a phasic variation of nitrogen retention. He described types A, B and C. In type A the illness was usually an akinetic stupor and began just before the end of nitrogen retention. In type B the illness began some time during the first half of nitrogen excretion, and in C it began just before the end of nitrogen excretion. The illness in types B and C was psychomotor excitement, which was more violent the later it began in the phase of nitrogen excretion. Slow activity has been found in the EEG during the illness.

Gjessing believed that the variation in nitrogen retention was due to phasic variations of thyroid function and that the illness could be cured by massive doses of thyroid.

PARANOID STATES

Paraphrenia

This term was first used to designate a group of delusional patients who showed practically no disorders of emotion and volition. The syndrome is now generally considered to be paranoid schizophrenia occurring later in life and without severe deterioration of the personality.

Paranoia

Kraepelin defined this as 'the insidious development of a permanent unshakeable delusional system resulting from internal causes, which is accompanied by perfect preservation of clear and orderly thinking'.

Circumscribed delusional psychoses without hallucinations, etc., are occasionally found but are not common. Some psychiatrists consider such illnesses to be schizophrenic. The commonest variety of this illness is the 'jealous husband syndrome'. The patient has delusions of jealousy about his wife, but no other signs of mental illness (*see* pp. 84, 106).

Process versus Development (*see* p. 84)

Some paranoid states can be considered to be understandable developments of abnormal personalities. On the other hand, in some paranoid patients there is a sharp break in the personality. Jaspers suggested that such a sharp irreversible change was due to a psychic process. As the only non-organic psychosis which produces such an effect is schizophrenia, then it can be assumed that schizophrenia has produced the paranoid state.

Paranoid Personalities and Delusional States

The Sensitive Paranoid Personality

This type is often a quiet, sensitive person who feels he is deserving of better things, but some disability such as physical deformity, masturbation, illegitimacy, etc., holds him back. Slowly the patient becomes more embittered, and some event which exposes his sensitive preoccupation may act as a key experience and release a paranoid state.

The Querulent Paranoid Personality

He is usually a suspicious, high-minded individual who is always defending his rights or supposed rights, for example, the 'barrack-room lawyer' spoiling for a fight. Sometimes a real or imagined injustice leads the patient to engage in litigation. He loses, but carries his case from one court to another, often abusing his opponents and being punished for contempt of court.

Organic Paranoid States

Acute Organic Paranoid States

Clouding of consciousness usually helps in diagnosis, but occasionally transient paranoid states occur due to organic disease, with only minimal degrees of clouding of consciousness. This may occur during physical illnesses such as coronary thrombosis, following minor operations or childbirth.

Chronic Organic Paranoid States

Patients with marked non-progressive brain damage may attribute their difficulties to others and believe that other people are treating them unfairly and persecuting them.

Paranoid Depressions (*see* pp. 70, 123)

Some anxious depressed patients believe they are being persecuted, protest about the persecution, and do not believe that they deserve such ill-treatment. If no other clear signs of schizophrenia are present then these patients are suffering from a paranoid depression. These symptoms should not be confused with delusions of guilt, in which the patients say 'I am wicked; I deserve to be punished; I am punished'.

Paranoid Schizophrenia

Classically, there is typical disorder of thought and affect, but the illness may begin as a paranoid state and typical schizophrenic symptoms may not occur for some time. If there is an obvious break in the personality, schizophrenia can be assumed.

Schneider has claimed that certain symptoms are diagnostic of schizophrenia in the absence of coarse brain disease. These are:

1. Certain hallucinations, for example, voices which talk about the patient in the third person, voices in the form of a running commentary, hearing one's thoughts spoken aloud.

2. Delusional perception.

3. Disorders of the possession of thought, for example, thought insertion, thought withdrawal and thought broadcasting.

4. Experience of influence, i.e. anything in the spheres of sensation, feeling, thinking, or somatic activities, which is experienced as due to foreign influences.

Summary

A paranoid state may be due to: (*a*) schizophrenia; (*b*) depression; (*c*) personality development; (*d*) a reaction to stress in a paranoid personality; and (*e*) coarse brain disease.

DIFFERENTIAL DIAGNOSIS

Adolescent Crises

The adolescent is in turmoil with depression, ruminations, philosophical ideas, irritability and difficulties of affective expression. Usually there have been difficult relations with parents for years, and these are made worse by the need for independence in adolescence. Although schizophrenia is popularly believed to be a disorder of late adolescence, the peak incidence is 23–30 years and about 15 per cent appear after the age of 40 years.

Hysteria (see p. 78)

A severe variety of this disorder sometimes occurs in adolescent or early adult females who show severely disturbed behaviour with violence to themselves and others, and who may claim to experience visual hallucinations. Rapport is extraordinarily well preserved throughout.

Mania

Some manics are irritable, interfering and paranoid. They misinterpret legitimate attempts to control their unpleasant behaviour and may insist even after discharge that they were unjustly detained. In acute mania incoherence of thought may be present because of the very rapid flight of ideas or intercurrent infection.

Epilepsy

A schizophrenic-like paranoid psychosis can occur in epilepsy, usually in the temporal lobe variety. In these cases the EEG may be normal but there is a history of attacks of some kind. Sometimes epileptic speech and circumstantiality are present. In other patients catatonic psychoses occur; then the EEG is usually abnormal with continuous spike-and-wave patterns or repeated sharp waves.

Other Organic States

Usually there is some indication of neurological disease in the schizophrenic-like organic states, and the EEG may be helpful. One must be aware of amphetamine psychosis which can mimic paranoid schizophrenia. A history of repeated paranoid psychoses with recovery is suggestive of amphetamine addition.*

COURSE AND PROGNOSIS

Course of the Illness

The majority of schizophrenics develop defect states which consist of varying degrees of personality impairment, but these terminal states may be arrived at in different ways.

*Amphetamine can be detected in the urine by means of a fairly simple laboratory procedure.

Shifts and Phases

A shift is an acute episode with new symptoms, which subsides to leave behind some general worsening of the illness, while in a phase the acute episode disappears, leaving no defect. Those authors who believe that schizophrenics never recover do not, therefore, use the word 'phase' in connection with schizophrenia. Sometimes the patient has a phasic illness, which later recurs, and runs a steady downhill course. Other patients may suffer from an illness which runs a shifting course, so that the defect is worse after each shift.

Process Course

The word 'process' is sometimes used to indicate a steady downhill course of illness.

Prognosis

This may be for a given attack, for the possibility of recurrence, or for the likelihood of deterioration. The individual features related to prognosis are:

1. *Age*

Onset in adolescence or over the age of 40 years indicates a poor prognosis for recovery, but in the later age-group the chance of deterioration is slight.

2. *Speed of Onset*

An acute onset has a good prognosis, while a slow ingravescent onset has a very poor prognosis.

3. *Personality*

A marked premorbid schizoid personality indicates a poor prognosis.

4. *Physique*

A pyknic physique suggests a good prognosis, while a dysplastic physique suggests a poor one.

5. *Clinical Features*

Marked depressive features indicate a good prognosis, and so does an acute catatonic episode. However, affective blunting is almost always associated with an unfavourable outcome. The simple and hebephrenic forms have a poor prognosis for social recovery.

6. *Social and Psychological Background*

If the parents can accept that the patient is ill and are prepared to tolerate minor behaviour disorders, then the arrested schizophrenic may be able to live in the community. Much depends on the tolerance of the family and the general social environment.

TREATMENT

In general, the aim is to maintain the patient in social life, to arrest the disease and alleviate the symptoms with drugs.

Psychological and Social Treatment

Doctors and nurses should obtain the best possible rapport with the patient. He should be reassured and every effort made to understand his difficulties and to help him solve his problems. All personal contacts should be encouraged and he should take part in group activity (*see* p. 205). The patient should be given a regular steady occupation and, when the disease is arrested, he should be persuaded to take a job suitable for his mental state and should be discouraged from overambitious projects. In some cases the patient may be sent out to work from the hospital; it is important to arrange discharge as soon as possible.

The illness must be explained to the family and they should be advised about the general handling of the patient. Usually he is admitted to hospital and is sent home on week-end leave as soon as he is well enough. His progress while on leave should be discussed with the responsible relatives. It is important to make certain that the patient is not being treated as an irresponsible child. The psychiatric social worker can often help the family with social and economic problems while the patient is in hospital and after his discharge. She can also help by enlisting all the possible social agencies to help him and his family. In some cases discharge can be hastened by allowing residence at home and attendance at the mental hospital or at a separate day hospital during the day. Social clubs for discharged patients may help in building up social relationships.

Physical Treatments

Neuroleptics (*see also* p. 210)

Many classes of drugs, i.e. of fundamentally different chemical composition, are now available. They all blockade dopaminergic neurones in differing potencies, but also have other effects which account for the differences among them. Side-effects differ and patients may have idiosyncratic reactions to them. The physician would therefore be well advised to make himself familiar with a few drugs, which will give him confidence in prescribing and provide alternatives should it be necessary to change.

The three groups which have been longest available and are therefore the most commonly prescribed are the phenothiazines, the thioxanthenes and the butyrophenones. The phenothiazines range in daily dosage from fluphenazine 2 to 10 mg, to chlorpromazine 150 to 600 mg. The dosage of thioxanthenes ranges from flupenthixol 3 to 12 mg, to chlorprothixene 50 to 300 mg. Two butyrophenone are currently available, trifluperidol 1 to 3 mg and haloperidol 1 to 12 mg. Some of these drugs are available in a form suitable for intramuscular injection, but as such injections can be painful they should be used only as a last resort. If the nurses are sufficiently encouraging and patient, they can usually persuade even the most excited and disturbed schizophrenic to take the drugs orally. For the acutely disturbed schizophrenic, it is customary to prescribe the sedative drugs chlorpromazine or thioridazine 400 to 600 mg daily, given in divided doses 4-hourly. If the patient does not respond or cannot tolerate phenothiazine, then haloperidol up to 12 mg per day should be given instead. If necessary, the chlorpromazine may be given intramuscularly in doses of 100 mg every 4 hours until sedation is achieved and then the patient changed over to oral medication. The commonest side-effects are the extrapyramidal reactions of pseudoparkinsonism, i.e. rigidity, tremor and akinesia. The best treatment for these side-effects is reduction of the dose of neuroleptic, but if this is not practicable then antiparkinsonian drugs should be added. The daily dosages are benztropine 2 to 6 mg, orphenadrine 100 to 400 mg. These two drugs can also be given intramuscularly. Procyclidine 5 to 60 mg can also be given intravenously.

The dosage of neuroleptics for chronic schizophrenics varies enormously. Some patients require almost as much as during the acute phase and others may not need any neuroleptics at all. Over the course of time, the dosage of neuroleptics or antiparkinsonian drugs required to control symptoms may diminish considerably, and for this reason it is advisable to test the requirements by reducing the dosage slowly. This should be done every 6–12 months.

Chronic schizophrenics who are treated as outpatients may take their drugs irregularly or not at all. In consequence they may relapse and have to be readmitted into hospital. Such patients can be adequately maintained by the intramuscular injection of fluspirilene weekly or the decanoate salt of fluphenazine or flupenthixol given every 2–4 weeks, but the problem of controlling side-effects requires continual supervision.

Electroconvulsive Therapy

This treatment will produce symptomatic relief of marked depressive symptoms and of catatonic stupor. Some acutely disturbed patients appear to be resistive to drugs until they have received ECT. ECT has only a temporary effect on symptoms and its use should therefore be avoided as much as possible. In a chronic condition such as schizophrenia, there is a constant temptation to repeat the treatment and the more treatments that are given the greater will be the impairment of memory.

Thyroid Extract
Large doses may prevent attacks in periodic catatonia.

Prophylaxis
As only one in ten children of a schizophrenic succumb to the illness, genetic counselling is of no value in prophylaxis. If would-be parents have a schizophrenic parent, they can be reassured, as only 3 per cent of grandchildren of a schizophrenic develop the disorder.

Among the children of schizophrenics who subsequently develop schizophrenia, a high proportion have a history of difficulties in the mother's pregnancy and labour. This would suggest that better antenatal and obstetric care would be of prophylactic value.

Evidence is accumulating that, among the children of schizophrenics, differences in behaviour and personality can be found between those who will subsequently become schizophrenic and those who will remain well. This raises the hope for individual prophylaxis.

Chapter 11

Psychiatric organic states: general principles

INTRODUCTION

These are mental illnesses which are caused by coarse brain disease; that is, anatomical and physiological changes can be demonstrated in the brain. The fact that psychotic illnesses resulting from coarse brain disease are called 'organic' does not imply that schizophrenia and manic-depressive disease could not be the result of some sort of brain disorder.

Schneider has called psychiatric organic states 'bodily based psychoses', but this term is too clumsy for use in English. This worker has divided symptoms in these conditions into obligatory, which always occur in a given organic syndrome, and facultative, which may or may not occur. In acute organic psychoses clouding of consciousness is the usual obligatory symptom, which in chronic organic psychoses deterioration of the personality and the intelligence are obligatory symptoms. While this is roughly true there are many exceptions. Disturbances of consciousness do not necessarily occur in acute organic states. Wieck has pointed out that these are 'transit syndromes' which are reversible and in which clouding of consciousness is not prominent.

Facultative symptoms were regarded as being the result of focal lesions or of individual predispositions. It was believed that the morbid process might accentuate personality traits or release a constitutional predisposition to a functional psychosis. The argument that clinical pictures of functional psychoses were due to the release of inborn predispositions was often circular. It may well be that certain combinations of lesions of the brain may be responsible for these clinical pictures. It must also be remembered that several transit syndromes resemble functional psychoses and there is no evidence that functional psychoses are more common in the families of patients with these transit syndromes.

On the whole, the kind of psychiatric illness produced by coarse brain disease depends on : (1) the speed of action of the morbid process; (2) the extent and severity of the brain damage; (3) the duration of the brain damage; (4) the presence of focal lesions; and (5) the individual predisposition.

Rather than talk of acute and chronic organic states it is better to divide these conditions into reversible and irreversible states (*see Fig.* 1).

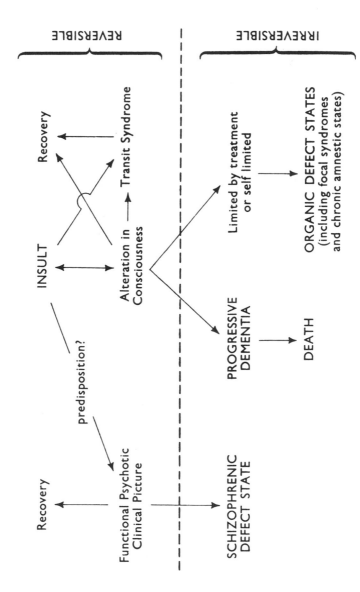

Fig. 1. Mental disorders caused by coarse brain disease.

The reversible states may be conditions in which there is alteration of consciousness, transit syndromes with no alteration of consciousness, or functional psychotic clinical pictures. The irreversible organic states may be progressive dementias which lead to death or organic defect states in which the morbid process has been arrested and left behind a permanent defect, e.g. an alcoholic Korsakoff state may not recover and a permanent memory defect with slight intellectual deterioration is left behind and is not progressive because the patient is in hospital and denied access to alcohol.

CLASSIFICATION
Reversible Organic States
1. Those with marked alteration of consciousness.
   a. Delirious states—acute and subacute.
   b. Organic stuporose states—apathetic confusional states.
   c. Organic twilight states.
2. Transit syndromes.
   a. Emotional hyperaesthetic syndromes.
   b. Depressive and manic syndromes.
   c. Organic paranoid states.
   d. Organic hallucinosis.
   e. The exogenous paranoid hallucinatory syndrome.
   f. Catatonic syndromes.
   g. Expansive confabulatory syndromes.
   h. Amnestic syndromes.
3. Functional psychotic clinical pictures.

Irreversible Organic States
1. Progressive dementia or the chronic brain syndrome.
2. Organic defect states.
   a. Non-progressive intellectual defect states.
   b. Chronic emotional hyperaesthetic syndrome.
   c. Chronic amnestic states.
   d. Focal syndromes.

REVERSIBLE ORGANIC STATES
1. Organic States with Marked Alteration in Consciousness
These are the commonest reversible organic states, but are not infrequently followed by a transit syndrome in which consciousness is not grossly disordered.

Acute Delirium
Here there is a dream-like change in consciousness in which memory images acquire the same importance as perceptions. Active and passive

attention are decreased. The patient is usually apprehensive and may even be terrified, believing that people are trying to kill him. Delirium tremens is a good example of delirium and has previously been described.

Subacute Delirium (the Confusional State)
Here there is a mild degree of clouding of consciousness and the level of awareness fluctuates considerably. The patient is perplexed and disorientated in time and place, but the extent of the disorientation varies markedly. The condition becomes worse at night with gross disorientation, restlessness and anxiety. Ideas of persecution may occur, especially at night. Isolated visual hallucinations may also occur at night. Incoherence of thought is usually present and can be marked. Sudden changes of environment bewilder the patient. This condition is most often caused by infection, trauma and electrolyte imbalance.

Organic Stuporose States (Apathetic Confusional States)
In some severe acute infections, such as typhus and typhoid, there is a general lowering of consciousness with only a few or no sense deceptions. In less severe brain disorders there may be a mild general lowering of awareness and difficulty in comprehension with no hallucinations. These patients are not restless or anxious, but somewhat apathetic. The clinical picture resembles that which is found in progressive dementia and may easily be mistaken for it. This apathetic confusional state is not uncommon following a slight cerebral thrombosis in cerebral arteriosclerosis. The unwary may mistake this condition for a severe irreversible dementia and to their chagrin the patient may make an excellent recovery in a few weeks.

Organic Twilight States
The field of consciousness is restricted, so that all thinking and acting is dominated by a small group of ideas, which totally exclude all others. In addition to the restriction of consciousness there is also some degree of clouding. Occasionally vivid visual and auditory hallucinations preoccupy the patient, although he gives no indication of this, but appears bemused and distracted. The degree of appreciation of the environment is always less than usual, but a few patients do not appear obviously abnormal to uninformed bystanders. Such individuals occasionally make long journeys or wander about for days.

2. Transit Syndromes
Emotional Hyperaesthetic Syndrome
This is a mixed neurotic clinical picture with anxiety, depression, irritability, difficulty in concentration and memory, feelings of exhaustion and restlessness, and emotional lability. It can occur in any variety of

coarse brain disease and in chronic physical diseases, such as pulmonary tuberculosis, which have a general debilitating effect. It may also occur as an irreversible state in non-progressive permanent mild brain damage.

Depressive and Manic Syndromes

Typical depressive illnesses can occur in cerebral arteriosclerosis, Addisonian anaemia, general paresis and other varieties of coarse brain disease. Manic syndromes are much less common in organic states, but they do occur, particularly in lesions affecting the hypothalamus.

Organic Paranoid State

This is a condition in which there is no clouding of consciousness but marked ideas of persecution occur with no hallucinatory voices. It is an acute condition which occurs after major surgery or severe physical illness, such as cardiac infarction. Often the previous personality is paranoid or otherwise abnormal. This illness occurs in general hospitals and usually lasts a few days.

Organic Hallucinosis

In this condition the outstanding feature is continuous hallucinatory voices in a state of clear consciousness and delusions of persecution which are a logical outcome of the voices. The commonest cause is alcohol (see p. 104), but it can be the result of chest infections, carbon-disulphide or carbon-monoxide poisoning, general paralysis of the insane, and epilepsy among other causes. This clinical picture is not always reversible and can become chronic in alcoholism, general paresis and carbon-monoxide poisoning.

The Exogenous Paranoid Hallucinatory Syndrome

This syndrome resembles acute paranoid schizophrenia. The previous personality is sometimes anankastic with some sensitive traits, but some patients are careless and neglectful. The mood at first is irritated and morose and later becomes suspicious and anxious. Delusions of persecution occur and the patient believes that he is about to be evicted, discharged from work, or shunned by the family. Clear hallucinatory voices occur in the form of a conversation and are attributed to real people in the environment. The patient angrily rejects the idea that the voices are hallucinations. The patient may hear voices talking about his thoughts, but he does not hear his own thoughts spoken aloud. Experiences of external influence do not usually occur. This syndrome occurs in amphetamine addicts and also is likely to occur in patients who are taking or misusing drugs for the treatment of chronic physical illnesses, such as bronchial asthma and Parkinsonism. The illness may occur as a transitional phase between delirium and complete recovery.

Catatonic Syndrome

Catatonic states of excitement or stupor may result from coarse brain disease, such as anoxia, encephalitis and epilepsy. Wherever possible an electroencephalogram and, if need be, a lumbar puncture should be performed on a patient with a previously normal personality who suddenly develops catatonic stupor. Another simple test is to administer intravenous sodium amylobarbitone very slowly and cautiously. If the catatonic stupor is due to coarse brain disease the stupor will become more profound, while if it is a schizophrenic catatonic stupor the mental state may improve dramatically or at least it will not worsen. Catatonic stupor may be the result of 'petit mal status' in which there is a continuous spike and wave discharge in the electroencephalogram.

The Expansive Confabulatory Syndrome

Classically this occurs in general paralysis of the insane, but it may occur after head injury and in typhus. For example, an 18-year-old youth sustained a severe head injury and after a few days he developed the idea that he was 'Batman' and had given birth to hundreds of 'bat babies'. He also gave garbled accounts of events involving the medical staff and his employer.

The Amnestic Syndrome

This condition has already been described in detail in the chapter on alcoholism (*see* p. 105). The characteristic features are disorientation for time and place, the loss of registration of new memories, retrograde amnesia of some degree, confabulation, 'tram-line thinking' and euphoria. A large number of different varieties of coarse brain disease can produce this syndrome. Apart from alcohol the commonest are brain injury, brain tumours, subacute inflammations of the brain and dementing processes.

3. Functional Psychotic Clinical Pictures

Depressive, manic, or schizophrenic clinical pictures may occur in coarse brain disease. Paranoid schizophrenic and catatonic symptoms tend to be associated with temporal lobe epilepsy. Flor-Henry (1969) has found that they are more common with foci in the left lobe, whereas affective symptoms are more related to foci in the right lobe.

IRREVERSIBLE ORGANIC STATES

1. Progressive Dementia

Definition

This is an irreversible intellectual deterioration caused by coarse brain disease. The term should not be applied to reversible organic states in which there is an apparent intellectual deterioration.

Aetiology
1. *Infection of the brain and its coverings:*
   a. Acute, as in encephalitis and meningitis.
   b. Subacute, as in encephalitis.
   c. Chronic, as in syphilis and encephalitis lethargica.
2. *Metabolic and biochemical disorders:*
   a. Anoxia, including hypoglycaemia.
   b. Vitamin deficiencies, for example, pellagra and Wernicke's encephalopathy.
3. *Toxins:* Heavy metals and other toxic substances.
4. *Gross physical damage to the brain.*
5. *Epilepsy:* This is probably due to the effects of repeated anoxia.
6. *Vascular disorders:* Arteriosclerosis is the most important vascular disorder which causes dementia.
7. *Degenerations of the brain:*
   a. Idiopathic, in Alzheimer's disease and senile dementia.
   b. Inherited, in Pick's disease, Huntington's chorea and other inherited disorders of the nervous system.
8. *Neoplasm.*
9. *Demyelinating diseases of the nervous system.*

Onset
In the early stages a confusional state or an amnestic syndrome may be present. The speed of development of the dementia determines the presenting symptoms. Changes take place in memory, intellect, emotions and personality.

Memory
Memory for recent events is worse than memory for remote events, and the loss of memory is often the earliest sign of illness. The patient may compensate for some time by using a notebook. A true amnestic state may occur.

Intellectual Changes
In the early stages the patient tires easily in tasks involving abstract thought. General information becomes faulty and the individual becomes slow and muddled in the simplest intellectual tasks. Perseveration occurs. Speech deteriorates and the word store becomes less. At first patients are often verbose and repetitive, but in the end only a few odd words may be left at their disposal. Delusions may be caused by lack of understanding of the environment, by the reaction of the individual to his loss of ability, by the mood change, and by hallucinations. Paranoid and hypochondriacal delusions are not uncommon. Grandiose delusions occur if the mood is manic (classically, of course, in GPI).

Emotions

In the early stages the patient may become anxious and depressed when he has some insight into his lack of ability. Depression is common at the onset of arteriosclerotic dementia and Alzheimer's disease. Mood changes are often fleeting, but sustained mania or depression may occur. The premorbid emotional behaviour of the patient may be accentuated. Usually there is a blunting of feeling with irritable behaviour. Emotional lability is common; tears or laughter (especially tears) are provoked by a slight emotional upset or by no obvious cause. Apathy or childish euphoria is the final result.

Personality Changes and General Behaviour

A loss of inhibition occurs, which may lead to crimes of sexual misbehaviour. Excessive sexual demands may be made on the partner, heavy drinking may occur, and brutality towards wife and children may be displayed on the slightest provocation. There is a lack of cleanliness and care in dress and hygiene. Urinary incontinence occurs sooner or later, and the patient may indulge in silly childish pranks.

Other Psychiatric Symptoms

Hallucinations of any kind may be present, depending on the basic morbid process. Orientation for time and place is always faulty.

Neurological Signs and Symptoms

Epileptic fits are frequent with other physical signs, depending on the pathological basis of the dementia.

Outcome

If the process cannot be arrested the patient will die in a period of years from intercurrent infection or vegetative extinction.

2. Organic Defect States

Non-progressive Intellectual Defect States

These are most likely to be found after treated general paralysis of the insane and severe head injuries. Often there is also a mild focal syndrome such as lack of drive due to a frontal lesion. The patient's previous personality may give rise to a psychogenic overlay. Thus a hysterical personality with chronic non-progressive brain damage may have gross conversion hysteria or behave in a very histrionic way, whereas a paranoid personality may develop ideas of persecution and blame others for the mistakes which are the result of his intellectual deterioration.

The Chronic Emotional Hyperaesthetic Syndrome

This does not differ from the clinical picture described above. It is not uncommon after head injury.

Chronic Amnestic States

The clinical picture is that described on p. 105. Intelligence tests show some degree of intellectual deterioration, but the memory disorder is much greater than that which would be expected from the slight intellectual defect. The commonest cause of this condition is alcoholism.

Focal Syndromes

FRONTAL LOBE SYNDROME

Acute lesions of the dorsolateral frontal regions may give rise to poverty of movement, which may increase to a catatonic-like immobility, with incontinence of urine and faeces associated with apparent indifference. Acute lesions of the orbital region of the frontal lobes lead to affective overexcitability, irritability and fearfulness. These patients tend to have angry outbursts, negativistic behaviour, a tendency to silly joking (*Witzelsucht*) and gradually lose all inhibitions. In chronic lesions there is a silly euphoric mood with little sense of illness. Disorders of volition also occur. These patients are unable to persevere, unable to make decisions, and lack foresight. Eventually they show deterioration of personality and sometimes even antisocial behaviour. It has been claimed that the dorsal part of the frontal lobes is concerned with spontaneous drives, and the basal part with emotional life. The cheerful euphoric moods of some cases of Pick's disease and GPI have been correlated with the presence of severe lesions in the orbital regions of the frontal cortex.

TEMPORAL LOBE SYMPTOMS

Hallucinatory phenomena are observed in temporal lobe lesions. *Déjà vu, jamais vu,* and various emotions may persist for short periods. Hallucinatory smells, visions, noises and voices may be present. Hallucinations of memory—so-called flash-backs, or psychical illusions —also occur.

PARIETAL LOBE SYNDROME

Deficits are aphasia, unperception, apraxia and agnosia, disorders of body image and problems of spatial orientation. Patients also have difficulty in concentrating and co-operating; their responses are slow and inconsistent. Because of this, patients may sometimes be diagnosed as suffering from hysteria.

THE AMYOSTATIC SYNDROME AND BRAIN-STEM SYNDROMES

The Parkinsonian picture of rigidity and mask-like facies is associated with oculogyric crises. These latter may be linked with perseveration of thoughts, compulsive thoughts, memory images associated with marked anxiety, or a diffuse anxiety. There is also a bradyphrenia, i.e. a slowing of all mental activity. This condition is produced by encephalitis lethargica affecting adults, but, if it attacks children, it produces severe disorders of the personality often without a severe amyostatic syndrome. These children become cold, callous and brutal, and often show sexual abnormalities.

Patients with lesions of the globus pallidus and the structure around the walls of the third ventricle may suffer from visual hallucinations. Some patients with midbrain lesions have repeated, vivid, hypnagogic hallucinations, while others may confabulate. Manic-like states with flight of ideas may be observed in association with hypothalamic lesions. Disorders of appetite, fluid intake, sexual behaviour and sleep may also occur in such lesions.

Psychiatric organic states: specific illnesses

ACUTE INFECTIONS OF THE BRAIN AND ITS COVERINGS

Acute meningitis and encephalitis cause delirium or a subacute confusional state. In tuberculous meningitis treated with streptomycin amnestic states are seen during the period when the patient is critically ill.

In acute encephalitis sometimes a catatonic clinical picture is produced. Encephalitis lethargica occupies a special position in psychiatry because of the unusual mental disorders which occur in the chronic state. The acute illness occurred in Britain from 1917 to 1930, and consisted of a large number of different clinical pictures, usually associated with sleep disorder.

In the chronic illness, Parkinsonism, in which the rigidity is more marked than the tremor, occurs. The other striking feature is the oculogyric crisis, in which the eyes are deviated in one direction, usually upwards, for periods of time ranging from a few seconds to several hours. These crises may be associated with forced thinking, and the patient is usually anxious and disturbed during the attack. General changes of behaviour also occur, such as impulsive aggression, self-mutilation, suicidal attempts, and sexual perversions and crimes. Post-encephalitic children become restless, aggressive and depraved in their behaviour. They show behaviour similar to the severely disturbed aggressive psychopath and are just as foresightless and uncontrollable.

GENERAL PARESIS

General Points

This illness has played an important part in the history of psychiatry, because it was the first serious psychological illness for which a definite cause and an effective treatment were found. Today, in Western Europe the disease is rare. It must be remembered that general paresis is diagnosed, not on the psychiatric picture, which is very variable, but on the serology and special findings in the cerebrospinal fluid. Although the primary cause is the *Treponema pallidum,* it is not clear why some infected patients develop general paresis and others do not.

The Clinical Picture

Prodromal Symptoms

General fatigue, disturbed sleep, headaches, intolerance of alcohol and other general neurotic-like symptoms may be present before signs of dementia become obvious.

The General Clinical Picture

The picture is that of a fairly progressive dementia, of varying tempo. Often memory is poor, even when there is still a reasonable amount of general knowledge. There is usually a general indifference to gross intellectual errors and a mild euphoria, often with marked lability of affect. Peculiar bemused states of consciousness occur in which the patient looks strange and may be thought to be drunk.

Accessory Symptoms

Slightly less common is the euphoric form in which the patient is cheerful and has ideas of self-importance. Even less common is the expansive variety in which there are fantastic delusions of grandeur. In the present author's experience the depressive picture is not uncommon in this disease. Occasionally the depression is indistinguishable from a primary depression and the positive blood Wassermann reaction is unexpected. Sometimes the illness presents as an acute confusion with or without severe excitement and rarely a typical paranoid schizophrenic clinical picture is seen. Focal symptoms and signs may occur rarely. Juvenile general paresis may follow congenital infection.

Physical Signs and Symptoms

Neurological Signs

Argyll Robertson pupils, progressive spastic dysarthria, tremor and upper motor neurone weakness are the characteristic features. Sometimes the knee- and ankle-jerks are absent and the plantar response is extensor, i.e. taboparesis is present. Occasionally aphasia, apraxia and agnosia are present early in the illness. Epileptic fits are common, but so are congestive or apoplectiform attacks. In these there is a brief period of unconsciousness followed by focal neurological signs which last for some days.

Disorders of Mimicry

The face loses its wrinkles and becomes expressionless. The general posture is slack, and movements become awkward and wooden. The normal play of mimicry and gesture disappears.

Treatment

Large doses of penicillin, such as 600 000 units of procaine penicillin per day for 20 days, are usually effective. This, of course, only arrests the dementia, and the patient is left with some degree of non-progressive brain damage. Therefore, apart from specific treatment, social readjustment and occupational retraining may be needed.

PSYCHIATRIC DISORDERS IN EPILEPSY

Auras
Sometimes the aura which ushers in the fit is a hallucination, or a mood. Sometimes the change in consciousness due to the fit is slight and unnoticed, and occasionally the aura occurs without the fit. In such cases the unwary examiner may assume that the strange psychological symptom is neurotic or simulated.

Psychological Attack Disorders

Ictal Moods
Some patients with temporal lobe foci have mood states lasting for a minute or so in lieu of a fit. The mood may be depressive, anxious, euphoric, or very unpleasant.

Psychomotor Attacks
These are short-lived episodes of abnormal behaviour associated with an epileptic discharge in the EEG. This disorder occurs in patients with temporal lobe foci. They are often aggressive, behave strangely, and may have hallucinations and delusions.

Uncinate Fits
The patient passes into a 'dreamy state' which is ushered in by a hallucination of an unpleasant taste or smell, such as burning rubber, paint, or stale cabbage water. During the attack visual and auditory hallucinations often occur, sometimes with so-called hallucinatory memory flash-backs. *Déjà vu* and *déjà vécu* experiences are commonly found in temporal lobe epilepsy, as are states of bewilderment, depression, anxiety and euphoria during the attack.

Post-epileptic Automatism
Some degree of confusion is nearly always present immediately after recovery from a fit. In a few cases the confusion is quite marked; the patient may carry out fairly complicated actions for a few minutes and is often surprised at the situation in which he finds himself when he fully recovers consciousness. Antisocial acts, such as stealing or indecent behaviour, may occur during such states.

Episodic Psychiatric States

Confusional States
Typical delirious and subacute delirious states can occur in epileptics. At times these patients may be very excited and violent. The confusion

may be due to repeated fits, which may be subclinical, or it may be due to continuous cortical dysrhythmia of the nature of a diffuse slowing of EEG background activity. In some patients clinical pictures resembling catatonic stupor may occur. Continuous spike-and-wave discharges in the EEG (so-called petit mal status) are usually associated with stupor. Petit mal status epilepticus presents with clouding of consciousness, constantly fluctuating in intensity and lasting for hours or even days. The EEG shows continuous generalized spike-and-wave discharges, atypical in form. Generally found in children and young adults, it has been reported in older patients.

Twilight States
These may follow on a fit or may begin suddenly and end with a fit. Consciousness is restricted (*see* p. 52) and dominated by a few ideas, delusions, or visual hallucinations. General behaviour is fairly well ordered, but the patient often appears somewhat dull and distracted. The patient usually suddenly recovers from these states and has an almost complete amnesia for the episode.*

Epileptic Dysthymia
Depressed, ill-humoured, irritable states in the absence of clouding of consciousness are common in epilepsy. The dysthymia may begin insidiously and increase in intensity until a fit occurs, after which the mood usually returns to normal. In some epileptics there is a reciprocal relationship between dysthymia and the number of fits, while in others the dysthymia appears to be associated with the degree of abnormality of the EEG.

Paranoid Psychoses
Sometimes epileptic confusional states have a marked paranoid colouring and hallucinatory voices are prominent. However, a typical organic hallucinosis (*see* p. 155) can occur in epilepsy. Sometimes the illness is very like paranoid schizophrenia. There are typical schizophrenic hallucinatory voices, primary delusional phenomena and paranoid delusions. The psychosis often occurs in the presence of a normal or slightly abnormal EEG. In some cases the paranoid psychosis becomes chronic.

Epileptic Personality Changes and Dementia
General Personality Change
Epileptics with frequent fits show a slowing down of intellectual activity and a loss of immediate memory. Perseveration of the theme of thought and marked circumstantiality also occur. Thought proceeds in a slow,

*There is a tendency to use the term 'twilight state' for any episodic psychosis in epilepsy.

sticky way which has been called 'adhesive'. Once they are engaged in a conversation patients tend to continue talking interminably and it is difficult for their victim to break off the conversation. They are self-centred, self-righteous, awkward, irritable people. Religiosity is common, and they are often oily, sanctimonious humbugs.

Dementia

Some degree of dementia is always associated with epileptic personality change, but some epileptics show very gross dementia and become virtually mindless.

The Temporal Lobe Personality

Many patients with temporal lobe epilepsy have an abnormal personality which is easily recognized by the expert but is very difficult to describe. They tend to be chronically uncertain and at times are unable to make decisions and are very easily influenced. There is a general attitude of mistrust and a difficulty in making personal contacts. These patients seem unable to relate themselves to the environment, to evaluate experiences, to fit them into their personality, and to elaborate their own thoughts and actions. It is as if all the necessary constituents are present for rational behaviour but somehow they do not manage to be integrated. Depression is often complained of, but the patient does not convey the feeling of depression to the examiner. Suicidal attempts which are usually difficult to understand and seem to have little relation to the alleged cause, are not uncommon. Hypochondriasis is common, but there is a lack of suffering. Taylor (1972) has provided evidence that antisocial behaviour in these patients tends to be associated with foci in the left temporal lobe and neurotic symptoms with the right lobe.

EFFECTS OF COARSE PHYSICAL INJURY TO THE BRAIN

The psychiatric sequelae of brain injury may be classified as follows:
1. Immediate sequelae:
   a. Acute confusional states.
   b. Amnestic states.
2. Late sequelae:
   a. Unequivocal organic states.
   b. Functional psychiatric disorders.

1. Immediate Psychiatric Sequelae of Brain Injury

a. Acute Confusional States

Following a head injury consciousness is often lost for some time. This state of concussion is probably due to the simultaneous discharge of all cortical neurones and a reversible change in the reticular system.

Consciousness may return suddenly or there may be a period of confusion before consciousness is absolutely clear.

b. Amnestic States

In severe injuries the confusional state may last for some days and be followed by an amnestic state which may last for days or a few weeks.

2. Late Sequelae of Brain Injury

a. Unequivocal Organic States

There are three types of unequivocal organic states:
  i. Personality change and dementia.
  ii. Epilepsy and epileptic psychoses.
  iii. Acute and subacute organic states due to chronic subdural haematomas.

i. PERSONALITY CHANGE AND DEMENTIA

Sometimes a typical frontal lobe syndrome occurs. Many patients become morose, irritable, depressed and bad-tempered, with aggressive outbursts. Others may show emotional lability.

Dementia may occur after severe head injury. Punch-drunkenness or traumatic encephalopathy is a dementia due to repeated brain damage inflicted in the course of boxing, which passes as a sport in the Western world. These patients have slurred speech, poor memory, defective intelligence, unsteadiness of the arms and legs, and tremor of the hands.

ii. EPILEPSY

This may follow closed head injuries but is more common after penetrating head wounds. It is no different from 'idiopathic' epilepsy and the usual psychiatric complications of epilepsy can occur (*see* p. 163).

iii. SUBDURAL HAEMATOMA

This is an accumulation of blood in the subdural space, produced by head injury, often of a trivial kind. It can occur in diseases which cause excessive bleeding. Symptoms may follow the injury immediately, but are often delayed for weeks or months, possibly when the head injury has been forgotten.

Acute deliria, amnestic states, or a chronic confusional state resembling dementia may occur. Headache and clouding of consciousness are the outstanding symptoms. The level of consciousness may fluctuate markedly, so that the patient may be comatose, but within a few hours may be fairly well. Even when consciousness is not obviously disturbed the patient is usually dull and apathetic.

Localizing neurological signs are usually absent, but pareses, pupillary abnormalities, mild aphasic disorders and papilloedema can occur. The protein content of the cerebrospinal fluid is usually raised, and so is the pressure, although this can be normal or low. In the EEG there may be an area of electrical silence, or an excess of slow activity over the haematoma.

Subdural haematoma should always be considered when there are fluctuating mental symptoms associated with severe headache or where there is a rapidly developing apparent dementia.

b. Functional Psychiatric Disorders

There are four types of functional disorder:
- i. The post-concussional syndrome.
- ii. Psychological reactions to the effects of brain injury.
- iii. Depression.
- iv. Schizophrenia.

i. THE POST-CONCUSSIONAL SYNDROME

These patients complain of headache, jumpiness, dizziness on stooping, depression, irritability and intolerance of noise. In many cases compensation is a complicating factor and, in fact, exactly the same symptoms can be found in compensation neuroses in which there is no head injury. It is possible that in some cases there is some generalized brain damage, but it is unlikely that it plays more than a minor part in the production of the symptoms.

ii. PSYCHOLOGICAL REACTIONS TO BRAIN INJURY

Refusal to accept the intellectual defect produced by brain injury may lead to a paranoid state (see p. 144).

iii. DEPRESSION

This may be a reaction to severe brain damage or a dysthymia due directly to the brain damage. Suicide is more common in the brain-injured than in the general population.

iv. SCHIZOPHRENIA

This can follow head injury, but must be distinguished from organic hallucinosis and epileptic paranoid psychosis. If schizophrenia follows the head injury immediately, or without an intervening period of normality, then it must be attributed to the injury.

THE PRESENILE DEMENTIAS

General Discussion

These dementing illnesses occur before the age of 60 years. Dementias are degenerative disorders of the central nervous system,

which can be classified from the psychiatric point of view in the following way:
1. Degenerations in which the psychiatric symptoms are most prominent:
   a. Alzheimer's disease.
   b. Pick's disease.
   c. Rare varieties of presenile dementia.
2. Degenerations in which neurological and psychiatric symptoms are of equal importance:
   a. Huntington's chorea.
   b. Creutzfeldt–Jakob disease.
   c. Hepatolenticular degeneration (Wilson's disease).
3. Degenerations in which neurological signs are outstanding, but which can be associated with dementia.

1. Degenerations in which the Psychiatric Symptoms are Most Prominent

a. Alzheimer's Disease

This is the commonest presenile dementia, usually occurring between 40 and 60 years of age, but is occasionally seen in adolescents and young adults, and very rarely in children. Many neuropathologists believe it is an early manifestation of senile dementia. It probably has a multifactorial genetic basis.

PATHOLOGICAL CHANGES
The brain is shrunken, with wide sulci and enlarged ventricles. Microscopical investigation reveals a decrease in the cells of the cerebral cortex, especially in layers 3 and 5. Degenerative changes are seen in the remaining cells. The outstanding features are argyrophilic plaques and Alzheimer's neurofibrillary changes, which are most pronounced in the temporal cortex and hippocampus. The plaques vary in size from 15 to 150 μm in diameter and contain granular or filamentous material which stains well with silver and has the staining reaction of amyloid. Varying degrees of proliferative and regressive changes may be found in the glial cells at the periphery of the plaques.

In the neurofibrillary change the fibrils of the nerve-cells become irregularly thickened and stick together. These altered fibrils stain very well with silver stains. Spirals, loops, strands and baskets of altered neurofibrils are seen.

It is the pre-synaptic cholinergic cells which are mainly affected, as shown by the reduction in choline acetyltransferase. Both are closely associated in extent with the amount of cognitive impairment.

PSYCHIATRIC CLINICAL PICTURE
The course of the illness can be divided into a stage of personality change, a stage of intellectual and speech disorders, and a terminal utter dementia. The clinical picture of dementia has already been described (*see* p. 156). The special features of Alzheimer's disease are: (1) depression and anxiety, often occurring in the early stages, but tending to be transient; (2) disorders of space and time, i.e. parietal lobe symptoms, usually occurring early in the illness; (3) aphasic disorders, which would be expected from diffuse parietotemporal lesions, marking the onset of the second stage; (4) reading and writing are more disturbed than speech; (5) echolalia and the senseless repetition of odd words or phrases are both quite common; and (6) palilalia and logoclonia (*see* p. 61) are usually present.

NEUROLOGICAL SIGNS
Muscle tone is often increased in the early stages, but the rigidity is neither clasp-knife nor cogwheel; epileptic fits occur in over 25 per cent of cases; extrapyramidal signs occasionally occur; the gait is often stiff, awkward and unsteady. In the final stages sucking reflexes, and forced grasping and groping are frequently present.

The EEG is almost invariably abnormal; the alpha rhythm is slowed or absent and diffuse theta rhythm may dominate. Irregular delta activity may appear.

COURSE OF THE ILLNESS
Death usually occurs from intercurrent infection within 2–10 years.

b. *Pick's Disease*
This is much rarer than Alzheimer's disease, but like that illness it is more common in females. It usually occurs in middle age, but can occur in youth and old age. It is widely held that it is due to an autosomal dominant gene.

PATHOLOGICAL CHANGES
Circumscribed atrophic areas are seen in the frontal and/or the temporal lobes. When the frontal lobe is involved the changes are usually more marked in the frontal basal region, i.e. in the gyrus rectus, in Brodmann's area II and in the inferior frontal convolution. Less commonly the convexity of the frontal lobe is most affected. When the temporal lobe is affected the changes are found in the pole and extend backwards to affect the whole of the middle and inferior temporal convolutions, but only the anterior third of the superior temporal convolution. In rare cases, where the parietal lobe is affected, the changes are found in the inferior parietal lobule. The areas affected are all those regions of the brain which were

the last to develop phylogenetically. Microscopical examination reveals a gross loss of cells in the three outer layers of the cortex of the affected area, which is associated with a cortical and subcortical gliosis. The remaining cells show the characteristic degenerative change, in which the cell enlarges, becomes rounded, and the cytoplasm becomes homogenous. Globular argyrophilic masses are also seen in the degenerating nerve-cells.

PSYCHIATRIC CLINICAL PICTURE
The usual signs of dementia appear, but as the morbid process affects the temporal and frontal lobes, the clinical picture is usually coloured by a frontal or temporal lobe syndrome. Social misbehaviour is often the first indication of the disease. Unlike those suffering from Alzheimer's disease, these patients are often silly and facetious, with a careless indifference to their own mistakes. Spatial and temporal disorders are rare, but aphasia of a sensory nominal or mixed type frequently occurs.

NEUROLOGICAL SIGNS
Epileptic fits are less common than in Alzheimer's disease. Disorders of gait are rare.

COURSE OF THE ILLNESS
It may last from 2 to 15 years, or even longer.

c. *Rare Varieties of Presenile Dementia*
Kraepelin described a rapidly developing dementia occurring in the fourth decade and after, in which incoherent excitement, restlessness, negativism, delusions and hallucinations were present. Stern described a presenile dementia associated with thalamic degeneration. Other obscure unclassifiable presenile dementias also occur.

2. Degenerations in which Neurological and Psychiatric Symptoms are of Equal Importance

a. *Huntington's Chorea*
This is inherited as an autosomal Mendelian dominant gene, so that it usually occurs in half the offspring of a patient. It may appear to miss a generation if the affected parent does not live long enough to develop the disease. The disease occurs in all races. The incidence is about 5 per 100 000 in Britain. The discovery of biological markers for the gene has given the first hope for treatment and effective prevention.

PATHOLOGICAL FINDINGS
There is generalized atrophy of the brain with enlargement of the ventricles. There is a marked loss of cells in the third, fifth and sixth

layers of the cortex, and a loss of nerve-cells, especially the small ones, in the caudate nucleus and the putamen. The red nucleus, the substantia nigra, the thalamus and the cerebellum may also be affected.

EEG
Low voltage records with little rhythmical activity are common and appear to be related to cortical atrophy. These changes do not predict which offspring will develop the disorder.

THE CLINICAL PICTURE
This is a slowly progressive dementia associated with jerky movements. The premorbid personality is usually abnormal. Depression, paranoid states, unpleasant psychopathic behaviour and atypical psychoses may precede obvious signs of dementia for some years. The illness becomes obvious about the age of 35 years, but can begin in the sixth or seventh decade. It has been seen in early childhood. The signs of dementia appear slowly and the patient gradually becomes intellectually incompetent. In some cases the patient may be able to live in the community for many years. Suicide and suicidal attempts are common in all stages of the illness, even when the dementia is profound. The involuntary movements develop insidiously and usually appear first in the face and upper limbs and are always more obvious there. The movements consist of abrupt stretching and jerking, which are irregular and uncoordinated, and most marked in the proximal parts of the limbs. The face and trunk are affected by writhing movements. Repeated sniffing movements are common. At first the movements are not obviously choreic and the patient gives the impression of being somewhat clumsy and fidgety. When the movements become more marked the patient may disguise them by turning them into voluntary movements. Thus a jerk of the arm may be turned into a movement of smoothing down the hair.

UNUSUAL CLINICAL PICTURES
Occasionally depressive, paranoid and paraphrenic clinical pictures occur. Sometimes the dementia is not accompanied by choreic movements, while some patients have minimal or no psychiatric symptoms.

COURSE OF THE ILLNESS
It usually lasts from 10 to 15 years and the patient dies before the age of 60 years.

b. Creutzfeldt–Jakob Disease (Cortico-striato-spinal Degeneration)
This is a rapidly developing dementia associated with extrapyramidal disorders and sometimes with lower motor neurone disorders. Ataxia, dysarthria, spasticity, choreo-athetoid movements, tremor, cogwheel

rigidity and muscular wasting occur. Death occurs within 6 months to 2 years of the onset.

The Nevin–Jones variant of this disease is characterized by rapid deterioration, pronounced myoclonus, absence of lower motor involvement, typical EEG changes at some time, and marked spongiform changes in the brain found post mortem. This form is transmissible to chimpanzees by inoculating brain-biopsy material (Roos et al., 1973).

EEG
Generalized bilaterally synchronous polyphasic sharp waves, and sharp and slow wave complexes are found. There is also present some irregular delta wave background activity.

c. Hepatolenticular Degeneration (Wilson's Disease)

This disease is the result of a biochemical defect which is usually considered to be inherited as a Mendelian recessive. The basic disorder is the failure of the alpha-globulin fraction of the plasma proteins to combine with the copper absorbed from the intestine. The copper becomes loosely attached to the plasma albumin and is taken up by the proteins in the brain and the liver. This excessive deposition of copper leads to widespread degeneration of the cells in the brain and the liver. The changes are most marked in the putamen and in the caudate nucleus. The liver becomes cirrhosed. There is also an increase in the urinary excretion of amino acids, but the origin of this anomaly is not known.

CLINICAL FEATURES
The first symptom is usually tremor and the illness tends to begin in the second decade. Muscular rigidity soon develops so that voluntary movements are impaired. Dysarthria and dysphagia frequently occur fairly early in the course of the illness. The facies may be Parkinsonian or there may be a silly vacuous smile. A diagnostic feature which is not always present is the Kayser–Fleischer ring of golden-brown pigmentation of the cornea near the limbus.

PSYCHIATRIC CLINICAL PICTURE
A mild dementia which progresses very slowly is the common psychiatric picture, but depression, mania, and even clinical pictures resembling paranoid schizophrenia are occasionally seen. Emotional lability and general loss of interest occur early in the illness. A little later these symptoms may alternate with periods of euphoria.

COURSE OF THE ILLNESS
If untreated, death commonly occurs within 1 to 6 years after the onset, although at least one patient survived for 30 years. The progress of the

disease can be arrested by administering chelating agents such as penicillamine in doses of 8–10 150 mg capsules per day.

3. Degenerations in which Neurological Signs are Outstanding, but which can be associated with Dementia

These are numerous and include such conditions as motor neurone disease and the cerebellar degenerations.

PSYCHIATRIC SYMPTOMS IN CEREBRAL NEOPLASMS

Walther-Büel (1951) found that 70 per cent of a series of 600 patients with brain tumours had psychological disorders. These could be classified as: (1) clouding of consciousness, 38 per cent of patients showing psychological symptoms; (2) the amnestic syndrome, 38 per cent; (3) symptomatic epilepsy with psychological symptoms, 12 per cent; (4) hypersomnia, 2–3 per cent; (5) functional psychiatric syndromes, such as schizophrenia, mania, depression, and neuroses, 4·5 per cent; and (6) combinations of groups (1), (2), (3); these combinations seemed characteristic of cerebral tumours.

Walther-Büel found that, on the whole, the psychiatric symptoms in brain tumours were an expression of general disturbances of brain function. Hypersomnia, uncinate fits and the frontal lobe syndrome were of localizing value, but this concerned only 5·5 per cent of the whole series.

PSYCHOLOGICAL ILLNESSES CONNECTED WITH CHILDBEARING

Pregnancy

Normal Pregnancy

Irritability and emotional lability often occur in the first 3 months. Morning sickness occurs during this period and has a psychological basis. After the third month most women have a sense of well-being; in fact, some inadequate neurotic women insist that they feel well only during pregnancy.

Hyperemesis Gravidarum

This has been alleged to be a hysterical exaggeration of normal morning sickness, supposed to occur in immature hysterical personalities who are unconsciously, if not consciously, rejecting motherhood. The evidence for this is no more than that emotional stresses may play a part in the causation. The treatment consists of psychotherapy and the administration of phenothiazines, such as perphenazine, 2–4 mg three times a day. The drug may have to be given intramuscularly at first. If there is loss of weight or haematemesis it will be necessary to admit the patient to hospital and correct fluid and electrolyte imbalance by i.v. therapy.

Neurotic and Psychogenic Reactions

In general, typical depressions are rare during pregnancy and most depressions during this time are psychogenic reactions of abnormal personalities to stress. Many unmarried pregnant women are unhappy, distressed, and threaten suicide. It is difficult to assess the seriousness of such threats. Depression can be treated with electroconvulsive therapy during pregnancy without undue risk to mother or child. Modified insulin therapy should not be given during pregnancy. The antidepressant drugs appear to be without risk in pregnancy.

The Puerperium

The puerperal psychoses are not a unitary group, but are constitutionally determined responses to physical and psychological stress.

Organic States

Many women are emotionally labile, irritable and somewhat anxious during the first few weeks of the puerperium. If labour has been prolonged and much sleep has been lost a transitory confusional state with auditory hallucinations may be seen. Delirium and subacute delirious states are less common since the introduction of the antibiotics.

Affective Psychoses

Depression is the commonest psychosis in the puerperium. If it begins soon after childbirth the clinical picture may be rendered somewhat atypical by a mild confusional element. If the depressive features are well marked in a puerperal psychosis the diagnosis of schizophrenia should not be made unless there are symptoms of the first rank (see p. 145). Puerperal depression responds to electroconvulsive therapy and the antidepressive drugs, such as imipramine, phenelzine and amitriptyline.

Schizophrenia

This does occur in the puerperium, but is not as common as depression.

MENTAL DISORDERS OF OLD AGE

Many different kinds of nervous illness occur after the age of 60 years. Since the number of old people in the Western world is increasing steadily, mental disorders in old age are becoming more important and therefore warrant separate treatment in a textbook.

The Psychology of Ageing

Practically every psychological function increases in efficiency in childhood and adolescence until it reaches its maximum value somewhere between 15 and 20 years of age, depending on the function and the methods of measurement. After this there is a slow decline which is usually unequivocal by the age of 35 years. This applies to such functions as intelligence, motor speed, reaction time and immediate memory. This decline of intelligence is compensated in the third, fourth and fifth decades by increasing emotional stability and knowledge. However, by the seventh and eighth decades the decline in intelligence is obvious, especially in the dullard. Personality traits tend to be enhanced by ageing. The only personality change which is always associated with ageing is rigidity, which increases steadily with age.

The Size of the Problem

Some 5–7 per cent of people over the age of 65 have dementia in some degree. The number of old people in the population of Great Britain is increasing. Thus 12·6 per cent of the population of England and Wales were of pensionable age in 1944, but with current population trends 19·1 per cent of the population will be of pensionable age in 1984. In 1937 the first-attack admission rate to mental hospitals for elderly patients in England and Wales was, for the age-group 55–64 years, 75 per 100000 for males, and 79 per 100000 for females. For the age-group 65+ the rate was 79 per 100000 for males, and 77 per 100000 for females. The admission rates for New York State are considerably higher than the English admission rates and show a marked excess of males over females. This difference is partly due to the admission of English psychiatric patients to social welfare and chronic sick institutions, and partly due to social factors. The admission rate of old people to mental hospitals probably varies inversely with the degree to which the aged are protected against insecurity by pensions and other benefits.

Classification of Mental Disorder in the Aged

More than 100 years ago Thomas Clouston (1883) pointed out that about one-third of the old people admitted to his mental hospital were subsequently discharged. In 1896 Kraepelin asserted that the majority of mental disorders of old age were depressive states. In Germany and the United States this fact was forgotten and severe mental disorders in old age were considered to be due to dementia, which might be present with depressive or paranoid features. More recently Roth (1955) has claimed that he was able to classify all but 14 of 464 senile patients admitted to a mental hospital into five groups. These were: (1) affective psychoses; (2) senile psychosis; (3) arteriosclerotic psychosis (now known as multi-infarct dementia); (4) delirious states; and (5) late paraphrenia.

1. *Affective Psychoses*

These were mainly depressive and accounted for about half the cases. Only a few of these patients subsequently became demented.

2. *Senile Psychosis*

This is a dementia, but Roth decided not to use the term 'senile dementia', because it had been claimed that there was no correlation between the brain changes and the degree of the dementia. This has subsequently been disproved, and this group will be referred to here as 'senile dementia'.

3. *Multi-infarct Dementia*

This is a dementia secondary to repeated small infarcts of the brain produced by arteriosclerosis.

4. *Delirious States*

These were rapidly developing states of clouded consciousness with or without a detectable physical basis.

5. *Late Paraphrenia*

Individuals suffering from this disorder had fairly well-systematized paranoid delusions and a well-preserved personality in the absence of coarse brain disease. Kay and Roth (1961) have claimed that these patients are really schizophrenic. Perhaps a better designation for this group is 'senile paranoid state'.

Note: Although most workers in this field would agree that Roth's five main groups include the majority of severe mental disorders in old age, at least two other workers have found rather more unclassifiable cases than Roth. The differentiation of multi-infarct from senile dementia is often not easy, and in many cases depends on the post-mortem examination rather than on the clinical findings.

Affective Psychosis

Aetiology

Roth found that senile depressives, who broke down for the first time after the age of 60 years, had more severe and more chronic illness than those who had broken down before that age, but the familial incidence of manic-depressive disease was the same in both groups. He concluded that those patients who became depressed for the first time over the age of 50 years had better personalities and were breaking down because of the severe stress of physical illness. Roth considered that bereavement, retirement and loneliness were only contributory factors of little significance.

Clinical Picture
DEPRESSION

Usually it is a typical agitated depression, but sometimes there is a simple depression with retardation, slowing down of all activity, and a difficulty in making decisions. This may lead the unwary to make a diagnosis of early senile dementia. Some patients present with neurotic-like states displaying anxiety and hypochondriasis.

MANIA

These patients are hyperactive with flight of ideas. They formed 5–10 per cent of Roth's series.

DIAGNOSIS

In senile dementia, there is a history of many months of poor memory, grasp and orientation, while in arteriosclerotic dementia lability of affect and neurological signs tend to occur. In paranoid states the delusions cannot be derived from the mood, and other symptoms, such as auditory hallucinations, are present (*see* p. 182). Clouding of consciousness occurs in some depressions as a result of malnutrition or concomitant physical disease. In such cases the symptoms of depression have clearly preceded the clouding of consciousness. Cognitive defects may be present in a depressive setting (depressive pseudodementia) but respond well to treatment.

Treatment

Inpatient treatment will be required in most cases. A thorough physical investigation, treatment of malnutrition and careful investigation of social background will be necessary.

ELECTROCONVULSIVE THERAPY

This may be advisable if there is no response to antidepressants or if the patient is severely depressed, with agitation, leading to exhaustion or feeding difficulties. Risks must be taken in the presence of physical illness, since the depression can kill from suicide or intercurrent infection.

DRUGS

Imipramine 60 mg per 24 hours. Side-effects due to this drug are much more frequent in elderly patients. Mono-amine oxidase inhibitors are useful in mild cases of depression (*see* p. 129).

MANIA

The treatment of mania is described on p. 120.

Senile Dementia

Aetiology

A hereditary factor is probable, but not proved. Brain changes are always present.

Morbid Anatomy

Signs of atrophy of the brain are usually visible macroscopically. Microscopically there is diffuse outfall of nerve-cells, but the cytoarchitecture is fairly well preserved. Neurones show shrinkage and chromatolysis. There is some macro- and microglial proliferation. Senile plaques and neurofibrillary changes are usually present, but these may be absent. Anterior frontal areas are usually severely affected, and the motor area and the cortex posterior to it are less affected. Plaques and neurofibrillary changes may occur in the periventricular grey matter of the third ventricle, in basal ganglia and in the thalamus.

The Psychiatric Clinical Picture

AGE AND SEX

Patients are usually over 70 years of age, and there is an excess of females.

ONSET

There is a gradual onset, but the disorder advances rapidly.

MEMORY

This is the first intellectual function to be noticeably affected. Recent memory fails, but memory for remote events is apparently intact.

BLUNTING OF EMOTION

This leads to petulant and irritable behaviour; finally to apathy or childish euphoria. Depression, with extravagant delusions of guilt, and depravity may occur. Usually the mood is shallow and transient. Mood changes of this kind are more common in multi-infarct dementias.

INTELLECTUAL DEFECTS

The patient tires easily and cannot follow the argument. He may get over difficulties for a time by rigid adherence to a routine. Slowness and perseveration are evident, and the individual becomes muddled with the simplest tasks. Speech deteriorates. At first it is verbose and repetitive, with stereotyped phrases, and the train of thought is easily lost, but finally it becomes a mere babble of words. Delusions arise from lack of grasp, failure of orientation and inability to interpret the environment. Thus, mislaid articles are alleged to be stolen and nurses are identified as the patient's children.

SLEEP

This is often disturbed. The patient potters about the house in the middle of the night and may wander about the streets.

URINARY INCONTINENCE

This occurs early. Faecal incontinence occurs sooner or later.

TOILET AND CLEANLINESS
These habits are faulty, and the patients will not wash.

ACUTE DELIRIUM
This may be provoked by infection, a fracture, or a sudden change in the environment. There is severe restlessness, with auditory and visual hallucinations and paranoid ideas. The patient may commit violent assaults or wander incessantly. The death-rate is high. Recovery from the episode leaves the patient more demented than before.

Outcome
Most of these patients are in an advanced state of dementia on admission to mental hospital and usually have a history of 1–2½ years of illness. Sixty per cent are dead in 6 months and 80 per cent are dead in 2 years following admission to mental hospital (Roth, 1955). Death is due to intercurrent infection or more usually to vegetative extinction. The weight falls, all activity declines, blood pressure drops and the temperature becomes subnormal.

Diagnosis
Tumour, general paresis, multi-infarct dementias and Alzheimer's disease must be excluded.

In multi-infarct dementias the course is more acute; the illness remits and fluctuates. Neurological signs and symptoms occur sooner or later, and there is a preservation of personality until the late stages.

Alzheimer's disease occurs in an earlier age-group; there is a discrepancy between physical and mental ageing.

Treatment
The patient should be kept at home unless his behaviour becomes too difficult. He should be kept out of bed and given general nursing care. Phenothiazines may be given for restlessness, but only small doses may be needed, as such patients are usually very sensitive to these drugs.

Multi-infarct Dementia
Aetiology
It usually begins in the sixth decade, but occasionally in the fifth, and hypertension is present in about half the cases. A severe cerebrovascular accident ushers in half the cases.

Clinical Features
The onset may often be a delirious episode which brings the patient to the doctor, but sometimes it is depression or a suicidal attempt.

PSYCHOLOGICAL SYMPTOMS
Memory for recent events is impaired, but may be relatively isolated, and the patient may compensate with a note book. Occasionally there is a full-blown amnestic syndrome. The intellectual functions are impaired; there is difficulty in concentration and the patient is slow to grasp situations, especially new ones. Judgement is relatively well preserved. Until a late stage the patient has insight into the change taking place in him. Emotion is often blunted and interests are diminished. The patients are often despondent and pessimistic due to awareness of their own decline. Emotional incontinence is characteristic. Depression is common, and severe, persistent, depressive mood changes occur in 5–10 per cent of cases; usually depressions are short-lived and often in the setting of the clouding of consciousness. Determined suicidal attempts occur in delirious episodes, but the patient may be euphoric on admission to hospital after the attempt.

SOMATIC SIGNS AND SYMPTOMS
Headache, giddiness, tinnitus and chest pains are common. Coronary artery disease is also common.

NEUROLOGICAL SIGNS AND SYMPTOMS
These occur sooner or later. Epileptic fits occur in 15–20 per cent of cases; usually generalized and less often Jacksonian. Occasionally there is loss of consciousness, no fit, but hemiplegia with recovery. Minor neurological abnormalities, such as sluggish pupils, unequal tendon jerks and extensor plantar responses, are often seen. Parkinsonism occurs in a small proportion of cases.

Course
Usually it is fluctuating with acute delirious episodes with clouding of consciousness which may give the impression of severe dementia. Recovery from these episodes occurs in days or weeks, but residual impairment is detectable afterwards. Social recovery is common. Fluctuation in severity may occur from hour to hour; the patient may be disorientated at one time, but lucid an hour or two later. Clouding of consciousness is often more severe at night. Finally the patient becomes fatuous, forgetful and develops faulty toilet habits, but even so some shell of the personality may remain. Death usually ensues from cerebro-vascular accident, pneumonia, or heart failure.

Prognosis
In Roth's series, 6 months after admission one-third were dead, one-quarter discharged, and the rest were inpatients. After 2 years 70 per cent were dead. These are mental hospital figures and may not reflect the true outcome.

Diagnosis
Cerebral tumour, general paresis and presenile dementia must be excluded. Subdural haematoma should be considered (*see* p. 166).

DIFFERENTIATION FROM SENILE DEMENTIA
In multi-infarct dementia the following features are distinctive:
1. Signs of a cerebrovascular lesion.
2. A markedly fluctuating or remitting course.
3. Preservation of insight and personality until a relatively late stage.
4. Explosiveness or incontinence of emotional expression.
5. Epileptic fits.

Treatment
Patients should remain at home where possible, and should be kept active. If the depression is severe electroconvulsive therapy can be given, or an antidepressant drug. These measures must be used cautiously since they can increase the degree of confusion.

Delirious States
Aetiology
Roth found that in 50 per cent of delirious patients there were acute infections, the commonest being pneumonia and acute bronchitis. He also found that the illness followed major operations, especially prostatectomy and cataract extraction. However, in 30–40 per cent of his cases Roth could find no specific cause and assumed that a toxic factor or vitamin deficiency was the cause. In a series of 93 senile patients admitted to a delirium unit Williamson and Fish found that 9 were misdiagnosed depressives and 1 was a senile paranoid state. Of the remainder, 38 were suffering from multi-infarct and/or senile dementia, 12 had cardiac failure which was frequently the result of a recent cardiac infarct, and 10 suffered from respiratory or urinary tract infection. The remaining patients suffered from miscellaneous conditions such as primary or secondary cerebral neoplasms, fat embolism, head injury, and so on. In 6 patients barbiturates appeared to have played an important part in the causation of the delirium. The tendency of the aged to become confused even on small doses of the quick-acting barbiturates is not sufficiently appreciated.

Clinical Features
The patient will have been mentally well until recently, and looks well preserved. The rapport, despite clouding of consciousness, is surprisingly good for short intervals except in severe cases. Marked fluctuations in the level of awareness are very characteristic. These patients give fairly elaborate, positive, wrong answers, whereas advanced multi-infarct patients and senile dements give vague answers or deny all knowledge.

There is a richness in the content of thought as compared with the well-established dement. Inconsistent orientation is fairly common, so that two incompatible orientations may occur side by side.

Diagnosis

Delirium in a senile dementia is characterized by contentless hyperactivity and incoherent excitement. Delirium in multi-infarct dementia may be difficult to distinguish in the early stages of the disease. The appearance of neurological signs and duration for months or weeks may decide in favour of multi-infarct dementia. On the whole the presence of clouding of consciousness excludes the functional psychoses, but a mania, depression, or a paranoid state may be complicated by a delirium produced by malnutrition or intercurrent disease.

Treatment

The underlying infection should be treated if possible, and antibiotics should be given if the patient is febrile or very ill. Parentrovite may be administered.

Senile Paranoid State

Aetiology

One-quarter have some defect of sight or hearing. Females predominate, and patients are usually isolated individuals living on their own (Roth). Some are probably cases of schizophrenia.

Clinical Features

Florid persecutory delusions are always present; the patient complains of being gassed and raped; people are alleged to enter the house and interfere. Hallucinations occur, which may be voices, noises, odours and lights. There is normal orientation and good contact with surroundings. No deterioration in toilet habits occurs. Judgement and reason are well preserved outside the delusions. Sometimes delusions of poisoning lead to malnutrition and a confusional state.

Diagnosis

Senile psychosis, multi-infarct dementia, delirious states and depression should be differentiated.

SENILE DEMENTIA

Loosely connected and ill-systematized persecutory delusions occur in this condition.

MULTI-INFARCT DEMENTIA

Persecutory delusions are occasionally closely knit, but they tend to fluctuate. Dementia is usually obvious and neurological signs may be present.

DELIRIOUS STATES
Clouding of consciousness occurs.

DEPRESSION
Some depressives have delusions of persecution, which they consider to be unjustified. If there are no other non-understandable symptoms the illness should not be called schizophrenic.

Prognosis

Roth found that only 5 per cent were dead in 6 months and 20 per cent within 2 years of admission. The mean age of these patients was higher than that of the affective group; there is an unusual longevity. Recovery before the introduction of phenothiazines was rare. Only 20 per cent of Roth's patients were out of hospital within 2 years of their first admission.

Treatment

By phenothiazines, for example, thioridazine 300–400 mg in 24 hours (*see* p. 210). Few of these patients fail to respond satisfactorily to high doses of phenothiazines.

Chapter 13

Sexual disorders

GENERAL DISCUSSION
Classification
Sexual disorders may be classified as follows:
1. Disorders of sexual function, for example, impotence, frigidity, etc.
2. Disorders of the direction of sexual drive.
   a. Deviation of the aim of sexual satisfaction. These are the perversions such as fellatio, anal intercourse, etc.
   b. Deviation in the choice of sexual partner, for example, homosexuality, bestiosexuality, and so on.

Normal Sexual Intercourse
This can be defined as 'sexual activity which has as its aim an orgasm in both partners, produced by the activity of the penis in the vagina'. The sexual activity which precedes the insertion of the penis is called 'foreplay'. This can take many forms, such as genital kissing, oral kissing, biting and manual stimulation of the penis, clitoris, or vagina. However, as long as the foreplay is only preparatory to the insertion of the penis in the vagina, it cannot be regarded as a sexual perversion.

Sexual intercourse begins with the man fondling the breasts and fingering the introitus. This and other foreplay bring about a readiness on the part of the woman for coitus. It also increases the man's desire and leads to an erection, which in turn excites the woman, who responds with increased vaginal secretion. This increase in secretion stimulates the man even more, reinforces his erection and leads to insertion of the penis. Coitus then follows and ends with the man ejaculating and the woman having an orgasm. The weakest point in the man's sexual performance is the achievement and maintenance of an erection, whereas the weakest point in the woman's coital activity is the achievement of orgasm. Thus the absence of orgasm in the female is the commonest disorder of coitus, while in the male inability to maintain an adequate erection is the most frequent disorder.

Sexual drive varies considerably. Many individuals lead happy and useful lives with a level of sexual activity which the average person (and average psychiatrist) would regard as grossly inadequate. Some persons have high sexual drive, but it is pointless to attach to their activities the labels of satyriasis and nymphomania as if they suffered from some disorder.

DISORDERS OF SEXUAL FUNCTION
Impotence
This is the failure of a man to have a satisfactory orgasm with his penis in the vagina.

Variations of Impotence
1. Inability to obtain an erection or to maintain it long enough to achieve penetration.
2. Ejaculatio praecox. Ejaculation occurs before or immediately after insertion, to the dissatisfaction of both partners.
3. Ejaculatio retarda. Coitus takes place, but ejaculation does not occur. All these may be *primary*—when the condition has always been present, or *secondary*—when they appear after a period of sexual competence.

Physical Causes
These account for no more than 1 in 10 cases. Endocrine disorders are important (e.g. Cushing's disease); among these must be included diabetes mellitus, which may lead to an intractable impotence, alleged to be related to a local neuritis. Liver disease may account for the impotence of alcoholics. Neurological diseases, e.g. multiple sclerosis may produce impotence. Hypotensive drugs, e.g. guanethidine, may produce difficulty in ejaculation.

Psychological Causes
The following psychological conditions may be responsible:

1. PSYCHIATRIC ILLNESSES
Diminution of sexual function may occur in all conditions, except hypomania. Loss of libido and impotence are common in depressive states. Severe anxiety from any cause will also lead to impotence.

2. THE EFFECTS OF THE IMMEDIATE SITUATION
Attempts at coitus in situations in which there is a possibility of discovery may fail, because the anxiety is sufficient to interfere with an erection. Fear of venereal disease or disgust make some men impotent with prostitutes or with very promiscuous women.

3. THE WOMAN
A wife may express her antipathy to sexual intercourse by being completely passive, permitting penetration, but refusing to stimulate the husband in any way. The lack of emotional response and the lack of physiological response, in the form of increased vaginal secretion, diminish the husband's desire. Impotence occurs and the wife blames the husband and laughs at him. The repeated failure and the wife's scornful

attitude convince the man of his impotence. Thus the basically frigid wife avoids coitus and is able to blame her husband for the lack of something which she does not want. This is really a 'double-bind' technique (*see* p. 136). Some wives, who are basically frigid, use their ability to allow or refuse coitus in order to control their husbands. The husband may be disgusted by this behaviour and some become impotent because of the lack of genuine feeling on the part of his wife.

4. UNCONSCIOUS PSYCHOLOGICAL CAUSES

Psychoanalysts believe that unconscious attitudes due to childhood difficulties are of fundamental importance, e.g. severe unconscious castration anxiety may cause impotence, because the man regards the vagina as a castrating mechanism. Latent homosexuality which is related to castration anxiety also plays a part in some cases. Sometimes the partner is identified with the 'pure' sister or mother, so that the impotence is a reaction formation produced by incest wishes. Often unconscious antipathy towards coitus can be found in both partners.

5. THE VICIOUS CIRCLE

Erection is a sign of manhood, so that failure to achieve an erection and have intercourse produces a sense of shame and marked anxiety. The next attempt at coitus is, therefore, approached with fear. This leads to a poor erection and failure to have coitus. This vicious circle of impotence—anxiety, further impotence, more anxiety—is very difficult to break.

Treatment

Although endocrine diseases are not very common causes of impotence, most patients with impotence are given testosterone before they are referred to a psychiatrist.

The circumstances in which impotence occurs must be carefully investigated by interviewing both the husband and the wife. The wife's attitude to sexual intercourse must be assessed. The patient should be told not to attempt coitus during the first few weeks of psychotherapy. If the causes of the impotence appear to be fairly superficial, the patient should be told to attempt sexual intercourse when he feels like it. If possible he should take a small dose of sedative, for example, meprobamate 200 mg, or amylobarbitone sodium 65 mg, half an hour before coitus. The reduction of anxiety produced by the sedative may permit satisfactory intercourse. This treatment is particularly useful in patients with premature ejaculation. If these measures fail, psychotherapy should be continued and sexual intercourse should not be attempted again for a few weeks. Intensive psychotherapy still has some support, based largely on faith and hope. A controlled trial (Ansari, 1976) found no significant difference between the results of 'simple' psychotherapy and the more elaborate procedures which have become popular in recent years.

Penile splints which allow the insertion of a flaccid penis have been used. It is claimed that coital activity with a splinted penis leads to an erection and an orgasm. This is not a very satisfactory form of treatment. The prognosis in secondary impotence is much better than in the primary type.

Priapism

This is a painful penile erection in the absence of sexual desire. It lasts for days and is usually associated with dysuria. The corpora cavernosa are engorged, but the corpus spongiosum and glans are not. It is often caused by diseases of the central nervous system and blood disorders. In about 25 per cent of cases it is due to leukaemia. Occasionally sudden interruption of coitus just before ejaculation produces priapism. If the condition is not due to disease of the central nervous system the corpora cavernosa should be aspirated with a wide-bore needle and washed out with normal saline.

Frigidity

General Problems

Frigidity is the absence of an orgasm in the female during sexual intercourse. It is more common than impotence, since the female has much more difficulty in achieving an orgasm than the male. The woman's first experiences of coitus are often painful and disappointing. Later, coitus is often unsatisfactory because the man does not indulge in sufficient foreplay and ejaculates somewhat prematurely. Thus the woman is not likely to have an orgasm until she has had some practice with a competent partner. While many men can have sexual intercourse with almost any woman, many women need to feel loved and wanted apart from the sex act. If such women feel that their partner is using them only for physical satisfaction, their enjoyment of coitus is diminished and they do not have an orgasm.

Varieties of Frigidity

1. TOTAL FRIGIDITY

The woman has no sexual desire, cannot be aroused sexually, and is nauseated by the idea of coitus. This is very rare.

2. PARTIAL FRIGIDITY

Sexual excitement develops slowly and the woman may need much love play. Even then orgasm may not be reached unless the circumstances are just right. Another form presents as normal response to external stimulation, even to the point of orgasm, but all excitement disappears at any attempt to insert the penis.

Physical Causes

Disorders of the endocrine glands and the nervous system can cause frigidity. Local causes of pain and discomfort are also important.

Psychological Causes

The following psychological causes may be responsible:

1. PSYCHIATRIC ILLNESSES

Depression is often associated with a decrease in sexual desire and a dislike of sexual intercourse. This may lead to disagreements with the husband and enhance the feelings of guilt. Frigidity appearing after childbirth may have this origin. Loss of libido and frigidity are common in schizophrenia.

2. THE EFFECTS OF THE IMMEDIATE SITUATION

Anxiety from any cause may produce frigidity. Sexual intercourse in circumstances in which it is likely to be interrupted, fear of pregnancy, domestic difficulties, bad news, and so forth can all lead to frigidity.

The most extreme effect of anxiety is vaginismus, in which any attempt at coitus produces spasm of the adductors of the thighs and arching of the back, making it impossible.

3. PRECONCEIVED IDEAS

Some women are brought up to believe that coitus is a wife's painful duty, which must be tolerated, but cannot be enjoyed. Such an attitude may be reinforced by an inconsiderate husband who makes no attempt to stimulate his wife.

4. THE MAN

If the husband fails to arouse his wife and ejaculates soon after insertion of the penis, the wife will be disappointed. This will enhance any antipathy towards intercourse, so that even if the husband's performance improves it is still not adequate to bring about an orgasm.

5. UNCONSCIOUS CAUSES

Psychoanalysts have claimed that oral fixation may produce frigidity, because frustration at this level may lead to the woman being unable to accept gifts and in particular to accept the gift of the penis. Anal fixation may also produce frigidity. It has also been suggested that penis envy may produce frigidity, which can be regarded as an attempt to retain the penis. Abraham suggested that vaginismus expressed an unconscious wish to break off and retain the penis.

Treatment

A careful investigation of the coital technique and the circumstances in which it is performed must be made and any faults discussed. The husband may need a sedative to prevent premature ejaculation. Good results have been claimed for tricyclics; their effect arises probably from their anticholinergic action. The patient's attitudes to sex must be carefully explored and any false ideas corrected. If these simple measures fail, more intensive psychotherapy is necessary. Marked aversion to sexual intercourse, in particular vaginismus, is very difficult to treat.

AETIOLOGY OF THE DISORDERS OF SEXUAL DRIVE

Constitutional Theories

It has often been claimed that perversions are inborn, but there is no good evidence to support this view.

Psychoanalytic Theories

In the perversions the Oedipal conflict is not resolved, so that the castration anxiety leads to the choice of a sexual object which disguises the incest fantasies and allows sexual satisfaction. Nacht has suggested that the pervert has such intense aggressive and libidinal drives that the ego has to put a safe distance between itself and the object which is both unconsciously desired and feared. This leads to the formation of a defence mechanism which is completely eroticized. Activation of this defence mechanism brings about an orgasm. Sometimes this activation produces severe anxiety and this leads to an orgasm. The eroticized defence mechanism is derived from earlier pregenital libidinal fixations. The ego is unable to make a genital investment of the object, which is feared and forbidden. This direct eroticization of the defences leads to marked therapeutic difficulties, since the symptom is not only the solution of a conflict but is also a conscious source of sexual satisfaction. This is in contrast to the neurotic symptom which does not produce direct satisfaction although it may result in considerable secondary gain.

CLINICAL FEATURES OF DEVIATION OF AIM (PERVERSIONS)

Often the opposite type of perversion occurs in association with a given perversion. Thus voyeurism and exhibitionism, for example, may occur in the same individual. Apart from this many different perversions may occur in the same individual.

Sadism (Active Algolagnia)

The pervert obtains sexual enjoyment from the suffering of others. The term 'sadism' is now used in a wider sense of enjoyment of the suffering of others without any frank sexual element. Usually the degree of suffering inflicted is limited, but the sight of blood may be necessary to produce an orgasm. The punishment may be carried out with whips, canes, backs of hair brushes, or the bare hands. Usually the sadist likes beating the buttocks, but the genitalia or the whole body may be beaten. Other perverts enjoy biting the sexual object. Sometimes the sadistic practices take the form of play-acting in which the victim is chained, bound with ropes, humiliated and degraded in some way. Other sadists enjoy watching sadistic practices, or, in other words, they are voyeurs and sadists. The sexual object may be of the same sex, the opposite sex, a child, or an animal. In general, males are more often sadistic and females masochistic. Thus two perverts may make a harmonious heterosexual sadomasochistic relationship. A few sadists obtain sexual satisfaction from violent murder and mutilation of the sexual object.

Masochism (Passive Algolagnia)
In this perversion sexual enjoyment results from pain and humiliation. Usually these perverts do not like to feel a lot of pain. However, some of them do have fantasies of being killed. Often the pain is used only to produce sexual excitement before vaginal or anal intercourse. Some patients need to be tied up or chained, while others need to be humiliated. Sometimes orgasm is achieved by being defecated upon or urinated on by someone else. This may be carried out by the partner defecating on a glass table with the subject lying underneath. 'The horse of love' is a complicated masochistic practice in which the pervert gets his enjoyment from being ridden like a horse. A saddle is strapped on the back and the partner wears boots and spurs and mounts the subject as if he were a horse.

Associated perversions may be present. There may be some elements of fetishism. The partner may be obliged to dress in shoes, boots, or furs while he or she beats the patient. Some male masochists like to be trodden on by a woman wearing high-heeled shoes. Oral perversions may be combined with masochistic practices so that the subject may lick his partner's feet or anus or may persuade his partner to micturate or defecate into his mouth.

Psychoanalytic Theories of the Origin of Sadomasochism
In young animals and children there is a primary erogenous masochism, since they appear to enjoy marked excitation, which leads to some discomfort and pain, so long as the pain is not too severe. Masochism could, therefore, be regarded as a preservation and elaboration of this 'primary masochism'. Witnessing and experiencing brutality in childhood is likely to produce sadomasochism.

Originally Freud explained sadism as being derived from the aggressive features of the libido and masochism as the turning back of the aggression on to the subject. Later, when he introduced the concept of

Thanatos or the death instinct, he suggested that in sadism the death instinct is eroticized by the libido. When it is externalized it produces sadistic behaviour, but when turned back on the self it produces masochism.

Sadism can be regarded as a defence against severe castration anxiety. The subject resolves the Oedipal conflict by symbolic castration. He acts on the basis of the formulation, 'I am not castrated. I am the castrator.' Masochism can also be regarded as a defence against castration anxiety or it may represent castration symbolically.

Voyeurism (Scoptophilia)

In this perversion the individual obtains sexual enjoyment from watching naked men, naked women, naked children, normal or perverse sexual acts, or excretory acts. Sometimes the subject watches himself having sexual intercourse in a mirror.

Psychological Theories

The child sees the mother and embraces her with his look. Since the mother frequently satisfies the child with food and affection, then seeing the mother is associated with pleasure. It this way the act of looking becomes libidinalized. Since many mothers are seen by their young sons in varying states of nudity it would appear that this behaviour is not the major cause of voyeurism. This perversion has been explained as a defence against castration anxiety. The sight of the female genitalia or sexual intercourse during the Oedipal stage of libidinal development accentuates the castration anxiety. The subject seeks to witness repetitions of the original frightening scenes in order to reassure himself that castration has not occurred.

Exhibitionism

Symptomatic Exhibitionism

Some epileptics, manics, schizophrenics and mental defectives exhibit their genitalia.

Clinical Features

This perversion is confined to males, although a few females exhibit their breasts. Most of these perverts are mild timid men who are married and have a fairly reasonable sex life. The pervert chooses a public place which is not too well frequented, and shows his penis to one or two women, girls, or, rarely, boys. A few of these subjects exhibit their buttocks. When the penis is demonstrated it may be flaccid or erect and the pervert may masturbate or even ejaculate in front of the victim.

Some authorities have divided exhibitionists into impulsive neurotic and perverse types. The former is not very common. These patients have depression and anxiety associated with an uncontrollable desire to exhibit the penis. Finally, after an unsuccessful struggle to control the impulse they exhibit a flaccid penis and the anxious depressed mood disappears.

The perverse exhibitionist enjoys the act and exhibits an erect penis while masturbating and, if possible, ejaculating in the presence of his victim. For pleasure to be complete the victim should react violently to the act with shock, fear, interest, or even pleasure. This type of pervert takes great care not to be caught. The penis is often out of the trousers underneath a buttoned-up coat, which can be quickly undone in a suitable situation. The two types are really the extreme ends of a continuum.

Psychoanalytic Theory
The perversion is regarded as a defence against castration anxiety. Thus by demonstrating his penis the subject is reassured that he is not castrated. The fear of the victim proves to him that he has power over others and therefore has no need to be frightened of anyone. Finally, it may be the expression of a wish to see a girl with a penis in order to assuage his castration anxiety. It is as if he is saying to his victim, 'I am showing you what I would like you to show me.'

Other Perversions of the Sexual Aim
Many other perversions occur and are often worked into elaborate routines with those already described. Thus there are oral perversions in which sexual satisfaction is obtained by licking, sucking, biting, or ingesting the object. Similarly there are anal and urethral perversions.

DEVIATIONS IN THE CHOICE OF SEXUAL PARTNER
Paedophilia
Here the pervert chooses a child as a sexual partner. Some mental defectives do this because their low intelligence leads them to select a partner with a similar intelligence, and also because of their lack of appreciation of the seriousness of the situation. The true pervert seems to identify with the child and treats it in the same way as he would like to have been treated at that age, so that this perversion appears to have a narcissistic basis. Occasionally the object is of the opposite sex but usually it is of the same sex. Various kinds of sexual activity may take place with the victim.

Gerontophilia
These patients need an elderly sexual partner, and this can be regarded as a displacement of incestuous wishes. Occasionally adolescents between the ages of 14 and 20 years make aggressive attacks on elderly women with a view to rape or with no obvious purpose.

Erotic Zoophilia (Bestiality)

These perverts use an animal as a sexual object. This is partly determined by the environment. Thus Kinsey found that whereas only 8 per cent of the men in his sample had had sexual relations with an animal, no less than 50 per cent of those brought up on farms had had such relations. It often occurs in mental defectives *faute de mieux*. Sometimes it appears that the pervert chooses an animal as a sexual object because he knows that it cannot dominate him. Some voyeurs prefer to observe zoophilic sexual behaviour, and brothels cater for this by staging exhibitions of this kind.

Necrophilia

This consists of sexual intercourse with the dead. Some authors have suggested that the choice of a chronically sick or severely crippled partner is really a modified variety of necrophilia.

Very few cases of true necrophilia have been investigated. In some cases it appears to be due to mild mental defect in a solitary shy gravedigger. In others it has been suggested that the perversion is due to the patient having had a parent who suffered from a prolonged fatal illness. One case has been reported of a very sadistic man who mutilated corpses and had sexual intercourse with them. In this way he spared human beings from the serious consequences of his sadistic perversion.

Fetishism

In this perversion sexual satisfaction is obtained from contact with an inanimate object. Some subjects need a partner with a particular feature, such as large breasts, a crippled arm, dwarfism, and so on. This abnormality has been considered to be allied to true fetishism.

The fetish object may be gloves, underclothes, shoes, handbags, pieces of material, fur, rubber sheeting, and so on. The fetishist may masturbate into the object or he may get the most sexual pleasure when he steals the object. Thus some patients steal female underclothes from clothes-lines, others cut off schoolgirls' plaits, and some cut pieces of material from women's coats and dresses. There are some fetishists who wear a fetish object or persuade their partner to wear it during coitus; for example, the rubber macintosh fetishist may want his partner to wear a rubber macintosh during intercourse.

Psychoanalytic Theory

Severe castration anxiety causes the subject to turn away from the desired object, so that the fetish represents a desired partial object which has been made unrecognizable. The fetish can also be regarded as a symbolic penis, which means that the patient is trying to control his castration anxiety by giving the woman a penis.

Transvestism

In this perversion the subject obtains relief from tension or sexual enjoyment from dressing in female clothes. He may admire himself in the mirror and may masturbate or copulate while dressed as a woman. Some of these patients get considerable enjoyment from walking about the streets in female dress. Transvestism is rare in females.

Psychoanalytic Theory

The transvestist deals with his castration anxiety by acting as a woman with a penis.

Transexualism

Patients with this abnormality have the over-valued idea that they have the mind of the opposite sex in the wrong body. The male patients may claim that they are changing their sex and are frightened of all male activity, including erections. They may claim that they are having periods and produce rectal bleeding to substantiate this claim. These patients are not always homosexuals. The cause of this condition is obscure. It is usually claimed that they have had an unhappy childhood, with a poor father figure and a disturbed relationship with the mother. This applies to many men who are not transexualists. Many of these persons ask for treatment by 'sex-change' surgery. The results are satisfactory when the necessary social readjustment can be achieved, but if not, the person is left very much worse off.

Auto-eroticism (Masturbation)

Practically all men masturbate to some degree during adolescence. It does no physical harm, but may produce much guilt and shame. In some rather primitive communities the belief that masturbation causes tuberculosis, insanity and softening of the brain still flourishes. Masturbation is a substitute for normal or perverse sexual activity. While it should not be encouraged it may be a convenient safety valve in some cases.

Male Homosexuality

Clinical Features

The subject feels himself sexually attracted by other males. This attraction may be exclusive or only preponderant. It does not exclude heterosexual activity and may be episodic. Kinsey found that 46 per cent of the men in his survey had had homosexual experience of some kind at some time in their lives. He put forward a seven-point scale of homosexuality, which ranges from the completely heterosexual Group O to the completely homosexual Group 6. The other groups are:

GROUP 1
Accidental homosexuality due to circumstances, including
drunkenness.

GROUP 2
Heterosexual activity predominates, but homosexual incidents are more
than accidental.

GROUP 3
These men are equally interested in both types of sexual activity,
but they are able to be completely homosexual given the right
circumstances, for example, in prison or in the armed forces.

GROUP 4
Mainly homosexual, but heterosexual activity is more than
accidental.

GROUP 5
Almost entirely homosexual, but may have occasional heterosexual
activity.
     The desired homosexual partner can be classified according to the
degree of femininity as follows: (1) the feminine man (the 'pansy'); (2)
the adolescent boy; (3) the adult male; and (4) the aged male.
     Some homosexuals can use any male object as a source of sexual
satisfaction. Some insist that their partner must be exactly like them and
cannot tolerate any difference in the behaviour of the partner. Others
need a virile male partner whom they can serve as a woman. This latter
attitude is not necessarily incompatible with heterosexual activity.
Homosexual activity covers the whole range of perversions and is by no
means restricted to anal intercourse.

Psychiatric Disorders and Homosexuality

Overt homosexuality is the extreme end of range of sexual orientation.
It is therefore abnormal only in Schneider's sense. Now that the social
pressures against homosexual men have been reduced, the proportion
who find difficulty in coming to terms with their orientation has
correspondingly been diminished. Some homosexuals are able to have
homosexual activity only while under the influence of drink or
drugs.
     Sexual behaviour and the choice of object may change after a cerebral
lesion. This has been reported in patients suffering from brain damage
following head injury, encephalitis, typhus, syphilis and senile
dementia.
     It has been stated that schizophrenia and mania may release
homosexual behaviour. If this does occur it is extremely rare.

Aetiology

Many psychiatrists have regarded homosexuality as an inborn defect or as an inherited disorder. Kallmann found 100 per cent concordance in a series of uniovular twins in which at least one member was a homosexual. Few workers in this field are convinced of the genetic basis of this disorder. Slater (1966) pointed out that there is an excess of subjects born to elderly mothers, but no chromosomal abnormalities have been found in homosexuals. After all, the youngest sons of large families often have intense relationships with their mothers.

Endocrine disorders have no relation to homosexuality and patterns of sexual behaviour are due to the nervous system. Hormones can only inhibit or excite the structures within the nervous system responsible for these behaviour patterns. Thus oestrogens do not produce homosexual behaviour in men but suppress libido irrespective of its direction.

Many homosexuals date their homosexuality from seduction in childhood. Isolated homosexual episodes in childhood probably have no effect on a normal child, but repeated homosexual activity must have. This particularly applies to disturbed children and children from broken homes.

Psychoanalytic Theories

Freud believed that about the fourth year of life the libido became concentrated on the genitalia and the little boy developed an Oedipus complex in which he loved his mother and hated his father. A realization of the difference between male and female genitalia leads him to regard the female as a castrated male and to believe that his penis may be cut off. Oral anxieties from an early stage of libidinal development may cause the boy to think that the vagina can castrate him by biting or tearing off his penis. The boy usually resolves the Oedipal situation by identifying with his father. Should he fail to do this his castration anxiety may lead him to insist that a sexual partner must have a penis. Apart from this, disappointment with the love object, in this case the mother, causes a regression from object love to identification, so that the boy identifies with his mother and can only love men.

Female Homosexuality

In Britain very few women ask for treatment for homosexuality. This is probably because homosexual practices by two adult females have never been a criminal offence in Britain. Apart from this, female homosexuality is not regarded by the community with such horror as male homosexuality. Havelock Ellis estimated that 4–10 per cent of English women were homosexuals, while Hamilton claimed that 25 per cent of American women had had homosexual liaisons. Kinsey and his group found that by the age of 35 years 19 per cent of American women had

had homosexual contact and 11 per cent had had an orgasm during homosexual activity.

Social Aspects of Male and Female Homosexuality
In Britain and in Western civilization generally homosexuals tend to create a homosexual subgroup. Thus there are clubs, journals and cafés which cater for homosexuals and function as contact organizations.

TREATMENT OF DISORDERS OF THE DIRECTION OF SEXUAL DRIVE
The Perversions apart from Homosexuality
Most perverts come for psychiatric treatment only when their perverse practices have brought them into conflict with the law. They are, therefore, not really seeking treatment, but are trying to find a way out of the social difficulties produced by perverse practices which they enjoy and are not prepared to give up. It is doubtful whether psychotherapy has ever cured a perversion apart from homosexuality.

Several different workers claim to have cured isolated perversions such as transvestism, rubber fetishism, and exhibitionism by means of aversion therapy. In view of the poor results of psychotherapy these aversion techniques are worthy of an extensive trial.

Where the perverse activity is liable to lead to severe prison sentences the patient may be willing to accept treatment designed to diminish or remove sexual drive. This can be achieved with the drug cyproterone, which is an androgen blocker without feminizing effects. It is given in divided doses of 100–200 mg per day, and takes several months to achieve its full effects. Oestrogens are unsatisfactory because of their feminizing effects.

The Treatment of Homosexuality
Indications for Treatment
If the homosexual comes for treatment it is important to discover why he is doing so. If it is because of criminal proceedings or pressure from relatives it is hardly worth attempting treatment.

Eclectic Psychotherapy
Psychotherapy is helpful in those young men between 18 and 25 years of age who have just begun homosexual activity, who have some heterosexual drive, and wish to have treatment for good reasons. In these cases the therapist behaves as a kindly, tolerant father figure, with whom the patient can identify. A careful detailed history must be taken. The therapist must try to create an atmosphere of trust and must not indulge in moral condemnation. In the discussion of the past all the factors which prevented the individual from making adequate contact with women

must be brought into prominence. In the therapeutic discussions the patient should come to understand the healthy concept of heterosexual love and marriage. He must also be persuaded to be completely honest with himself about his homosexual tendencies and to be constantly on the watch for the 'unconscious' development of homosexual attachments. It is amazing how these patients, apparently unwittingly, can put themselves into a homosexual milieu. The patient should make every effort to live as much as possible in a heterosexual environment. He should be encouraged to join mixed social clubs, to learn ballroom dancing, and so on. His difficulties in handling his relationships with women must be discussed. Relaxation exercises may help him to overcome shyness and gaucherie in female company.

It is important to remember that marriage in itself is not a cure for homosexuality. The well-meaning doctor who advises a homosexual to get married should remember that he is exposing the wife to the risk of marital disharmony.

Endocrine Treatment

Oestrogens and cyproterone diminish libido but do not affect its direction. These treatments should be used only in very exceptional circumstances.

Chapter 14

The treatment and management of psychiatric disorders

GENERAL PRINCIPLES OF MANAGEMENT

1. The Interview

An attempt should be made to obtain a reasonable outline of the history of the illness, the family history, the personal history and the personality, at the first interview. Wherever possible this should be supplemented by information from a relative or friend.

In some illnesses, such as acute schizophrenia or severe depressive illness, the diagnosis may be made at the first interview and physical treatment of some kind can be started immediately. This does not absolve the psychiatrist from obtaining a fairly detailed account of the patient's personal history and environmental conditions. In the present state of our knowledge we cannot afford to neglect any factor which logically seems to have played a part in the causation or prolongation of a psychiatric illness. The task of the good psychiatrist is twofold. In the first place he must do his utmost to help his patient, and to achieve this end he must not neglect anything which may conceivably alleviate his patient's condition. In the second place he must continually submit his concepts to close scrutiny and careful investigation. In other words, he has to have one attitude as a doctor and another as a scientist, though he need not regard them as incompatible, for they strengthen each other.

The art of interviewing can only be acquired by experience. Every effort has to be made to put the patient at ease and to create a feeling of true sympathy, which enables the patient to talk about his difficulties freely. It is important for the examiner not to appear censorious, although he must not agree with delusions or false beliefs or appear to condone grossly immoral behaviour. It may be necessary to assure the patient that one does not doubt the reality of his experiences, but one believes that they have been caused by a nervous illness.

The doctor should not encourage the patient by admitting that he too suffers from the same symptoms. This cannot help the patient and is likely to undermine his confidence. It should be remembered that the patient is coming for professional help, not for an afternoon's chit-chat.

Criticism of fellow practitioners should never be made by the examiner. If a patient expresses criticism of this kind, it should be made clear to him that the examiner does not agree and does not wish to hear any more criticism. The patient who is criticizing one doctor when talking to another will be criticizing the latter in the near future.

It may be difficult to keep the patient to the point, but a balance must be struck between giving the patient his head and interrupting him after every sentence. Embarrassing topics, such as sexual behaviour and hallucinations, must not be avoided, but approached in a natural manner. If there is an indication that the patient is depressed the examiner must ask him if he has suicidal thoughts. The easiest way of approaching this subject is to ask the question: 'Do you ever feel that life is not worth living?' If the answer is 'Yes', then the next question must be: 'Have you ever thought of doing something about it?' This will allow the patient to give details of any proposed or half-hearted attempts at suicide in the recent past. Relatives often become annoyed when they discover that the doctor has been asking the patient about suicide, and may say that the doctor is putting ideas into the patient's head. This is not true since most depressed patients have toyed with the idea of death as a solution to their problems, although they may not have actively contemplated suicide. In fact many of these patients are relieved by discussing their suicidal ideas, which they have not dared to mention to their relatives. If the patient is suffering from a depressive illness he should be told that he will recover and that he is suffering from a well-known nervous illness from which recovery is the rule. It is neither possible nor even desirable to institute day-and-night supervision of every patient with suicidal thoughts. If the patient is in hospital the doctor in immediate charge should make every effort to win the patient's confidence and establish a good relationship with him. The patient should be persuaded to ask for help from the nearest doctor or nurse as soon as he feels so depressed that suicide seems to be the only way out. Admission to a reasonable hospital environment often helps the suicidal patient, because he has been removed from a situation with which he cannot cope and put into a protective environment in which few demands are made of him.

2. Defining the Complaint

The psychiatrist must always ask himself the question: 'Why did this patient come for help at *this* time?' The initial complaint may bear little relationship to the actual reason for the patient's attendance at the clinic. For example, when a lifelong homosexual comes to a clinic to ask for treatment for his deviation it may be because he is depressed, or because he is involved in criminal proceedings, or because a close relative has discovered his deviation and is insisting that he be treated.

3. The Assessment of the Individual

An unbiased assessment of the patient's personality assets as well as all his faults and failings must be made as early as possible in the illness and reviewed from time to time as new information emerges. Some doctors become so involved with their patients that any reasonable assessment of their patients by another doctor is regarded as a personal insult. A dispassionate assessment of a patient is not a moral judgement but an attempt to separate the patient's psychic reality from the true state of affairs.

It is very important to discover any interests or hobbies which the patient has, because these may be developed in order to compensate for irremediable situational difficulties. An interest in religion or a sense of social service may be very valuable assets, particularly in alcohol addicts.

4. The Environment

The domestic, occupational and general social situation confronting the patient should be carefully investigated for problems which may be causing or aggravating the nervous illness. Where possible an account of the environmental difficulties should also be obtained from a relative. Sometimes a visit to the home or to the place of work by a psychiatric social worker is extremely valuable.

5. Control of the Therapeutic Situation

In hospital the patient is being cared for by a well-defined team, of which the psychiatrist is the leading member. When the patient is living in the community a large number of different social agencies may play some part in treatment and they must be properly co-ordinated. Some patients are able to involve every possible agency in their case and to play off one against the other. The therapeutic team must, therefore, always be properly defined, so that there is no wasted effort and all members of the team know the part they have to play.

Where admission to hospital is essential for the proper treatment or for the safety of the patient or others the psychiatrist must not hesitate to recommend compulsory admission if the patient refuses to agree to admission. Should the relatives refuse to consent to compulsory admission, legal action can be taken in Britain (*see* p. 229) to take the matter out of their hands. Where such action cannot be taken the relatives should be left in no doubt about their responsibility and the fact that any other treatment is second best. It is not uncommon for severe depressives to agree to outpatient electroconvulsive treatment and to refuse admission to an acute psychiatric unit. It should be made clear that outpatient treatment is a poor substitute for proper inpatient care.

Neither the patient nor his relatives should be allowed to dictate the type of treatment required. The psychiatrist should carefully explain the nature of the treatment and why it is necessary. If the patient refuses the treatment recommended and wishes to leave the hospital, the psychiatrist should explain the consequences to the patient and relatives and then discharge the patient. He should make it clear that if there is a change of mind in the patient or relatives he will be happy to readmit the patient for treatment. A sick person has the right in general to decide whether he prefers the illness or the treatment, but if his judgement is disturbed by illness, the situation should be made clear to the relatives. Their wishes should not be disregarded except in situations of real danger.

Control of the situation does not mean that the doctor dominates the treatment situation. The patient must not be regarded as the personal possession of the psychiatrist, the nurse, or the psychiatric social worker. Relatives of the patients should not be regarded as troublesome interlopers who interfere with the control which the hospital staff has over the patient. Many trained mental nurses need to possess their patients rather like overprotective mothers. This tendency can be corrected tactfully during group discussions. The psychiatrist should make sure that each member of the treatment team and the key relatives know what parts they have to play in the overall plan of treatment.

A common form of domination is the 'father-knows-best' attitude, when the doctor decides on the solution of the patient's problems and tries to impose his plan for the reorganization of the patient's life without bringing the patient to realize the need for these changes. This type of behaviour is often found among kindly but ill-informed general physicians, who naively believe that once the patient has been given a logical solution to his problems he will naturally accept it and carry it out.

The psychiatrist and other members of the therapeutic team must be on their guard against being manipulated by the patient or his relatives. Sometimes domestic unhappiness is turned into an illness which is used as a weapon against the spouse. In general, unhappy marriages are due to faults on both sides and it is difficult, if not impossible, to apportion the amount of responsibility for the situation between the two partners. A 'double-binding' wife may convince the doctor that she is in no way responsible for her long-suffering husband's bad behaviour. Once this has been done the doctor may be used to bully the husband. Some patients try to enlist everyone in their cause. The doctor or the social worker should not become a partisan on his patient's behalf, particularly in marital problems.

Another common form of manipulation is the resort to illness by the petty criminal when arrested for a minor crime. Some criminals, when in trouble, can produce clinical pictures indistinguishable from a depressive illness; others develop severe anxiety states, while some react with severe excitement and senseless violence. If the illness has developed after arrest and before trial it should be regarded as a psychogenic reaction which, because it is a reaction to the arrest, cannot be held to mitigate the offence.

Some patients try to invade the therapist's private life. This must be resisted at all costs. Patients are treated in the consulting room, not over the dinner table.

6. Diagnosis

Although occasionally emergency treatment may be necessary before the diagnosis is certain, the old maxim, 'Diagnosis precedes treatment', is just as relevant in psychological as in internal medicine. It was once fashionable in 'psychodynamic' circles to decry formal diagnosis, but this attitude is now uncommon: a formal diagnosis may suggest an adequate line of treatment and a prognosis. Thus the diagnosis of a depressive illness suggests a definite treatment such as electroconvulsive therapy or an antidepressant drug. Nevertheless, a formal diagnosis does not exhaust all the possibilities of treatment. It is also necessary to make a diagnostic formulation which takes into account all the environmental difficulties and the abnormal personality traits which, it is reasonable to assume, have some bearing on the patient's illness. To put the matter in another way, one must try to produce a comprehensive answer to the threefold question: 'Why did *this patient* break down in *this way* at *this time?*'

7. The Plan of Treatment

The diagnostic formulation indicates the plan of treatment. For example, if the domestic and occupational situations are partly causative then one line of attack will be social readjustment. However, if a depressive illness is also present, physical treatment will also be indicated.

The plan of treatment should be reviewed from time to time and modified as the patient's condition changes and new facts emerge.

INSTITUTIONAL CARE

Reasons for Admission to a Psychiatric Hospital

The reasons for hospital admission are to obtain treatment which cannot be given as an outpatient or because the patient is a danger to himself and others. Occasionally, it may be helpful for the patient, or his relatives, if he is away from home for a short while. The mere presence of delusions or hallucinations is not in itself a reason for detention in a mental hospital. The aim of the mental hospital is the earliest possible discharge of the patient which is consistent with his well-being and with that of the community.

The Acute Patient

Acute mentally ill patients should be nursed well away from chronic patients. Many lay people believe that there is only one mental illness which may be mild or severe. Thus, when a depressed patient in a mental hospital sees a chronic, somewhat dilapidated patient cheerfully passing his water on to the flower bed, he feels that within a few years he will be just as dilapidated.

Shortly after the patient's admission a plan of treatment should be worked out. The psychiatric social worker, the nurses, the occupational therapists and other auxiliaries must know what the treatment plan is and what part they are expected to play. The plan must be reviewed at regular intervals of two or three weeks. This is best done by holding regular weekly ward meetings which are attended by all members of the therapeutic team.

The Subacute Patient

If after 6–9 months following admission the patient is not fit for discharge, he should be transferred to a ward in which there is active occupational therapy and group activity. Where possible the patient should be placed in a ward in which the patients are about his age and have roughly the same behaviour problems.

The Chronic Patient and Rehabilitation

Owing to faulty mental hospital administration in the past many chronic schizophrenics have been allowed to deteriorate in gloomy unpleasant surroundings. In order to deal with this problem it is necessary to process such patients through a rehabilitation ward, which will encourage them to work at the highest possible level consistent with their schizophrenic defect. These patients should be organized into groups in charge of one nurse and be put to work on some task which has a useful end-product and a reasonable financial reward. Every effort must also be made to restore the patient's sense of personal identity. He must be given his own clothes and have adequate wardrobe and locker space to store his personal effects.

The General Principles of Mental Hospital Organization

Segregation on the Basis of Behaviour

Patients should be allotted to wards, not on the basis of formal diagnosis, but on the basis of their need for supervision. Turbulent patients, and those lacking in initiative and faulty in their toilet habits, should be nursed in small wards with a high nurse–patient ratio. Those requiring little supervision can be nursed in larger ward units, preferably with a large number of separate single rooms which will give those patients who can appreciate it a reasonable amount of privacy. Such wards have a low nurse–patient ratio. Intermediate wards with a moderate number of patients and a moderate nurse–patient ratio can accommodate those patients needing some degree of supervision.

If it is mental hospital policy to admit senile patients then geriatric wards must be organized. There should be one such ward for admissions and the physically ill and another long-stay ward for arteriosclerotic and senile dements. The geriatric wards should be on the ground floor with easy access to a garden.

Work

Where possible every patient should be gainfully employed on work with a definite end-product and which yields a reasonable financial incentive. In Britain it is possible to obtain contract work which can be carried out in the hospital workshops. One senior member of the nursing staff should act as 'Works Officer'. He should obtain suitable contract work and organize suitable occupations within the hospital. He should also be responsible for supervising the patients who are working in the hospital services such as the kitchens, the maintenance services, and so on.

Self-government

The patients should be given as much responsibility for the organization of their social life as is possible. Ward committees of patients should be set up. These can organize the ward chores and social activities, such as whist drives, beetle drives, play readings, discussion groups, and so on. A central patients' committee should be organized to arrange social activities for the whole hospital. The different committees will, of course, need help from the doctors, the nursing staff, the occupational therapists and the psychiatric social workers, but as far as possible the patients should be encouraged to use their own initiative.

The Therapeutic Community

All the measures so far discussed form a part of the 'therapeutic community'. This term means the organization of the hospital in such a way that every influence to which the patient is subjected is brought into the general plan of his treatment. The most important result of a well-organized therapeutic community in a hospital with an enthusiastic medical and auxiliary staff is the effect on the morale. The optimism and enthusiasm which are communicated to the patients and their relatives help them tremendously.

Day Patients

Some patients, especially young schizophrenics, may learn to readjust to the outside world by living at home and working in the hospital by day.

Night Patients

Some patients with difficulties at home may find it easier to live in the hospital at night and go out to work during the day. Once they have made a reasonable occupational adjustment they should be encouraged to find suitable lodgings. This principle can be extended and separate night hospitals or hostels may be organized in or near the mental hospital or in a nearby large town. In Britain the local authorities are obliged to establish hostels for patients fit to live in the community. With few exceptions, such provisions have been woefully inadequate.

The Day Hospital

This is best sited in a large centre of population away from the mental hospital. It is organized to give the various forms of treatment such as electroplexy, psychotherapy, drug treatment, occupational therapy, and so on. The patients attend the day hospital for 5 days a week.

In large centres it may be necessary to have three different types of day hospital or three major divisions of a day hospital, in order to deal with the three groups of patients suitable for day hospital care. These are the acute patients, the chronic schizophrenics and the geriatric patients. Where possible the latter group should be accommodated in a special section of an ordinary geriatric day hospital. In some parts of the world the same building has been used as a day and as a night hospital.

The General Hospital Psychiatric Unit

The modern trend in Britain is to build no more mental hospitals, but to establish acute psychiatric units in the general hospitals. These are envisaged as consisting of 40–60-bed units with day hospital facilities and an outpatient service. These units should help to bridge the gap between psychiatry and the other specialties. However, it is important that the work of these units should be closely co-ordinated with the work of the mental hospital, so that there is a properly integrated community mental health service.

The Community Mental Health Service

Ideally the mental hospital should be regarded by the community which it serves as the centre of the mental health services. A close relation between the hospital and the community must be built up. It is partly brought about by the hospital organizing extramural services, such as outpatient clinics, in the general hospitals throughout the area served by the mental hospital and also by domiciliary visits by doctors from the mental hospitals. Open days at the mental hospital when anyone can visit the hospital and get to know the work which is being carried on are very useful. So are mental health exhibitions held in conjunction with the local authority. The organization of an association of friends of the hospital can be very useful in establishing good relations between the hospital and the community. These associations can be formed with the help of ex-patients, the relatives of patients and people anxious to serve others in some way.

In Britain the local authorities, apart from duties in connection with the admission of patients to mental hospitals, have duties in connection with after-care and are obliged to provide adequate hostel accommodation for mentally handicapped patients who are fit to live in society. This means that close co-operation between the department of community medicine and the mental hospital is essential. A central co-ordinating committee of representatives from the hospital services, the department of community medicine and the general practitioners of the area should help to produce an integrated community mental health service.

Clubs for Patients

These can be organized by the mental hospital, the psychiatric unit of the general hospital, the local authority, or a voluntary organization. To obtain the best results a psychiatrist should attend the club, but the patients themselves should organize their own activities. Apart from social evenings, extramural activities, such as rambles and visits to art galleries and theatres, may be organized. Sometimes attendance at a club for patients discharged from the mental hospital is a very useful way of following up the patient. The club provides a link with the hospital and the patient can ask for help as soon as he feels the need. Naturally the club may be an essential part of the treatment of a shy, isolated patient.

SYMPTOMATIC TREATMENT

1. Excitement

This can be due to catatonia or mania or any number of organic states, such as delirium, epilepsy, pathological intoxication, and so on. The treatment is obviously that of the underlying disease, but it may be difficult to get near enough to establish a diagnosis.

Oral Sedation

If the excitement is not too severe, and particularly if it seems to be due to anxiety, the patient may be persuaded to take a substantial dose of a quick-acting barbiturate, such as 200–400 mg of quinalbarbitone, amylobarbitone sodium, pentobarbitone, or diazepam 30 mg.

Chloral mixture B.P.C. (1·3 g in 15 ml mixture), in a dose of 15–30 ml, may be very effective in excited old people, but should not be repeated very frequently. Trichloryl is a derivative of chloral which is presented in 0·5 g tablets. The dose is 2–4 tablets.

Chlorpromazine is a very useful tranquillizer, but if given orally for excitement it should be given in the form of the elixir (50 mg in 30 ml elixir). The initial dose should be 75 mg and this should be followed by 200 mg 4–6-hourly, depending on the effect.

Parenteral Administration of Sedatives

DIAZEPAM INJECTION (10 mg 4-HOURLY)
This can be given intramuscularly. While it is valuable in status epilepticus it is of less value in excitement.

CHLORPROMAZINE

An injection of 50–100 mg intramuscularly can be given 4–6-hourly. This is the best intramuscular sedative for excitement. Careful watch must be kept for hypothermia and the drowsy apathy typical of chlorpromazine poisoning. As soon as the excitement is under control the minimum amount of the drug necessary to control the excitement should be given over the next 48 hours. At the same time oral administration of the drug should be begun and the dose rapidly increased until the patient is receiving 400–500 mg per day during the third day of treatment (*see* p. 148). Haloperidol 5 mg i.m. is an alternative.

2. Agitation and Anxiety

In depression the accompanying agitation is relieved by the specific treatment for depression so that in inpatients there is no need to treat the anxiety symptomatically unless it is very severe. Difficulty in the assessment of the improvement produced by the specific antidepressive measures may be encountered when the patient has been given heavy sedation for the anxiety. If treatment is needed for this symptom then diazepam 3–30 mg daily in individual doses, or lorazepam in half these quantities, should be given.

As a method of treatment during an acute bout of anxiety these drugs are very effective, but they should be avoided for long term management. For this purpose, teaching the patient the techniques of relaxation is much better and can sometimes be very effective.

Some reasonably stable personalities under severe strain may find that their anxiety is so pronounced that they cannot cope with the problems of everyday life. These patients may be kept going with small doses of sedation, such as meprobamate 400 mg three or four times a day. Chlordiazepoxide 10–30 mg, diazepam 5–10 mg or oxazepam 15–30 mg three times a day are very effective anxiolytics. The drug should be withdrawn as soon as the patient's difficulties have been resolved or if there is a tendency to increase the dose.

3. Insomnia

General Treatment

As far as possible neurotic patients should be persuaded to try to sleep without hypnotics. If they cannot sleep they should not read or get out of bed, but lie in bed with their eyes closed. Some patients can be taught relaxation techniques, such as autogenous training, which can be carried out in bed before going to sleep.

Müller-Hegemann has devised a simple relaxation technique for insomnia. The patient is instructed to concentrate on his breathing. As he breathes in, he concentrates on the word 'breathe' and as he breathes out on the word 'peacefully'. On his next breath in he concentrates on the words 'let it' and as he breathes out on the word 'stream'. He continues to concentrate on these words: 'Breathe; peacefully; let it; stream' keeping the words in step with inspiration and expiration. In some severe neurotics a mild hypnotic may be given to allow the patient to settle down into this technique. At the end of the week the drug can be withdrawn and the patient instructed to continue with the concentration on the words on retiring.

Depressives and very agitated patients should be given hypnotics, but the drugs should be withdrawn as soon as possible.

Hypnotics

If a drug is an effective rapidly acting sedative and hypnotic it is potentially an addictive drug. Chloral hydrate addiction is well known, so that it is likely that the newer chloral derivatives will be addictive, particularly because they are more pleasant to take.

CHLORAL HYDRATE
This can be taken as a mixture, such as 15–30 ml of chloral mixture B.P.C. It has a rather unpleasant taste which is not easy to disguise; it also tends to act as a gastric irritant.

DICHLORALPHENAZONE
In 600 mg tablets this is an excellent hypnotic especially for old people. The dose is 2–4 tablets.

TRICHLORYL
This is a metabolite of chloral, which is less irritant to the stomach and is presented as a 500 mg tablet. The dose is 2–4 tablets.

CARBROMAL
This is a derivative of urea. It is presented in 325 mg tablets. The dose is 1–3 tablets. It may cause skin rashes, including purpura.

BENZODIAZEPINES
It is very difficult to commit suicide with these drugs and they have therefore replaced the barbiturates. Nitrazepam 10–20 mg and flurazepam 15–30 mg are currently fashionable, but there is little to choose among this class.

4. Depression

Amphetamine, dextroamphetamine and methylamphetamine have all been used to relieve depression. Their action is short-lived and they give rise to addiction very easily. For these reasons, they must be regarded as obsolete for psychiatric purposes. Milder euphoriant drugs such as methyl phenidate, pipradol, and, the most recent, pemoline are available, but their role in the treatment of depression has not been defined.

THE PSYCHOTROPIC DRUGS

Classification

In the past quarter century many new non-sedative drugs have been introduced which have profound effects on the central nervous system. It is difficult to classify these drugs on either a chemical or a pharmacological basis. The following classification is useful:

1. Neuroleptics.
    a. Phenothiazines.
    b. Thioxanthenes.
    c. Butyrophenones.
    d. Diphenyl-butyl-piperidines.
    e. Others.
2. Sedatives.
    a. Hypno-sedatives.
    b. Tranquillo-sedatives.
    c. Benzodiazepines.
3. Thymoleptics.
    a. Amphetamine-like drugs.
    b. Tricyclic compounds.
    c. Tetracyclic compounds.
    d. Mono-amine oxidase inhibitors.
    e. Others.
4. Psychotomimetic drugs.

1. Neuroleptics

a. Phenothiazines and Allied Compounds

The basic chemical structure of this group consists of two benzene rings held together with one atom of nitrogen and one of sulphur, thus:

Different radicals can be attached in the 2 and 10 positions. These drugs can be divided into the following three groups depending on the side chain attached in the 10 position: (1) compounds with an aliphatic side chain ending in a dimethyl amine group; (2) compounds with a side chain ending in a piperidine ring; and (3) compounds with a side chain ending in a piperazine ring.

Chlorpromazine is the most well-known representative of the first group. The drug is an antiemetic and tends to cause drowsiness in large doses. Pseudoparkinsonism occurs, but not usually when moderate doses are given. Pyrexia and hypothermia may occur and severe hypothermic crises may be provoked in myxoedematous patients. Skin rashes may occur in nurses handling the drug and patients taking the drug may become very light-sensitive and easily become severely sunburnt. In about 1 in every 500–600 patients a severe obstructive jaundice develops. Very rarely the drug causes agranulocytosis.

Thioridazine is a typical member of the second group. It has no anti-emetic effect and does not usually produce pseudoparkinsonism. Common side-effects are dizziness, drowsiness, dryness of the mouth and stuffiness of the nose. Amenorrhoea, suppression of lactation and loss of sexual desire may occur when moderate doses are given. In exceptionally large doses of 2–3 g in 24 hours retinal pigmentation has been reported, but there is no indication that this occurs in a dosage of less than 600 mg daily.

All the members of the third group tend to produce pseudoparkinsonism, akathisia and spasm of the neck and shoulder-girdle muscles resembling torsion dystonia.

Trifluoperazine and perphenazine are representative of this group. The pseudoparkinsonism usually occurring on moderate dosage can be treated with antiparkinsonian drugs, such as orphenadrine hydrochloride 50 mg three times a day or benztropine methanesulphonate 2 mg three times a day.

Fluphenazine decanoate is a long-acting drug which can be given intramuscularly in doses of 25 mg (1 ml) every 14–28 days. A test dose of 12·5 mg is given at first and if there are no untoward effects, 25 mg is given in 1 week's time and at 2-weekly or 3-weekly intervals thereafter. This drug is very useful because chronic schizophrenics, whose symptoms are well controlled by phenothiazines, often refuse to take drugs after discharge from hospital and subsequently relapse. Such patients' symptoms may well be controlled with injections of fluphenazine decanoate given at appropriate intervals. As this drug causes marked pseudoparkinsonism, patients usually have to be given antiparkinsonian drugs.

b. *Thioxanthenes*

This group of drugs has a structure closely resembling that of the phenothiazines but with the nitrogen atom in the central ring replaced by carbon. Clinically they resemble their phenothiazine analogues closely in dosage and effect, but they are very useful for patients who cannot tolerate phenothiazines.

c. *Butyrophenones*

The first of this group of drugs to be introduced was haloperidol and it has been found to be particularly useful in the treatment of excitement due to mania or schizophrenia. For severe excitement 5 mg may be given intramuscularly or even intravenously and repeated 6-hourly until the excitement is under control. Pseudoparkinsonism is a common side-effect but responds well to antiparkinsonian drugs.

d. Diphenyl-butyl-piperidines

Pimozide is the first of this new class of compounds and will doubtless be followed by many others. It is a selective antagonist of cerebral dopaminergic transmitters and has a low incidence of extrapyramidal reactions. It is claimed to be of special value for schizophrenics who are apathetic and inert.

e. Other Neuroleptics

The dibenzothiazepines are potent neuroleptics and it has been claimed that they have minimal extrapyramidal reactions. The benzamides, e.g. sulpiride, are said to have no sedative action and to have an antidepressant effect as well. These two groups of drugs are still relatively new and their role in the treatment of, especially, schizophrenia has not yet been fully evaluated.

Reserpine is an alkaloid from the plant *Rauwolfia serpentina* which has been used for centuries by the Ayur-Vedic practitioners of India for the treatment of insanity. This drug produces hypothermia, hypotension, water retention and an increase in appetite. It may also sometimes produce a typical depressive illness which can be very severe. For these reasons it must be regarded as obsolete in psychiatric use.

2. Sedatives

a. Hypno-sedatives

Members of this group allay anxiety in small doses and in larger doses act as hypnotics. The well-known hypnotics have already been considered in the section on symptomatic treatment (*see* p. 209).

b. Tranquillo-sedatives

These substances block polysynaptic reflexes. The most widely used of this group of drugs is meprobamate. It is presented in 200- and 400-mg tablets and the dose is up to 400 mg four times a day. It is very effective in controlling anxiety and 400 or 800 mg taken one hour before retiring may relieve insomnia due to anxiety. It tends to produce gastric discomfort, diarrhoea and skin rashes. Like the quick-acting barbiturates it is addictive.

c. Benzodiazepines

These drugs are anxiolytics and are now widely used in the treatment of anxiety. They have replaced barbiturates because it is so very difficult to commit suicide with them. Many of them have already been described (*see* pp. 208, 209).

3. Thymoleptics

a. *Amphetamine-like Drugs*

Amphetamine and its derivatives have already been considered (*see* p. 209).

b. *Tricyclic Antidepressive Drugs*

Imipramine was the first drug of this kind to be used for the treatment of depression and since then many derivatives and analogues have become available.

All of these drugs have side-effects which are related to their anticholinergic properties. The commonest and most prominent is dryness of the mouth. Less common are excessive sweating, postural hypotension, difficulty in visual accommodation, constipation and retention of urine. They also affect the heart, as shown in the electrocardiogram by a prolongation of the QT interval, and clinically by some irregularity of heart action. This is of little practical importance except in patients suffering from cardiac disease. In general, the side-effects are less prominent in the case of the more recently introduced drugs but there is much individual variation in the response of patients to them. In any case, most patients find that the side-effects diminish over time. In general, these drugs take 2–3 weeks for their therapeutic action to take effect, and this may sometimes be even as long as 6 weeks. Patients show continuous improvement for 2–3 months. It is said that protriptyline can take effect within a week but unfortunately it produces marked autonomic effects.

One subgroup of these compounds, which includes amitriptyline, doxepin and dothiepin, has a sedative effect which is of value for those patients who show anxiety, agitation and initial insomnia.

The standard dose is 150 mg per day and patients who do not respond to a dose of 250 mg are unlikely to respond to a higher dose. The full dose can be taken at night or it can be divided into a morning and evening dose. It is unnecessary to give the drug more frequently.

c. *Tetracyclic Compounds*

Two drugs are currently available in this series, maprotriline and mianserin. It would appear that they are as effective as the standard tricyclic compounds but they have less side-effects, especially the latter. Dosage is of the same order.

d. *Mono-amine Oxidase Inhibitors*

These compounds inhibit mono-amine oxidase enzymes thus preventing the destruction of noradrenaline and increasing the activity of adrenergic neurones in the central nervous system. At one time, many drugs in this class were available, but the number has dwindled. The most commonly used are phenelzine, which is a hydrazine derivative, and tranyl-cypromine, which is not. The former is given in a dosage of 60–90 mg a day, and the latter in a dosage of 20–30 mg. Side-effects are dizziness, swelling of the ankles, excitement and confusion, but they are very uncommon. A rare but important side-effect is the appearance of excitement and mania.

These compounds may cause very severe reactions when given together with certain other drugs. The blood pressure becomes extremely high and the patient experiences a prostrating headache. This 'hypertensive crisis' may culminate in intracranial haemorrhage, coma and death. Such crises can be produced by tyramine compounds found in certain foods. The commonest is cheese, but these compounds are also found in meat and yeast extracts, and also in bananas. An injection of phentolamine 5 mg will promptly reduce the blood pressure.

e. *Other Antidepressive Drugs*

One recent introduction is viloxazine, which is of interest because it is a bicyclic compound. The first trials suggest that its therapeutic effect comes on quickly. It is important because it is the first of a new class of compounds.

Tryptophan is a naturally occurring essential amino-acid and has been demonstrated to have a slight but definite antidepressive effect when given in doses of up to 4 g daily. It potentiates the effect of mono-amine oxidase inhibitors and probably also of tricyclic compounds.

Lithium is of some value in the treatment of depressive illness, and it has been clearly demonstrated that it has a prophylactic effect in recurrent depression, increasing the intervals between attacks and shortening the length of attacks. It can be combined with other antidepressive treatments.

Psychotomimetic Drugs

This is a steady growing group of drugs with many different chemical structures which produce a confusional state when given to human subjects. These drug-induced psychotic states are known as 'model psychoses' and are characterized by disorders of mood, thinking and perception, especially visual, which are often mistakenly compared with the symptoms in acute schizophrenia. Some are interesting since they resemble the catecholamines and 5-hydroxytryptamine which are normally found in the mammalian nervous system. They are of no therapeutic interest.

PHYSICAL TREATMENTS
1. Modified Insulin Therapy
Technique

The patient fasts from 8 p.m. and is given 20 units of insulin intramuscularly at 7.30 a.m. the following day. After 3 hours he is encouraged to eat a hearty breakfast. The dose of insulin is increased by 10 units every day until a maintenance dose of 60–100 units is reached. The maximum dose of insulin should produce moderate sweating and slight drowsiness. If the patient passes into moderate or deep sopor he should be given sugared tea and encouraged to eat a good breakfast as soon as he is able to do so.

Indications

This is a useful treatment for severely disturbed neurotic patients who are so distressed that they require to be removed from their domestic environment. The increase in weight tends to cause a sense of bodily well-being and the physical effects of the insulin have a marked suggestive effect.

2. Electroconvulsive Therapy
Procedure

The patient should be kept off sedatives, especially benzodiazepines, for at least 24 hours. ECT is generally given in the mornings and the patients should not have eaten since the previous night, but may have a drink not less than an hour before the treatment. Before giving treatment, the patient's clothing should be loosened, the bladder emptied and dentures removed. The best machine to use is the Maxwell–Macphail 'Phasotron' which gives a sharp-fronted wave of current for a period of 0·5 seconds. This produces the best effect with the minimum of current (Maxwell, 1968).

The sites of application of the electrodes are then washed with ether soap and dried. A sphygmomanometer is applied to the arm not used for the injections and the systolic blood pressure determined. Light anaesthesia is then induced by i.v. injections of methohexitone (1 per cent solution) 80–120 mg or thiopentone 125–250 mg, together with 0·6 mg of atropine. An airway should then be inserted. The cuff is then inflated to above systolic pressure and the syringe changed to one containing 40–80 mg of succinylcholine which is then injected. Pure oxygen is then administered by positive-pressure inflation during depolarization and continued for half a minute after the onset of respiratory paralysis. The electrical stimulus is then applied through electrodes moistened with 5 per cent solution of sodium bicarbonate. As soon as the seizure is evident, in the forearm, the cuff is deflated. When the convulsion is over, ventilation with oxygen should be resumed until spontaneous respiration is re-established.

This method of detecting the convulsion (sometimes known as the 'Hamilton manoeuvre') is only slightly inferior to EEG recordings. Some method of detecting the convulsion should always be used.

Treatment should be given by a trained anaesthetist who is prepared to intubate if necessary, and an adequate apparatus for artificial breathing should be available.

Unilateral ECT has been introduced as having less effect on the memory than the older method. It is given on the non-dominant side, i.e. on the right side in right-handed patients. Left-handed patients should be carefully tested to ascertain from which side language is controlled, otherwise memory defect may be replaced by difficulties with speech. It is a good precaution to test even right-handed patients. An alternative is to use the technique of bifrontal ECT as recommended by Abrams and Taylor (1973).

Convulsions can also be induced by the inhalation of flurothyl vapour. In a sense it is a return to the original technique of inducing the convulsion by drugs. It does not have any obvious therapeutic advantage over ECT.

For depressives, treatment should be given twice weekly for 6 treatments. Clinical experience suggests that early relapse follows a lesser number. In general, patients should not be given more than 12 treatments; if they have responded poorly to 12, they are unlikely to do better with more. Even going beyond 8 or 9 should be considered carefully. It is a common belief that when the patient has made a good recovery, then 2 more treatments should be given, but the evidence indicates that there is no value in this (Barton, Mehta and Snaith, 1973).

Older patients may show some confusion after a treatment and should be kept in hospital for the rest of the day, if treated as outpatients.

Patients should be warned that there is some loss of memory after ECT. The deficiency is very small with a standard course. In most cases, memory deficit decreases to trivial proportions by 3 months and has usually gone by 6 months. The effect on memory increases rapidly with increasing numbers of treatments. The sinister reputation of ECT in the USA is based largely on a number of instances in which badly trained psychiatrists have given an excessive number of treatments, presumably on the principle that 'if a little is good for you, a lot is a lot better'.

Some patients become very fearful of the treatment and this is a sure sign that they are not responding. The psychiatrist should then consider very carefully whether ECT is indeed the right treatment and only if he is quite sure of what he is doing should he encourage the patient to continue with the treatment.

Some patients make a slight or temporary recovery with electro-convulsive treatment, but after a further period of a few months electroplexy may produce a complete recovery.

Indications

In severely depressed suicidal patients electroplexy is the treatment of choice; it will benefit depressives who have made no response, or only a partial response to drugs.

It is also indicated in the cycloid psychoses (*see* p. 142). In acute schizophrenia in which there is catatonic stupor or marked depression, electroplexy will remove these unpleasant symptoms and make the patient more accessible.

This treatment has also been used in the past to control violent unruly schizophrenics and has euphemistically been called 'maintenance ECT'. This is likely to produce brain damage. Since the introduction of the phenothiazines and other tranquillizers there is even less justification for this type of treatment.

In some centres ECT has been given extensively to outpatients. This should be regarded as a second-best line of treatment. If the depressive is left at home he will find it difficult to cope with his environment because of the increasing confusion; female patients may be expected to continue with most of the domestic chores. If outpatient ECT is given it must be carefully explained that the patient is ill and should be treated as an invalid during, and for 3 weeks after, the treatment. There is, of course, less objection to the administration of ECT to a day hospital patient as he is in a reasonably well-controlled environment and can obtain reassurance very easily.

Contraindications

Congestive heart failure, cardiac infarction within the preceding 6 weeks, and a previous history of subarachnoid haemorrhage are all important contraindications. If the patient has active tuberculosis or has had active tuberculosis in the preceding year ECT can be given, but antibiotics, such as para-aminosalicylic acid (PAS) and streptomycin, should be given and continued for at least 6 weeks after the electrical treatment is stopped.

Old age is not a contraindication to ECT as long as the patient is otherwise physically fit.

3. Prefrontal Leucotomy (Lobotomy)

Technique

This operation consists of severing the fibres which connect the orbital and medial surfaces of the frontal lobe to the thalamus.

Complications

Haemorrhage and the usual complications of a surgical operation may occur. The other important complication is epilepsy which occurs in 1–2 per cent. To avoid this the patient should be given phenobarbitone 30 mg twice daily for the year following the leucotomy. If at any time after the patient has been leucotomized it is necessary to prescribe a phenothiazine drug, then the patient should also be given phenobarbitone, because phenothiazines are likely to produce epileptic fits in the predisposed.

Indications

Clinical experience with the modern forms of leucotomy indicates that it is of value in the treatment of the more severe and chronic forms of anxiety and obsessional states and also depressions. The patients who respond best are those with a well-adjusted personality, whose illness started in the second half of life with rapid onset, previous good remissions, marked depression and previous good response to ECT.

General Considerations

Leucotomy should never be regarded as the first line of treatment but should be thought of when all other methods have failed and the patient has been ill for some years. The risks of operation have to be balanced against the serious disabilities of the patients, their suffering and their high risk of suicide. Fortunately, the development of new treatments is steadily diminishing the need for this treatment.

It seems paradoxical to destroy a part of the brain to cure a mental disease which may be due to a disease of the brain. The psychiatrist would do well to remember the words of Isaac Judaeus, who wrote: 'Treating the sick is like boring holes in pearls, and the physician must act with caution lest he destroy the pearl committed to his charge.'

PSYCHOTHERAPY

1. General Discussion

Physical versus Psychological Treatment

In order to organize our knowledge it is necessary to use an empirical dualism and to look upon the mind and body as separate entities when, in fact, they are merely different ways of looking at a living organism. This naive dualism is often carried over into psychiatry, so that psychotherapy is regarded as dealing with a bodiless mind and physical treatments with a mindless body. It is tempting to regard the complete change of the personality claimed to be produced by psychoanalysis as a physiological change and to compare it with the permanent changes in animal behaviour which Pavlov and his pupils produced during conditioning experiments. On the other hand, it seems just as likely that many of the successful results of physical treatments are due to suggestion. The distinction between psychotherapy and physical treatment in psychiatry is not as sharp as would appear at first sight.

The Problem of Transference

Freud pointed out that during psychotherapy the patient identifies the therapist with a parent or some other person who has played an important part in the patient's childhood. The patient, therefore, transfers to the therapist all the emotions which he had in relation to this person. The neurotic symptoms and attitudes become attached to the treatment situation so that the illness becomes a transference neurosis. During the analysis the patient works through his emotional difficulties and is finally cured when they have disappeared. When this happens the transference situation is resolved and the patient no longer has any emotional dependence on the therapist.

Since ambivalence, or positive and negative feelings towards the same object, occurs in all emotional relationships, the patient both loves and hates the therapist. As the treatment progresses the negative aspect of the relationship may become very pronounced, or, in other words, negative transference occurs. The therapist also develops a transference and identifies the patient with some important person in his life. This is called the 'counter transference' and it too can be positive or negative.

Transference and counter transference occur to some degree in all doctor–patient relationships and every doctor must train himself to be fully aware of the transference situation. Many patients improve immediately with any kind of treatment because they wish to please the therapist and to preserve the love and attention which they receive from him. The improvement is therefore dependent on the maintenance of the transference situation, so that the improvement is only temporary. Any attempt to break off the treatment at this point leads to a marked worsening of the symptoms.

The handling of the transference situation is the major problem in psychotherapy. The psychoanalyst, who himself has had a successful personal analysis, is theoretically more able to carry out psychotherapy, because he has had experience of working through a transference situation. The counter transference raises difficulties for the therapist because he may derive satisfaction from the love and affection which he receives from the patient and this may make it difficult for him to resolve the transference situation. It is well to remember that the aim of psychotherapy is to treat the patient and not the therapist!

2. Psychoanalysis

The Classic Technique

The patient lies on a couch and is told to 'free associate', while the analyst sits watching the patient. The analyst is completely passive and merely exhorts the patient to let his thoughts wander and say everything which comes into his mind without hesitation. Despite the protestations of the psychoanalysts there is no doubt that the patient is encouraged to produce certain types of material which fit in with the analyst's preconceived ideas. Changes in the analyst's breathing, the way in which he says an encouraging word, or the way in which he fidgets, can all influence the patient's line of thought although the analyst is unaware of doing so.

A psychoanalytic session lasts an hour, and five sessions are carried out each week. In theory the most suitable cases for psychoanalysis are young patients under 40 years of age, with an acute neurosis with little or no secondary gain and no marked character disorder.

Modified Techniques

Some analysts have attempted to shorten the treatment by giving the patient psychoanalytic explanations of his symptoms. This is frowned on by the purists, who point out that the interpretations given to the patient are really a form of suggestion. They seem to be worried that the patient may be cured by the wrong technique.

Jungian Analysis

This is usually carried out face-to-face and the analyst plays a more active part than the Freudian analyst.

3. Group Therapy

Many different forms of group therapy can be organized. On the one hand, there are the large activity groups in mental hospitals in which the patients are given didactic instructions and carry out simple group activities; while, on the other hand, there are small groups of six to eight neurotic patients led by a psychoanalytically trained therapist who helps the patients to analyse themselves in the group situation. The members of the small intensive psychotherapy group must be chosen with care. They should be of roughly the same social class, have the same cultural background, and suffer from fairly similar psychological disorders. It is important not to include someone who is in any way radically different from the other members of the group, because he is liable to become the scapegoat. The group discusses the problems of its members under the leadership of the therapist. The amount of active intervention and direction of the group by the therapist depends on his theoretical concepts and on his personality.

Group therapy is very useful for patients who tend to act out their difficulties, because they can learn to recognize and to modify their behaviour in the social milieu provided by the group.

Psychodrama is a form of group therapy in which the patients are allotted parts to play; by acting they learn to understand and modify their behaviour disorders.

4. Suggestion and Hypnosis

General Principles

If the patient is no longer deriving much primary or secondary gain from his symptoms then a direct attack on the symptoms with suggestion or hypnosis will usually lead to an improvement. If the patient is still in conflict then suggestion will fail and hypnosis may remove the symptoms and leave behind a severe emotional disturbance.

Suggestion

This can be carried out in many different ways, such as by the administration of inert tablets, highly coloured medicines, or mild electric shocks.

The Technique of Hypnosis

The patient lies on a couch and is made as comfortable as possible. The room should be dimly lit and reasonably quiet. The patient is told to focus on a pocket torch or the point of a pencil, which is held about 3 cm above and 8 cm away from the bridge of the nose. As it is fatiguing to keep the eyes in the right position the patient soon develops a sense of fatigue in his eye muscles and in particular in the levatores palpebrae. When the patient fixes his eyes on the object the hypnotist begins to say repeatedly, 'You are sleepy; you are feeling sleepy', and a little later he adds the words, 'Your eyelids are heavy, you cannot keep your eyes open'. These words are said in a soft persuasive voice or in a confident domineering way, depending on the personality of the hypnotist. The suggestion that the eyes are closing is repeated, and, as the eyelids begin to droop, the words, 'Your eyes are closing' are repeated insistently. Once the eyes close the hypnotist clinches the matter by suggesting that the arm will rise up of its own accord. He does this by saying, 'You are quite calm. As you lie there perfectly relaxed you feel your right arm is becoming lighter than usual. It is feeling lighter; it is rising up'. The words, 'It is feeling lighter; it is rising up' are repeated, and as soon as any movement begins the hypnotist becomes even more insistent, saying, 'It is rising up; you cannot stop it; it is rising up', and so on. Once the arm has become more or less vertical there is no doubt that the patient is in a moderately deep hypnotic trance. The patient is then told that the arm is heavy and will sink back on to the couch.

Hypnotic Treatment

Once a trance has been induced it can be used in the following ways:

a. A hysterical symptom can be removed and the patient told that when he recovers the symptom will have disappeared.

b. Unconscious memories can be recovered and used in psychotherapy.

c. The patient can be persuaded to relive a traumatic experience, i.e. he is abreacted.

d. Post-hypnotic suggestion can be made. The patient is told that he will do something after recovery from the trance.

In order to bring the patient out of the trance the hypnotist tells him that on the count of five he will wake up or that when the hypnotist snaps his fingers he will wake up.

The Value of Hypnotic Treatment

Hypnosis may be useful as a part of a general plan of psychotherapy, but it must be used with caution. It may be very useful to win a breathing space when the patient is extremely anxious and not accessible to psychotherapy. In some psychosomatic disorders, such as bronchial asthma, anxiety triggers off the psychosomatic disorder which in turn creates more anxiety, thus producing a vicious circle. In such a case hypnosis may produce relaxation, breaking the vicious circle and leading to an improvement in the psychosomatic disorder.

5. Narcoanalysis and Abreaction

Intravenous injections of thiopentone or sodium amylobarbitone have been used to obtain unconscious material which would otherwise take a long time to emerge with ordinary psychotherapy. There is no particular value in this technique but it may be useful because it gives the patient an excuse to produce material of which he is ashamed. These drugs are sometimes called 'truth drugs', but what a patient says when under the influence of barbiturates is not necessarily true. Despite the old tag *in vino veritas,* every barman knows that drunk men can lie!

This use of intravenous barbiturates to recover unconscious memories was at one time called 'narcoanalysis' and may be useful when a patient is unable to talk freely during psychotherapy. Apart from this these drugs can also be used in abreaction, when the patient is persuaded to relive a traumatic experience. Abreaction can also be induced by hypnosis, the intravenous injection of 10–30 mg of methylamphetamine hydrochloride (Methedrine), or the inhalation of small quantities of ether. In theory the patient is being disturbed by the pent-up emotions associated with the traumatic experience, so that if he relives the event with a full expression of the associated emotions he will be cured.

Abreaction is the treatment of choice in acute anxiety states caused by a terrifying experience in which the patient's life has been threatened. Such experiences are common in warfare, but are relatively infrequent in civilian life where, even if they do occur, they are often complicated by the possibility of compensation. Abreaction can also be used as a variety of suggestion, when the patient is told that the reliving of certain experiences will bring about a cure.

6. Relaxation Therapy

Some tense and anxious patients benefit considerably from learning to relax. The therapeutic effect of relaxation comes from the breaking of the vicious circle of anxiety, leading to muscular tension, leading to further anxiety, and so on. Apart from teaching patients general schemes of relaxation which lower the general level of tension, patients can be taught to relax in very stressful situations. There are two main methods of relaxation: that of Jacobson and that of Schulz.

In the Jacobson method the patient is taught to relax one group of muscles at a time until he is able to relax them all. In the Schulz method the patient learns to control his voluntary and involuntary muscles by concentrating on certain thoughts. For example, he is taught to relax his voluntary muscles by concentrating on the thought that his body is becoming heavy. This method is called 'autogenous training'.

7. Behaviour Therapy

This is the application of learning theory to psychotherapy. The fundamental idea is that neurotic behaviour is made up of learned patterns of behaviour which must be modified by the treatment process. Sometimes the therapy is very simple, as, for example, in the treatment of nocturnal enuresis, in which there is no organic cause. Here the patient sleeps on two tinfoil sheets which are placed under the bed sheet. The upper tinfoil sheet is perforated and is separated from the lower one by a thin cotton sheet. As soon as the patient wets the bed the two tinfoil sheets are connected electrically by the wet cotton sheet; a circuit is completed which trips a relay, which in turn rings a bell and wakes the patient up. The tension in the bladder at which nocturnal enuresis usually occurs becomes associated with the bell and waking up. After a few weeks the patient learns to wake up when the pressure in his bladder reaches the point at which enuresis usually occurred.

In other disorders, aversive stimuli such as electrical shocks or chemically induced nausea are associated with the undesirable behaviour pattern. This technique has been used for many years in the treatment of alcohol addiction. More recently it has been applied to the treatment of sexual perversions.

Wolpe has introduced 'psychotherapy by reciprocal inhibition'. The basic idea is that an anxiety response will be diminished if another more satisfying response is also present when the anxiety occurs. This technique is particularly valuable in the treatment of phobic states. The patient is taught to relax and then a hierarchy of 'stressors' is worked out, so that there is a graded series of situations known to the therapist, which produce little anxiety, some anxiety, and so on to maximum anxiety. The situation which produces least anxiety is taken first and the patient is encouraged to relive it. As soon as anxiety appears the patient is told to relax. A recent modification of this technique is the use of methohexitone sodium (Brietal sodium) as a relaxant. One ml of a 1 per cent solution of the drug is injected as soon as the patient becomes anxious when he is thinking about a stressful situation. After each injection the patient is encouraged to relax and the therapist waits 1 minute during which he continues to tell the patient to relax. Then the patient is persuaded to relive the anxiety-provoking situation and given 1 ml of 1 per cent methohexitone sodium as soon as anxiety occurs. This procedure is repeated ten times in one treatment session. Methohexitone sodium produces a pleasant relaxation which wears off fairly quickly because the drug is rapidly broken down in the body. This treatment can be used in the outpatient clinic, but patients should be advised not to drive a motor-car within a few hours of the treatment.

8. Practical Short Term Psychotherapy

With the exception of psychoanalysis nearly all of the techniques so far described can be used in short term psychotherapy, which aims at producing a substantial improvement in the patient's condition within a period of 6 months. The treatment which will be outlined can only be used in patients with average and superior intelligence, who are sufficiently sophisticated to accept the idea that some illnesses are psychologically determined and can be cured with psychological treatment. In simple-minded and dull patients one has to rely on a mixture of firm reassurance, simple explanation of symptoms, environmental manipulation, and suggestion.

Defining the Problem

The first step is to determine the precise reason which has brought the patient to ask for help. This can only be done as a result of a few careful preliminary exploratory interviews with the patient and his relatives.

Establishing the Facts

A clear account of the patient's personality, symptoms, and environmental difficulties must be made from information derived from all possible sources. In psychoanalysis the patient's own evaluation of himself and his environment, so-called psychic reality, is accepted by the therapist. In short term eclectic psychotherapy it is essential for the therapist to know the real situation, because he must help the patient to make the best possible adjustment in the shortest possible time.

It is important not to allow anxiety symptoms due to a real-life difficulty to be turned into an illness. In such circumstances the patient must be told that his nervous upset is the natural consequence of his situation and will improve when his personal difficulties are resolved. In marital disharmony it is quite common for one of the partners to turn his or her natural unhappiness into an illness, which is then used as a weapon against the spouse.

The Role of the Personality in the Illness

The therapist must always try to answer Clouston's first question, 'What sort of man was this when he was reckoned well in mind?' One must get a clear idea of the patient's previous personality in order to distinguish between the symptoms which are new and those that are exaggerations of long-standing anomalies of the personality. It may be necessary to explain to the patient that he has an abnormal personality in Schneider's sense (*see* p. 68) and that he must recognize the weak spots in his personality, so that he can avoid putting himself in stressful situations. This is particularly important in 'episodic psychopaths' who manage to get themselves into difficulties from time to time. It may be necessary to persuade the patient to tolerate certain abnormal personality traits in the same way in which one has to tolerate minor physical deformities such as a large nose or an asymmetrical face.

General Psycho-pathological Explanations

The patient should be given a simple explanation of the psychological causation of the illness and a psychological and physiological explanation of his symptoms at the onset of the treatment. If he has somatic symptoms of anxiety he should be asked to try to remember how he felt in the past when he was frightened. It is then explained to him that anxiety is fear for no reason and that his physical symptoms are the result of a constant state of fear. As the psychotherapy proceeds the therapist uses the material which emerges to illustrate the mental mechanisms (*see* p. 26) which are involved.

Putting the Onus on the Patient

Once it is decided to begin psychotherapy it is important to be sure that the patient accepts his illness as being psychological and that he realizes that psychotherapy aims at helping him to help himself. He must never be allowed to forget that psychotherapy is a joint effort by the patient and the therapist. It is always important for the therapist not to allow himself to be forced into a position where he is making decisions for the patient. Whenever the patient asks the question, 'What should I do?' the therapist must reply, 'What do *you* think you should do? Let us discuss all the pros and cons and then *you* must make up your mind.'

Setting the Goals to be Achieved

At the end of the preliminary exploratory interviews the therapist decides that there are several areas of conflict and ranks them in order of importance. He begins treatment by discussing what seems to be the most important area of conflict. When the patient has gained reasonable insight into his problems in this area then the next most important topic is dealt with. As the treatment proceeds new information emerges which may lead the therapist to modify his initial ideas about the nature and importance of the different areas of conflict.

Resistance

The patient may refuse to deal with anything except trivialities or he may say very little during the interviews. This is resistance and is produced by an unconscious wish to retain the neurotic symptoms because this appears to be the least stressful solution of the conflict. The nature of the resistance must be pointed out to the patient and may be overcome by persistence on the part of the therapist. Sometimes it may be necessary to direct the discussion away from a painful topic and then to approach the topic more obliquely. Another method of overcoming resistance is abreaction with ether, intravenous methylamphetamine, or sodium amylobarbitone.

Another less obvious form of resistance is the production of large amounts of interesting sexual material that conforms nicely with psychoanalytic theory. The therapist may unwittingly be deflected from his task and devote many sessions to fascinating psychoanalytically orientated discussions that are entirely beside the point.

Social and Environmental Changes

During psychotherapy it may become obvious that the patient should make changes in his environment, such as changing his job, joining a club, or altering his domestic arrangements. Once the patient decides to make such a change the therapist must help him to carry it out, but the help should never be more than the minimum necessary.

Consolidating the Insight

The patient is usually seen once a week for an hour. At the end of each interview the therapist summarizes what has been learned in the session. The patient is then asked to repeat this and the therapist makes any necessary corrections.

At the beginning of the next interview the patient is asked to explain what he has learned at the previous one. The therapist corrects any mistakes and then asks the patient to repeat the corrected version.

Periodic Review of Progress

Every 6 weeks the therapist reviews the progress so far and decides on his strategy for the next 6 weeks. One session is devoted entirely to a discussion of the patient's understanding of his illness.

At the end of 6 months the case is reviewed in detail and one of the following decisions is made:

1. To continue psychotherapy for a further limited period of 3 or 6 months.

2. To discharge the patient as cured, improved, or unlikely to benefit from further treatment.

3. To transfer the patient to supportive psychotherapy.

Supportive Psychotherapy

Some patients, particularly obsessional neurotics, seem to be helped by half-hour interviews every few weeks. The patient gets relief from being able to talk about his symptoms to a sympathetic listener who can reassure him. This supportive psychotherapy should, where possible, be carried out in evening clinics so that the patient does not lose work.

The Use of Drugs in Psychotherapy

Drugs may be used at the same time as the patient is receiving psychotherapy, but it must be made clear to the patient that the drug is merely a crutch and not a cure. Thus if anxiety is severe the patient may be given a sedative to allay the disturbance and allow the psychotherapy to get under way. The sedative should be given for a limited period so that the patient does not become habituated. Similarly, in the treatment of the perversions the libido may be suppressed with cyproterone or thioridazine in order to keep the patient out of temptation during the early weeks of treatment.

Chapter 15

Psychiatry and the law

The disciplines of psychiatry and the law meet in several areas and the psychiatrist needs some knowledge of the legal process, its relationship to mental illness and how it affects patients in both the criminal and civil aspects of the law.

The Mental Health Act 1959 and the Mental Health (Scotland) Act 1960 heralded a new era in the treatment of the mentally ill. It made provision for the mentally ill to be treated in a similar way to the physically ill on an informal or voluntary basis and it laid emphasis on the care of the patient in the community. It removed the legal aspects from the admission of patients and allowed medical practitioners to admit informally or by compulsion.

Over the course of time, certain deficiencies became apparent and an attempt has been made in the Mental Health Act 1983 to overcome them, although some of the new provisions have aroused considerable controversy. The Mental Health Act 1983 (England and Wales) first defines those categories of mental abnormality which would fall within its orbit and in Part I it defines a general category of mental disorder which is subdivided into mental illness, arrested or incomplete development of mind, psychopathic disorder and other disorders or disabilities of mind. It then defines the categories of severe mental impairment, mental impairment and psychopathic disorder as follows:

Severe Mental Impairment means a state of arrested or incomplete development of mind which includes severe impairment of intelligence and social functioning and is associated with abnormally aggressive or seriously irresponsible conduct on the part of the person concerned.

Mental Impairment means a state of arrested or incomplete development of mind which includes significant impairment of intelligence and social functioning with abnormally aggressive or seriously irresponsible conduct on the part of the person concerned.

Psychopathic Disorder means a persistent disorder or disability of mind (whether or not including subnormality of intelligence) which results in abnormally aggressive or seriously irresponsible conduct on the part of the person concerned.

Promiscuity or immoral conduct, sexual deviancy, or dependence on alcohol or drugs, by themselves, do not fall within the categories of mental disorder.

ADMISSION PROCEDURE UNDER THE MENTAL HEALTH ACT 1983: PART II

Informal Admission

The 1983 Act continues the aim of the 1959 Act which was to encourage the admission of patients on a voluntary basis and, by so doing, bring the treatment of the mentally ill into line with the physically ill. The new Act provides extra safeguards to protect the civil rights of patients admitted under compulsion.

Compulsory Admission

Compulsory admissions under Sections 4, 2 and 3 are respectively for a maximum duration of 72 hours, 28 days and 6 months and for the purpose of emergency assessment, assessment with or without subsequent treatment, and for treatment. Application must be made either by the nearest relative (as defined in Sections 26 and 29) or an Approved Social Worker (as defined in Section 13). The applications must be accompanied by medical recommendations. Only one is required for emergency under Section 4 (preferably by a medical practitioner who knows the patient), but two are otherwise required, one of which must be by an 'approved' practitioner. The two doctors must be independent as defined in Section 12. The recommendations must state clearly that the patient must be detained because of the nature or degree of mental disorder, or for his or her safety or that of other persons.

Admission for Assessment in Case of Emergency—Section 4

The application must be acted upon within 24 hours from the time the applicant has seen the patient or the medical examination is carried out, whichever is the earlier. The patient must be discharged after 72 hours, unless a second recommendation is made to bring the detention under Section 2.

Admission for Assessment—Section 2

The applicant must have seen the patient within 14 days of making the application. The Social Worker must inform the nearest relative who can, however, lodge an objection to the order with the local health authority. If the nearest relative asks for a Social Worker to make an application and this is not done, the reason must be recorded and sent to him.

If the two medical examinations and recommendations were not made at the same time, they should not have been separated by more than 5 days. The recommendations should make clear why voluntary admission is not possible.

A patient admitted under Section 2 has the right to apply to a Mental Health Review Tribunal within 14 days of admission. The nearest relative, the managers of the hospital or the Responsible Medical Officer can discharge the patient, although the last can bar the discharge by the nearest relative on certifying that the patient is dangerous. The patient must be discharged after 28 days unless he or she has been further detained for treatment.

Admission for Treatment—Section 3

The applications and the medical recommendations must conform to the requirements under Section 2. In the case of mental impairment or psychopathic disorder, the grounds for admission must state that these conditions are treatable, i.e. by giving the patients relief, assisting them to adjust better in the community or by preventing a worsening of the condition.

The duration of detention is for 6 months, renewable for another 6 months and yearly thereafter. The patient may appeal against the admission to a Mental Health Review Tribunal. If the detention is extended for a second 6 months, the managers of the hospital must automatically refer the case to the tribunal.

The nearest relative may discharge the patient, on giving 72 hours notice, unless the Responsible Medical Officer certifies that the patient is dangerous.

Patients already in Hospital—Section 5

This provides for the detention of informal patients already in a hospital (for whatever reason) if it should appear that the patient may be a danger to himself or others. The doctor in charge of the patient (or his appointed deputy) makes a report in writing to the managers of the hospital giving full information and explanation. The patient must be discharged after a maximum of 72 hours unless further powers of detention have been taken.

In the absence of the doctor, a psychiatric nurse (specially designated) may hold the patient for 6 hours until the arrival of the doctor. The application must be recorded and given to the hospital managers. The 6 hours will be included in the 72 hours of detention under this section, but the patient will be discharged immediately if no order is made by the doctor.

Applications for Guardianship—Section 7

Guardianship is designed to ensure that vulnerable persons are properly cared for and not exploited, ill-treated or neglected. It gives powers analogous to that of a parent over a child, but applies only to persons over 16 years of age.

Applications are made by the nearest relative or Approved Social Worker and must be accompanied by two medical recommendations under conditions similar to those for Section 2. The application must state that the person is over 16 years or give the exact age, that he is suffering from mental disorder and it is in the interests of his welfare that he should be received into guardianship. The application will be sent to the local social services authority which will be the guardian, or where the named guardian resides.

The guardianship may specify where the patient resides, where and when he should attend for treatment, occupation or training, and to give access to him of a specified medical practitioner, Approved Social Worker or other person. The duration is for 6 months unless renewed for a second 6 months and thereafter annually, by the Responsible Medical Officer or nominated medical attendant (usually the family GP).

The patient may be discharged by the nearest relative, Responsible Medical Officer or authority. The patient may appeal to a Mental Health Review Tribunal at any time within the first year. If the patient absents himself he may be retaken only before 28 days have elapsed.

Leave of Absence from Hospital—Section 17
Leave of absence from hospital may be granted to detained patients by the Responsible Medical Officer. To facilitate temporary transfer of a patient to another hospital, any officer on the staff of that hospital may take responsibility for the patient. If the patient fails to return he must be given notice in writing that his leave has been withdrawn. He cannot be recalled if his detention order has expired or if he has been continuously absent for 6 months.

A patient who has been absent without leave can be taken into custody and returned to the hospital, but not if he has been continuously absent for 28 days or orders under Sections 2 and 4 have expired.

PART IV: CONSENT TO TREATMENT

Treatment Requiring Consent and *a Second Opinion—Section 57*
This applies both to informal patients (including outpatients, etc.) and those detained under the Act for treatment. The treatments specified are surgical operations on the brain and surgical implantation of hormones to reduce male sexual drive.

Before the treatment can be given the patient must have given his consent. In addition two (duly appointed) non-medical persons must certify that the patient has consented and fully understands the treatment and its implications. Furthermore, an independent doctor must first consult a nurse and another person (not a nurse or a doctor) who have been involved in the treatment of the patient and on this basis certify that the treatment should be given.

Treatment Requiring Consent or *a Second Opinion—Section 58*
This applies only to those patients detained under the Act for treatment. The treatments specified are electroconvulsive therapy and continuation of drugs beyond 3 months.

The patient must first give his consent and the Responsible Medical Officer or an independent doctor (who has made the necessary consultations as in Section 57) must certify that he has done so and understands fully what is implied. If the patient has not given his consent, the independent doctor must certify to this and that the patient is not capable of understanding fully the nature and purpose of the treatment, but that it is necessary that it should be given.

'Treatment' implies a course of treatment and this should be specified (Section 59). If the patient withdraws his consent, then continuation requires the certification required under Sections 57 or 58 (Secton 60).

Treatment given under Sections 57 and 58 must be reported by the Responsible Medical Officer to the Secretary of State whenever the latter requires it, and on the next occasion when the detention is renewed. If the patient is subject to a restriction order the report must be given at the end of the first six months and whenever required by the statute.

Urgent treatment required to save the patient's life or prevent serious deterioration does not require consent or independent opinions, provided it is not irreversible or hazardous.

MENTALLY ABNORMAL OFFENDERS: PART III

A court may remand an accused person (liable to imprisonment) to a specified hospital for a psychiatric report or for treatment. Both the defence and the prosecution may ask for such an order. If the accused has been found guilty (except in the case of murder) the court can issue hospital or guardianship orders as the most appropriate method of disposal.

Remand to Hospital for a Report—Section 35
A Crown Court may issue this order for an accused person before trial or before sentence, but a Magistrates' Court may do so only if satisfied that the accused committed the offence or consents to the order. The grounds are that it would appear that the person accused is suffering from mental disorder.

The court must first receive evidence from the hospital managers or a medical practitioner that the person can be admitted within 7 days of the remand. The remand is for 28 days initially, renewable for 28 days up to a maximum of 12 weeks on application from the medical practitioner who will make the report. If the person absconds he may be re-arrested without a warrant for the court to deal with him as appropriate.

The psychiatric report may be made by any medical practitioner and the person may arrange for an independent report. While in hospital, the person may be given treatment as for an informal patient.

Remand to Hospital for Treatment—Section 36

If an accused person (of the type described in Section 35) is in custody awaiting trial, and it would appear that he is suffering from mental disorder such that it would be appropriate for him to be detained in hospital, a Crown Court may remand him to a hospital for treatment. A prison medical officer may also apply for such a remand.

Medical recommendations must be received from two doctors (one of whom is an 'approved' doctor) and assurance that the person can be admitted from the hospital managers or the doctor who would be in charge of treatment.

Further remands, re-arrest after absconding and independent reports can be made as in Section 35.

Hospital or Guardianship Order—Section 37

This applies to persons of the same type as those in Sections 35 and 36, after conviction by a Crown Court, when it considers that a hospital order is preferable to any alternative disposal. In the case of persons suffering from mental impairment or psychopathic disorder, the requirement is that treatment is likely to alleviate or prevent deterioration. If the offender is over 16 years of age, the court may make an order for guardianship if this is appropriate.

The court must receive evidence from 2 medical practitioners (one of whom is 'approved') who must agree on the diagnosis of the type of mental disorder and also receive assurance that arrangements have been made for admission either by the doctor who will be in charge of the treatment or from the hospital managers.

The order is for 6 months, renewable for 6 months and thereafter at 12-monthly intervals. The person may be detained in a suitable place for 28 days if a place in hospital is not immediately available. The order lapses if the person is not admitted in that time.

A Magistrates' Court may make a hospital order after conviction or, if satisfied that the accused committed the offence, without convicting the accused. The court must receive the usual evidence that the person can be admitted. The patient may appeal against the order to a Crown Court.

The patient may be discharged by the Responsible Medical Officer at any time, but not by the nearest relative. The latter and the patient may apply to a Mental Health Review Tribunal in the second 6 months of the order and in any subsequent 12 months. In the case of a guardianship order, the patient may apply to a tribunal within the first 6 months. The nearest relative may make application in the first 12 months and any subsequent 12 months.

Restriction Orders

The judge of the Crown Court may restrict the discharge of the patient, for an unlimited or a specified period, in order to protect the public. He will do so after hearing evidence from one of the two doctors making the recommendations, and preferably from the receiving doctor. He may make the restriction order despite the doctor's objections.

The patient cannot leave the hospital, be transferred or discharged without the consent of the Home Secretary, who may also remove the restrictions if he thinks they are no longer necessary. The Home Secretary may also discharge the patient, with or without conditions, e.g. that the patient lives at a specified address, is supervised by a probation officer or attends a psychiatrist. A patient who has been discharged under conditions may be recalled at any time (while the order remains in force) if it should be thought necessary, and must then be referred to a tribunal within one month.

A restricted person may appeal to the Court of Appeal (Criminal Division) against the order. A restricted patient may appeal to a Mental Health Review Tribunal in the second 6 months of the restriction order and thereafter every 12 months. The Home Secretary may refer the case to a Mental Health Review Tribunal at any time, and in any case, if the tribunal has not reviewed the case in the past 3 years.

Transfer to Hospital of a Sentenced Prisoner—Section 47

If a detained prisoner is suffering from mental disorder which requires treatment not available where he is, the Home Secretary may transfer the person to a hospital for treatment, with or without restrictions. Application is made usually by the prison medical officer. Medical recommendations consists of two reports from doctors, one of whom must be 'approved'. The person must be transferred within 14 days, or the transfer direction lapses. The person transferred may appeal to a Mental Health Review Tribunal within the first 6 months. If subject to a restriction order he may also appeal during each subsequent period of detention.

When the patient no longer requires treatment or no effective treatment can be given, he can be referred, by the Responsible Medical Officer, any doctor or a tribunal, to the Home Secretary who can then decide to order him back to prison, release or discharge him. At the date on which the prison sentence would normally expire, the patient reverts to the status of a patient under a hospital order.

Transfer to Hospital of other Detained Persons—Section 73

This applies to persons remanded in custody. The procedure is the same as in Section 47.

MENTAL HEALTH ACT COMMISSION

The Commission consists of a Chairman, and 12 each of lawyers, nurses, psychologists, social workers and laymen, together with 22 psychiatrists. Its functions are to provide second medical opinions relating to 'consent to treatment', to review the treatment of long term detained patients, to visit detained patients and to interview them in private. The visits will be once a year, but once a month for Special Hospitals (which provide special security for dangerous, violent or criminal patients).

MENTAL HEALTH REVIEW TRIBUNALS (ENGLAND AND WALES)

Mental Health Review Tribunals are set up for every Regional Health Authority. The jurisdiction of a tribunal may be exercised by three or more of its members usually comprising a legal representative (who must be a circuit judge or lawyer of equivalent rank) as the president, a medical member and a lay member who may also have experience in administration or a knowledge of social services. Such members are appointed by the Lord Chancellor. Where appropriate, application can be made by the patient, his nearest relative or the Secretary of State at the Home Office.

THE MENTAL HEALTH (SCOTLAND) ACT 1960

This Act has been modified by the Mental Health (Amendment) (Scotland) Act 1983 and in due course these changes will be consolidated into a new Act. The following description takes into account the amendments. Part 1 Section 6 defines mental disorder in the same way as the English Act.

PART IV: ADMISSION TO AND DETENTION IN HOSPITAL OR GUARDIANSHIP

Informal Admission

The aim of this Act is to encourage the admission of patients on an informal basis.

Section 31—Emergency Admission

In cases of urgency, an emergency admission may be made by one medical practitioner who has personally examined the patient on that day and who states that, by reason of mental disorder from which the patient suffers, and for his health or safety or for the protection of other persons, an urgent admission is necessary for the patient to be detained under Section 24 of this Act but compliance with full procedure would cause undesirable delay. Such an admission should not be made unless the consent of the nearest relative or the mental health officer has been obtained and a statement should accompany the patient to the effect that consent has been obtained or giving the reason why it cannot be obtained.

The removal of the patient to hospital can occur at any time within three days of the making of such a recommendation and lasts for a period not exceeding 72 hours. The board of management of the hospital must, where practicable, inform the nearest relative of the patient. The patient cannot be detained further under this section.

Section 24—Admission and Detention of Patients

Application under this section is founded on and accompanied by two medical recommendations which shall be in the prescribed form and shall include a statement of opinion—giving the grounds for the application on the same lines as in Section 3 of the English Act for 1983. Each medical recommendation shall describe the same mental disorder and may, or may not, also describe other forms of mental disorder.

Section 23—Patients Liable to be Detained in Hospital or Subject to Guardianship

A person who suffers from any mental disorder can be admitted to hospital or received into guardianship under Section 23 if the requirements for the recommendations are satisfied, including that the person has reached the age of 16 years, but no person over the age of 21 years shall be admitted or received into guardianship unless his mental handicap is such that he is incapable of living an independent life or guarding himself against serious exploitation, or he is suffering from mental illness other than a persistent disorder which is manifest only by abnormally aggressive or seriously irresponsible conduct.

A person (having reached the age of 16 years) can be received into guardianship under Section 25 if the prescribed form known as 'guardianship application' is approved by the Sheriff. After approval, the application is forwarded to the local authority where the patient resides.

The person named in the guardianship application may be the local authority to which the application is addressed, a person chosen by such an authority or any other person who has been accepted as being suitable to act as guardian. Such an application shall be accompanied by two medical recommendations based on the opinion that the patient is suffering from mental illness or mental handicap or both and that such a disorder requires or is susceptible to medical treatment and is of a nature or degree which warrants the patient's reception into guardianship and that such a procedure is necessary in the interests of the health or safety of the patient or for the protection of others.

Such an application may be made by the nearest relative or a mental health officer. The relative of such a patient should be informed of the steps taken if it is practicable and the applicant shall have seen the patient within 14 days of making the application.

When an application for admission is approved by the Sheriff, the patient can be removed to the hospital named in the application and the application is forwarded to the board of management of the hospital within seven days. The board of management of the hospital or local authority shall notify the Mental Welfare Commission of such an admission or reception into guardianship and the application and medical recommendations shall be forwarded to the Commission within seven days.

When a patient has been admitted to hospital or received into guardianship, it is the duty of the Responsible Medical Officer to examine the patient or to obtain from another medical practitioner a report on the condition of the patient. This must be undertaken within a period of seven days ending on the twenty-eighth day after admission or reception. If the patient is not discharged, the Mental Welfare Commission, the patient's nearest relative and the board of management or the local authority must be informed.

The duration of authority for detention or guardianship and discharge of patients is dealt with under Section 39. The period of detention must not exceed six months beginning on the date of admission to hospital or reception into guardianship.

Renewal of authority for detention in hospital or guardianship can be made for a further six months and, following this, for further periods of one year.

Two months before the expiry of the period, it shall be the duty of the Responsible Medical Officer to obtain from another medical practitioner, a report on the condition of the patient. This shall be done in the prescribed form and assessment of the need for further detention should be made. Such reports are forwarded to the board of management and the Mental Welfare Commission. Similar provisions are made for the renewal of guardianship orders.

Section 32—Detention of Patients already in Hospital

An application for admission or emergency recommendations can be made for a patient who is already in hospital. Such an application shall come into force on the day it is forwarded to the board of management.

In the absence of the appropriate medical practitioner, the patient may be detained by a nurse of the prescribed class for a maximum of two hours. The nurse shall make a written report stating that the patient has been detained, the reasons for doing so and the time, and give this to the board of management. A copy shall be sent to the Mental Welfare Commission.

PART VIIIA: CONSENT TO TREATMENT

This Part is a new addition to the principal Act. A copy of the certificate given under the following two sections must be sent to the Mental Welfare Commission within seven days.

Urgent treatment required to save the patient's life or prevent serious deterioration does not require consent or independent opinions, provided it is not irreversible or hazardous.

Treatment Requiring Consent and *a Second Opinion—Section 93B*

This Section requires consent to treatment corresponding to Section 57 of the English Act.

Treatment Requiring Consent or *a Second Opinion—Section 93C*

This Section corresponds to Section 58 of the English Act.

PART V: DETENTION OF PATIENTS CONCERNED IN CRIMINAL PROCEEDINGS

Section 54—Power of Court to Commit to Hospital

Where a court remands or commits for trial a person charged with any offence who appears to the court to be suffering from a mental disorder, and the court is satisfied that a hospital is available for his admission and suitable for his detention, the court may, instead of remanding him in custody, commit him to that hospital.

The hospital must be specified in the warrant. If the Responsible Medical Officer is satisfied that he is suffering from mental disorder, he can be detained under Part IV of the Act for the period of remand or the period of committal, unless he is liberated in due course of law.

The result of the examination shall be reported to the court either in writing or orally. Where a report indicates that the person is not suffering from mental disorder, the court shall have the power to commit him to prison or other institution.

A person convicted of an offence punishable by imprisonment in the High Court of Justiciary or the Sheriff Court, other than where the sentence is fixed by law, may be admitted to hospital or received into guardianship if the court is satisfied by the written or oral evidence of two medical practitioners, one of whom must have special experience in the diagnosis and treatment of mental disorder, that the offender is suffering from mental disorder of a nature or degree which, in the case of a person under 21 years, would warrant his admission or reception under Part IV. If, having regard to all the circumstances including the nature of the offence, the character and antecedents of the offender, the court considers that the most appropriate way of dealing with him would be admission or reception, the authority for this can be made.

Under Section 55, when a patient is found to be insane at the time of trial and the court cannot proceed, an order can be made by the Sheriff Court to detain such a patient in hospital. There is no need for conviction to be proven as long as the court is satisfied that the person did the act or made the omission.

A Court of Summary Jurisdiction, other than a Sheriff Court, which finds a person guilty of a crime which is punishable by imprisonment and it appears that he is suffering from mental disorder, shall remit him to the Sheriff Court for a hospital order. It is the duty of a prosecutor in any court to bring the court evidence of mental disorder if he suspects the accused is suffering from mental disorder.

A hospital order cannot be made unless a bed is available.

A State hospital shall not be specified in the order unless the court is satisfied, on the evidence of a medical practitioner, that the offender requires treatment under conditions of special security because of his dangerous, violent or criminal propensities and that he cannot be suitably cared for in an ordinary psychiatric hospital.

A similar order under Section 56 can be made in the case of a juvenile brought before the court who is in need of care or protection or whose parent or guardian is unable to control him, if he is suffering from mental disorder as defined in the Act.

Section 58—Effects of Hospital Orders and Guardianship Orders

The effect of such an order is the same as a person detained under Part IV of the Act except that subsection (2) of Section 23 and Section 40, relating to the duration of orders, shall not apply.

If a bed is not immediately available, the patient can be conveyed to a place of safety for a period of up to twenty-eight days to await admission.

Restriction of discharge of patients is dealt with under Section 60. The court can restrict the discharge of a patient for a limited period or without limit of time if it is satisfied that the nature of the offence and the antecedents of the patient are such that there is a risk that due to his mental disorder he is liable to commit further offences if at large and that it is necessary for the protection of the public. In such a case, the medical practitioner must give oral evidence to the court.

Under this section, the granting of leave of absence or the transfer of the patient cannot be carried out unless the Secretary of State has given permission.

The Secretary of State has the power to remove the restriction order if he thinks that the patient is not a danger to the public and he can discharge the patient subject to certain conditions or he can discharge him absolutely. He can also recall a patient who has been conditionally discharged.

Section 63

Where a person charged on indictment with the commission of an offence is found to be insane so that the trial cannot proceed or, if in the course of the trial, it appears to the jury that the person is insane, the court shall direct a finding to that effect to be recorded. If evidence is shown that a person was insane at the time of doing the act or making the omission constituting the offence with which he is charged, he shall be acquitted on account of his insanity. A person so dealt with shall be detained in the State hospital or other such hospital the court may specify and such detention shall have the like effect of a hospital order with an order restricting discharge without limit of time.

Persons charged summarily in the Sheriff Court can be dealt with in this manner and the findings recorded. Such a person shall be dealt with under Section 55 of the Act. If it appears to the court that it is impracticable for the person charged to appear before the court then, unless there is an objection on behalf of the accused, the court can proceed in his absence.

Section 65

If a person who is remanded in custody awaiting trial appears to the Secretary of State to be suffering from mental disorder of a nature or degree which warrants his admission to hospital under Part IV of the Act an application may be made to a Sheriff for an order of removal and detention in hospital. Such an order is based on the opinion of two medical practitioners. Such an order shall cease to have effect at the expiration of fourteen days from the date of the order unless the patient is transferred to hospital. If such an order is acted upon, it shall have the like effect of a hospital order with a restriction without limit of time.

Section 66

Under this Section, prisoners who are found to be mentally ill after conviction may be removed to hospital. Prisoners serving a sentence, civil prisoners and aliens detained in prison are covered by this section if they fulfil the necessary medical requirements.

It shall be the duty of the Mental Welfare Commission generally to exercise protective functions in respect of persons who may, by reason of mental disorder, be incapable of adequately protecting their persons or their interests. It is also the duty of the Commission to enquire into cases where there may have been ill-treatment and also to visit patients who are detained in hospital or subject to a guardianship order as often as they think appropriate. It shall also be their duty to bring to the notice of the board of management or the local authority any ill-treatment, deficiency in care or treatment or improper detention of patients.

MENTAL ILLNESS AND THE CIVIL LAW

In general, a mental disorder prevents a person from giving evidence under oath but a judge may decide a given person may do so. A jury may be obliged to determine what credence should be placed on such evidence. A valid contract cannot be made by a person of unsound mind.

Testamentary Capacity

This is the power of a person to execute a will. The psychiatrist may be asked to examine a patient who is about to make a will and give an opinion about his mental state. In the case of a patient who has recently died, the psychiatrist may be asked to give an opinion about the patient's mental state at the time of making the will. This opinion is given from the patient's history.

When a psychiatrist is asked to give an opinion about the state of mind of a person making a will, he should carry out a comprehensive psychiatric examination and the patient should be alone when such an examination is conducted. He should then obtain a full history including all the relevant facts about the patient's family, etc., separately from one or more relative. Details of the patient's estate, relatives and dependants should, if possible, be obtained from the patient's legal adviser. When such an examination is carried out, the fullest notes should be made in case of future need. If there is any doubt about any aspect of the case, a second opinion should be sought.

From such an examination, the doctor should satisfy himself that the patient is able to understand that he is making a will and the implications of such an act. He should ascertain that the patient is aware of the nature and extent of his property and that he is aware of those who have a claim on his estate. If he wishes to exclude anyone who has such a claim, he must be able to give a good reason for this.

A 'testor' should have a 'sound disposing mind' in that he has no insane delusions or suspicions about his relatives which would influence his judgement and that his memory is intact in that he can recount the contents of his will with reasonable accuracy.

A person who is of unsound mind, whether he is informally or compulsorily detained in hospital, is still able to make a valid will providing the psychiatrist is of the opinion that the testor has a 'sound disposing mind'.

Marriage and Divorce

Insanity can be grounds for nullity and divorce under the Matrimonial Causes Act 1965 (England and Wales) and the corresponding Scottish Act.

If, at the time of the marriage, either party was of unsound mind or a mental defective, or subject to recurrent fits of insanity or epilepsy, the marriage is voidable providing it can be shown that, at the time of the marriage, the petitioner was not aware of these facts. Such proceedings must be started within a year of the marriage. Following discovery of these facts, the petitioner must not have consented to sexual intercourse with the partner.

A petition for divorce may be presented on the grounds that the respondent is incurably of unsound mind and that he has been continuously under care and treatment for a period of at least 5 years. The definition of 'under care and treatment' is that the person is liable to be detained in hospital, mental nursing home or place of safety under the Mental Health Act 1983, that he is detained in pursuance of an order for his detention or treatment as a person of unsound mind or suffering from mental illness made under any law which deals with such matters including the law relating to criminal lunatics, or that he is receiving treatment as a voluntary patient.

In determining whether the period of care has been continuous, any interruption for a period of 28 days or less would be discounted.

No petition can be presented to the court until a period of 3 years has elapsed from the date of the marriage.

CRIMINAL RESPONSIBILITY

A cardinal principle of English law is embodied in the maxim *actus non facit reum, nisi mens sit rea* (an act does not make a person guilty unless his mind is guilty). A crime is composed of two elements: (1) the act—*actus reus* and (2) the mental element—*mens rea*. The psychiatrist may be asked to report on the mental element of a criminal act. It is for the prosecution to show that the necessary mental state was present at the time of the act.

The law presumes that everyone is sane until it is proved otherwise and the defence against a criminal prosecution can be shown if the accused was labouring under such a defect of reason, due to disease of the mind, as either (1) he did not know the nature and quality of his act or (2) he did not know the act was wrong. The question of the accused's mental state may be at issue on arraignment, on conviction or after sentence.

The onus of proof of insanity rests on the accused; this is against the general principle of English law where the onus of proof rests always on the prosecution.

In a defence of insanity, the accused must show that he was suffering from a disease of the mind when he did the prohibited act. He must then show that he was suffering from a defect of reason due to his disease of the mind and that this defect of reason must be such as to affect his legal responsibility in that he did not appreciate what he was doing nor that what he was doing was lawfully wrong.

The concept of diminished responsibility has been part of the law of Scotland for over a century and was admitted to the law by usage. The admission of this concept reduces murder to culpable homicide. Although earlier references are found to diminished responsibility, it was at the trial of Dingwall in 1867 by Lord Deas that the concept became established. Some confusion appears to have arisen as to whether this concept was only restricted to murder but, in 1963 the Lord Justice General stated, '... diminished responsibility is a plea applicable to murder. It is not open in the case of a lesser crime such as culpable homicide. ...'

This concept later became part of English law.

In 1957 the concept of reduced responsibility was introduced into English law under the Homicide Act of 1957. Under Section 2 of this Act, a person who has killed or been party to a killing shall not be convicted of murder if it can be shown that he was suffering from abnormality of mind (whether arising from a condition of arrested or retarded development of mind or any inherent causes, or induced by diseases or injury) as to substantially impair his mental responsibility for his act and omission.

It is for the defence to show that the person's responsibility is reduced. If this is shown, a person charged with murder will face a charge of manslaughter. It is worth pointing out that the sentence for murder is laid down by statute and is life imprisonment. The sentence for manslaughter is at the discretion of the judge.

The question of criminal responsibility in children is that children under the age of 10 years have no *mens rea,* are presumed to be *doli incapax* and therefore they are not liable for punishment by a criminal court. Children between the ages of 10 and 14 years are presumed to be *doli incapax* but evidence can be brought before the court that the child knew he was doing wrong. The court must be satisfied on two counts: that the child committed the act and that at the time he had guilty knowledge that he was doing wrong. Over the age of 14 years, the child is fully responsible unless proved to be otherwise.

Acts or omissions which are crimes can be classified in several ways: (1) according to source statutory (a crime which is defined and regulated by an Act of Parliament) and common law (that part of the law which is governed and ruled by common custom); (2) by the method of trial (indictable crimes or summary offences); and (3) as crimes against the person, crimes against property, and crimes against public order and the safety of the State.

Crimes against the person are considered by most people as the more serious crimes, in particular the crime of murder. Homicide is defined as the killing of a human being by another and it may be lawful (e.g. killing in self-defence). Unlawful homicide is murder, man-slaughter, causing death by dangerous driving and infanticide.

A psychiatric opinion is sought in all cases of unlawful killing and it has to be shown that, not only was the act of killing done, but the necessary mental element was present for such a killing to be defined as murder.

The psychiatrist has to pass an opinion about the state of mind of the accused at the time of the offence. He has also to give an opinion whether the man should stand trial and whether he is fit to plead.

A person who is found by a jury to have committed an act or omission but according to law was not responsible at the time, would have a verdict returned of 'not guilty by reason of insanity'. This verdict must be returned under the Criminal Procedure (Insanity) Act 1964.

The criteria for such a verdict to be applied were laid down by the House of Lords in the case of McNaghten in 1843. The basis of these rules states that at the time of committing the act or omission the accused was labouring under such a defect of reason from disease of the mind as not to know the nature and quality of the act he was doing or, if he did know, that he did not know it was wrong. For the accused to be fit to plead he must be able to understand the nature of the charge, be able to challenge a juror, know the difference between a plea of 'guilty' and 'not guilty', be able to follow the evidence, and be able to instruct his legal advisers.

The Psychiatrist as a Witness

Evidence falls into two broad areas. The evidence given by the majority of witnesses is the evidence of fact. A psychiatrist may be called to give evidence of fact. He is also called as an expert witness to give evidence of opinion usually based on his examination of the accused. An expert witness is allowed to give an opinion on his experience and can use other sources such as textbooks, reports, etc. He is also asked, from his examination, to deduce an opinion about the mental state of the accused.

MENTAL ILLNESS IN RELATION TO CRIME

Mental disorder, as defined in the Mental Health Act 1983, is only found in a comparatively small number of the criminal population. The figures that are available are from Home Office statistics and a number of reports on the prison population. Such surveys vary according to the population. A survey on a group of habitual prisoners showed that one-third or over were considered to be mentally disordered and a survey on a group of prisoners serving 4 years or over showed that a quarter were mentally disordered or handicapped.

The numbers found to be disordered varied with different samples. The Home Office statistics show those who are found to be mentally disordered on remand and who are dealt with under the Mental Health Act. A number of mentally disordered prisoners remain in prison either because it is felt they do not require active treatment or because a place cannot be found for them in a psychiatric hospital.

In 1971, 12 969 people were remanded in custody. Of these, only 1285 (9·9 per cent) were found to be suffering from a mental disorder and were dealt with under Section 60/65 of the Mental Health Act. Similarly, in 1972, 11 953 people were remanded in custody and of these, 1130 (9·4 per cent) were dealt with under Section 60/65.

The problem of personality disorders is complicated by the different criteria used when assessing personality. Of those in prison, it has been estimated that between 40 and 60 per cent suffer from personality disorders. In 1971 and 1972, 135 (1 per cent) and 87 (0·7 per cent) respectively were dealt with under Section 60/65 as suffering from psychopathic disorder and were considered to require or be susceptible to treatment. There may have been others who could have been diagnosed as suffering from psychopathic disorder but who were not considered to require or be susceptible to treatment and were, therefore, given a custodial sentence.

From this, it can be seen how difficult it is to give any precise figures about mental illness in criminals.

It becomes more difficult when the relationship between mental illness and crime is considered. The mental disorder may have a direct relationship to the crime, for example, a person may commit an offence as a result of a delusion or in response to hallucinations. In other cases, the offence may not be related to the mental condition, for example, a schizophrenic may steal food because he is hungry and not because of his delusions or hallucinations. It could be said that if he had not been suffering from schizophrenia he would have been able to earn money to buy food, so there may be an indirect relationship.

Clinical Conditions in Relation to Crime

It can be seen that certain clinical conditions may predispose to certain crimes, but it should be remembered that the reverse is not true.

The schizophrenic who suffers from delusions of persecution may feel that his life is being interfered with by his neighbours and he may commit a violent offence against them or even kill them. Similarly, he may attempt to burn down their property and so commit arson. Schizophrenic hallucinations may cause a patient to strike out and hit another patient. The chronic schizophrenic may be found amongst the petty criminals who commit 'nuisance' crimes because they are unable to cope in society.

Violent crimes such as murder may be committed by a depressed patient in response to his delusional ideas. He may kill a member of his family because of a delusion that they are suffering from some incurable disease. This may be followed by a suicide attempt or even suicide. A small number of depressed patients commit quite violent crimes against both people and property and the damage they cause is usually severe. When the patient is examined, he is found to be severely depressed or even stuporosed and it appears that, at the time of the offence, he suddenly became overactive. This overactive period lasts during the period of the offence, but, soon after, the patient returns to his depression and it becomes difficult to understand how he could have committed such violence.

Depression in parents who, during such episodes, threaten to kill their children must not be dismissed without a complete psychiatric examination. In such cases, it may be necessary to admit the parent to hospital, or arrange for a relative to be constantly with the parent and child, or to take the child into care. A number of cases of infanticide occur in such a depressive setting.

Minor crimes such as shoplifting may be seen to occur in middle-aged, depressed women but not all such offences are due to depression.

Acts of violence against the person or property can be caused by a toxic confusional state and, in cases where there is organic brain damage, by such lesions as temporal-lobe epilepsy or brain tumour and also in brain injury. Drugs such as alcohol can cause crime due to short-lived confusional states such as intoxication. A crime committed during such an episode would be dealt with as a normal offence since there is no lack of mental intent where alcohol has been self administered. Crimes can be committed when a person suffers from an alcoholic paranoid state.

A number of sexual offences are found in relation to the use of alcohol and assessments have been made which suggest that between 20 per cent and 40 per cent of all criminals have an alcoholic problem. This does not mean there is any direct relationship between their crime and their drinking.

Dementia can be associated with such crimes as indecent exposure, shoplifting, and arson. The act may be committed because of failing memory. A person may leave a shop forgetting to pay for the goods he has selected.

People suffering from personality disorder may revert to crime because of the difficulties they have relating to other people. They may commit crimes such as theft and those associated with the possession and use of drugs. They may also commit sexual offences such as rape, often associated with the use of alcohol. Heterosexual and homosexual offences against children may also be committed by such people.

Parents with personality disorders may commit violent acts against each other or their children.

The psychopath who is dealt with under the Mental Health Act will often have committed severely aggressive or irresponsible behaviour and such behaviour will have been present for a considerable period of time. When the history of such a patient is taken, it should be realized that he may have indulged in aggressive or irresponsible behaviour for a prolonged period although no official record of such behaviour may have been made. It may have been felt that no police action was necessary until a serious offence was eventually committed.

When a crime is committed by a middle-aged person and the act seems to be out of character, a complete and comprehensive examination should be carried out to exclude organic diseases such as brain tumour.

Offences committed by subnormals show a very wide variety from minor nuisance offences such as breach of the peace to major offences such as arson. Some of the offences may occur in relation to the subnormal's ability to cope in society. He may be unable to find or maintain employment and will steal to obtain money, food, etc. Because of his difficulty in making relationships, particularly with members of the opposite sex, he may commit a sexual offence.

The severely subnormal rarely commits offences but a number of cases have been reported such as murder, arson, assault and sexual offences such as indecent exposure. Occasionally, a severely subnormal person may mimic an offence he has witnessed.

Sexual Offenders

The Sexual Offences Acts of 1956 and 1967 list the following deviances which are punishable by law:

1. Rape: sexual intercourse with a female by threat, by intimidation, by false pretences or false representation and by causing to be administered a drug with intent to stupefy.

2. Intercourse with a girl under the age of 16 years.

3. Intercourse with defectives or the procurement of such persons.

4. Incest: sexual intercourse or cohabitation between persons related within the degree within which marriage is prohibited by law.

5. Unnatural offences: buggery with a human or animal.

6. Indecent assault on a man or woman.

7. Assault with intent to commit buggery.

Several other offences such as abduction are also dealt with in the 1956 Act.

The 1967 Act deals with male homosexual behaviour. Such an act is not an offence providing the parties consent and have attained the age of 21 years. Such an act is an offence when more than two persons take part or are present and if done in a public place. If one of the parties is severely subnormal within the meaning of the Mental Health Act 1983 his consent is not valid in law, but, if the other party was not aware or did not suspect that the man was severely subnormal, this is a defence against conviction. Male staff working in hospitals for the mentally disordered or who have responsibility for such patients would be dealt with under the 1967 Act if they committed buggery or gross indecency.

Homosexual acts, whether between consenting parties over the age of 21 years or not, are not permitted on British merchant ships. Such acts are covered by Army, Air Force and Naval disciplinary codes.

A number of sexual deviances are not dealt with as sexual offences but may be dealt with as other offences such as causing a breach of the peace, etc.

Sexual offenders can be divided into four broad groups:

1. The offender, normally well adjusted both mentally and sexually, who commits an offence because of circumstances such as excessive use of alcohol or drugs or because of a stressful situation in a normal sexual relationship. For example, the offender may commit an offence such as rape following the breakdown of his marriage.

2. The offender who shows sexually deviant behaviour but is psychiatrically non-deviant. He appears to be a well-adjusted individual who participates in abnormal sexual behaviour.

3. The offender who is both sexually deviant and psychiatrically deviant. Such an offender exhibits a personality disorder.

4. The offender who is sexually non-deviant but who suffers from a psychiatric disorder which is the primary cause of his sexually deviant behaviour. For example, the schizophrenic may commit an offence because of his delusions, or the subnormal may offend against children because of his inability to relate with adults.

Cases which show a psychiatric disorder should be treated with the appropriate medication for their psychiatric condition but a period of treatment with a libido-reducing drug may be indicated. Such drugs may be used in other cases either on a short or a long term basis. Behavioural techniques and psychotherapy all have a place in the treatment of sexual offenders.

SUPERVISION OF PATIENTS SUBJECT TO SPECIAL RESTRICTIONS

The report, 'The Review of Procedures for the Discharge and Supervision of Psychiatric Patients Subject to Special Restrictions' (the Aarvold Report) recommended that when a patient is admitted to hospital and is subject to a restriction order, the Home Office should, within 3 months, enquire whether the patient requires special care and assessment. The report suggested that, when such a patient is considered for discharge or transfer to a hospital within the National Health Service, the recommendation of the medical officer responsible should be supported by the recorded views of other professional personnel and that such cases should be referred to an advisory body independent of the treatment hospital. Such a body should be established by the Home Secretary. When such a patient is discharged, there should be a continuing after-care and continuous liaison between all those involved in such after-care. When discharge is considered, the patient should be asked for his written consent to the disclosure of relevant information to people who may be involved with him in the community (e.g. landladies) who are not part of the professional after-care team. The patient must be informed what information is to be disclosed and to whom.

A further report was published by the Committee on Mentally Abnormal Offenders (the Butler report) which covered all the aspects of the mentally abnormal offender from the time he is first concerned in a criminal act to the court proceedings, hospital treatment and after-care facilities. Special aspects of the report deal with such procedures as the establishment of regional secure units, alteration of the law with regard to fitness to plead, care and treatment of dangerous offenders, the establishment of special units for aggressive psychopaths, and consent to treatment.

Although the report has been accepted, many aspects of it cannot be brought into operation until the necessary legislation has been passed.

Court Reports

These are prepared by psychiatrists on many patients and there are several basic principles which should be observed. A full and comprehensive physical and psychiatric examination should be carried out. If there is a previous psychiatric history, the relevant notes should be fully scrutinized. The report should state from where the examiner has obtained his facts. The report should give all the relevant information but should not describe at length any information which has no relevance. It should not discuss the crime unless it has some bearing on the mental state of the accused. It should not decide on the guilt or innocence of the accused. It should clearly state an opinion from the facts obtained and should not be clouded by jargon. Finally, the report should advise the court of any medical or other disposal which the psychiatrist feels will help in dealing with the case.

ABORTION

The psychiatrist, in his practice, will see patients who require a therapeutic termination of pregnancy. Such terminations are carried out under the Abortion Act 1967. If, in the opinion of the psychiatrist, the following conditions can be satisfied, a recommendation can be made for the termination of the pregnancy:

1. The continuance of the pregnancy would involve risk to the life of the pregnant woman greater than if the pregnancy were terminated.

2. The continuance of the pregnancy would involve risk of injury to the physical or mental health of the pregnant woman greater than if the pregnancy were terminated.

3. The continuance of the pregnancy would involve risk of injury to the physical or mental health of the existing child(ren) of the family of the pregnant woman greater than if the pregnancy were terminated.

4. There is a substantial risk that if the child were born it would suffer from such physical or mental abnormalities as to be seriously handicapped.

The Act says that in determining the risk to the patient 'account may be taken of the pregnant woman's actual or reasonably foreseeable environment'.

This Act allows the total social, psychological and medical background of the patient to be taken into account when determining the need for a therapeutic abortion.

Chapter 16

Method in psychiatric case-taking

A short scheme for use in psychiatric case-taking is described below, and it is convenient to record the information obtained under two headings: (1) history, and (2) psychological examination.

1. HISTORY

Under this heading the following particulars should be obtained: (1) name, age, civil status; (2) source of information, i.e. patient, name of relative, letters from doctor or from social agencies; (3) complaint, or reason for seeking medical advice; (4) family history; (5) previous personal history; (6) history of present illness; and (7) treatment so far given.

Person giving the Information (if other than the patient)
Impression of Informant's Reliability, etc.
Relatives should be asked to give a history of the patient's illness as they have seen it. This should be set down separately from the history given by the patient.

Main Complaint or Reason for Admission
Give a brief statement and put in inverted commas words said by the patient.

Family History
Race, social group and general efficiency of family. Familial diseases, alcoholism, abnormal personalities, mental disorder, epilepsy.

Father
Health, age, or age at time of death and cause of death; kind of personality; occupation.

Mother
Health, age, or age at time of death and cause of death; kind of personality; occupation.

Siblings
Enumerated in chronological order of birth with Christian names, ages, marital condition, personality, occupation, health, or illness. Miscarriages and stillbirths should be included.

Home Atmosphere and Influence

Any salient happenings among parents and collaterals during patient's early years; relationship of patient to parents, relatives and others in the home.

Personal History

Date of birth and place; mother's health during pregnancy; attitude of parents towards pregnancy; full-term or premature? Was delivery normal? Breast- or bottle-fed?

Early Development

Precocious or retarded? Time of teething, talking and walking; cleanliness as to excreta. Delicate or healthy baby?

Neurotic Traits (in childhood)

Inquire regarding chorea, convulsions, night terrors, walking in sleep, tantrums, bed-wetting, thumbsucking, nail-biting, faddiness about food, stammering, mannerisms, fears, notable behaviour, or escapades.

Play

Make-believe, organized games, types of children preferred.

School

Age of beginning and finishing, schools attended, any special medical or psychological examinations, standard reached, evidence of ability or backwardness, aggressive or submissive at school? Attitude to authority, homework, etc.

Occupations (in full detail)

Age of starting work, jobs held, in chronological order, with wages, dates, reasons for change. Satisfaction in work, present economic circumstances.

Menstrual History

Age at first period; attitude of patient and mother; regularity, duration, and amount, psychic changes, climacteric symptoms.

Sexual Inclinations and Practices

Sexual information, how acquired? Masturbation, guilt, sexual fantasies, homosexuality, heterosexual experiences apart from marriage, marital relations.

Marital History

Duration of acquaintance before marriage and of engagement, partner's age, occupation, personality, compatibility, sexual satisfaction or frigidity? Contraceptive measures, common interests, differences and arguments, in-laws.

Children
Chronological list of children, giving ages, names, personality. Mention miscarriages.

Habits
Alcohol, tobacco, drugs; specify amount taken recently and earlier. Type of drinker—gregarious or solitary, continuous or 'spree'?

Medical History
Illnesses, operations, accidents, in chronological order.

Previous Psychological Illness
Obtain a detailed account; dates, duration, symptoms of attacks, in what hospital or outpatient department? Find out where records are likely to be obtainable.

Previous Personality
In describing the personality before the illness do not use technical terms, but give illustrative anecdotes, statements, or other evidence. Aim at a detailed picture of the individual, giving his own words when necessary. The following is a collection of headings, indicating the kind of information to be sought.

1. Social Relations: Adaptation
To family: Degree of independence from relatives.
To friends: Societies, clubs. Was he inclined to take the lead or to follow?
To highly organized activities: Religion, politics, art.
To work and workmates: Success.
What are his hobbies? How does he use his leisure? Does he indulge in romantic or imaginative fantasy or daydreaming? Has he a great desire for attention? Is he easily influenced? Wilful? Is he timid? What interest has he in dress and habits generally? Is he sociable or seclusive? Is he reserved, shy, self-conscious, sensitive, suspicious, resentful, quarrelsome, over-conscientious, strict, excessively orderly, irritable, impulsive, jealous, eccentric, selfish? Mannerisms. Attitude in moral issues.

2. Intellectual Activities
Observation, memory, judgement, alertness, reading, types of books and papers preferred? Special abilities. Inquisitive? Thoughtful, prone to ruminate?

3. *Mood*

Generally cheerful, despondent, pessimistic, anxious, worrying, self-depreciative or satisfied? Confident? Fluctuating with or without occasion? Emotionally demonstrative?

4. *Energy*

Output sustained or fitful? Rhythm, initiative. Resolute or undecided? Ambitious?

5. *Habits*

Eating, sleep. Attitude to health; interest in body regular or changeable?

Present Illness

Give an account, in chronological order, of the development of the illness from the earliest time at which a change was noticed until admission to hospital. Give data permitting the sequence of various symptoms to be dated approximately. (Write in the third person.)

2. PSYCHOLOGICAL EXAMINATION

Under this heading the following particulars should be noted: (1) general appearance and behaviour; (2) talk (with verbatim samples, if these convey the best impression); (3) mood; (4) orientation and attention; (5) special preoccupations and interests; (6) delusions, hallucinations, and obsessions; (7) memory; and (8) insight and judgement.

General Behaviour

Give a description as complete, as accurate and as life-like as possible of what you can observe in the patient's behaviour. Does the patient look ill? Is he in touch with his surroundings in general, and in particular? What gestures, grimaces, or other motor expressions, tics, or mannerisms are present? Does he display much or little activity? Is it constant, abrupt, or fitful, spontaneous, or how provoked? Is the patient free or constrained? Is he slow, stereotyped, hesitant, or fidgety? Note tenseness, scratching mannerisms, degree of attention. Do movements and attitudes have an evident purpose or meaning? Do real or hallucinatory perceptions seem to modify behaviour? Does the patient, if inactive, resist passive movements, or maintain an attitude, or obey commands, or indicate awareness at all? Note habits of eating, sleep, and cleanliness in general and as to excreta. Ascertain his way of spending the day. If the patient does not speak the description of his mental state must be limited to a report of his behaviour.

Talk

The form of the patient's utterances rather than their content is considered here. Does he say much or little? Does he talk spontaneously or only in answer; slow or fast, hesitantly or promptly, to the point or wide of it, coherently, discursively, loosely, with interruptions, sudden silences, changes of topic, comments on happenings and things at hand, appropriately or using strange words of syntax, rhymes, or puns?

Sample of Talk

A sample of conversation should be recorded verbatim. It should be representative of the form of his talk, his response to questioning, and his main preoccupations. Its length will depend on its individual significance.

Mood

The patient's appearance may be described so far as it is indicative of his mood. His answers to, 'How do you feel in yourself?', 'What is your mood?', 'How about your spirits?', or some similar inquiry, should be recorded. Many varieties of mood may be present; not merely happiness or sadness, but such states as irritability, suspicion, fear, unreality, worry, restlessness, bewilderment and many more, which are convenient to include under this heading. Observe the constancy of the mood, the influence which changes it, and the appropriateness of the patient's apparent emotional state to what he says.

Delusions and Misinterpretation

What is the patient's attitude to the various people and things in his environment? Does he misinterpret what happens, give it special or false meaning, or is he doubtful about it? Does he think that anyone pays special attention to him, treats him in a special way, persecutes or influences him bodily or mentally, in ordinary or scientific or preternatural ways? Does anyone laugh at him, shun him, admire him, or try to kill, harm, or annoy him? Does he depreciate himself in any regard; his morals, possessions, health? Has he grandiose beliefs?

The patient may wish to conceal these matters and may have to be patiently pressed.

Hallucinations and Other Disorders of Perception

These may be auditory, visual, olfactory, gustatory, tactile, or visceral. The source, vividness, reality, manner of reception, content, and all other circumstances of the experiences are important; the content, especially if auditory or visual, must be reported in detail. When do these experiences occur? At night, when falling asleep, when alone? Are there any peculiar bodily sensations, for example, a feeling of deadness?

Compulsive Phenomena

Does the patient have any obsessional thoughts, inclinations, or acts? Are they felt to be from without, or part of his own mind? Does their insistence distress him? Does he recognize their inappropriateness? What is their relation to his emotional state? Does he repeat actions such as washing unnecessarily, to reassure himself? Note phobias and anxiety.

Orientation

Record the patient's answers to questions about his own name and identity, the place where he is, the time of day, and the date. Is there anything unusual in the way in which time seems to pass for him? Disorientation is very often missed if these inquiries are not made.

Memory

This may be tested by comparing the patient's account of his life with that given by others, or by examining his account for evidence of gaps or inconsistencies. There should be special inquiry for recent events, such as those of his admission to hospital and happenings in the ward since. Where there is selective impairment of memory for special incidents, periods, or for recent or remote happenings, this should be recorded in detail and the patient's attitude towards his forgetfulness and the things forgotten should be specially investigated. Record the patient's success or failure in grasping, retaining, and being able to recall spontaneously or on demand 3 or 5 minutes later a number, a name and address, or other data. Give the patient a short story to read (*see* p. 49) and ask him to repeat it in his own words. Record his repetition of the story verbatim if possible and whether he sees the point of it. Give him digits forwards and then backwards and record how many he can repeat immediately after being told them. The Inglis Paired-associate Test may also be used (*see* p. 257–258). In describing the state of the patient's memory do not merely record the conclusions reached but give the evidence first, in full, and describe at appropriate length such facts of behaviour as seem to indicate whether he was attending, trying his hardest, or being distracted by other stimuli, etc.

Grasp of General Information

Tests for general information and grasp, as well as for ability to calculate, should be varied according to the patient's educational level and interests, but the answers to the following should be sought in all cases: name of the Queen and her immediate predecessors; names of the Prime Minister and Chancellor of the Exchequer; the capitals of France, Germany, Italy, Spain, Scotland; date of the beginning and end of the two world wars; the names of six large cities in Britain; subtractions of serial sevens from 100. (Note down the answers and time taken.)

These tests are not intended so much as a test of general intelligence as to see whether there has been any falling away from the patient's former presumptive level of knowledge and capacity.

Insight and Judgement

What is the patient's attitude to his present state? Does he regard it as an illness; as 'mental' or 'nervous'? Does he feel he is in need of treatment? Is he aware of mistakes he has made spontaneously or in performing tests? What is his attitude to his previous experiences, mental illness, and to the interview? What is his attitude towards social, financial, domestic and ethical problems? What does he propose to do when he has left hospital? Does he appear to be able to make sound judgements about his own future?

Simple Memory Test

1. *'The Donkey and the Salt'*

The following story may be read by the patient:

'A donkey loaded with salt had to ford a stream. He stumbled and fell into the water. It took him a few minutes to get to his feet, and when he did so he found that the load was much lighter, because the salt had dissolved in the water.

'He had to cross the stream the next day, when he was loaded with sponges. He remembered what had happened the day before, so he deliberately stumbled and fell into the water. The sponges soaked up so much water that he could not get to his feet again and he was drowned.' The moral is: 'The same remedy does not apply in all cases.'

2. *The Name and Address*

This should be read to the patient and he should be asked to repeat it immediately. If he fails to do so it must be repeated until he can reproduce it accurately. The number of repetitions necessary should be recorded, as this may give some idea of the degree of anxiety. Once the address has been learned the patient should be asked to reproduce it after 5 minutes. The following name and address can be used: 'Mr Robert Johnson, 53, Beechmont Drive, Manchester, 5'.

3. *The Inglis Paired-associate Test*

The test itself is of the ordinary paired-associate learning type, employing verbal presentation and the simple recall form of reproduction. Two alternative sets of stimulus–response material (whose statistical equivalence has been demonstrated) have been used, as follows:

| | Form A | | Form B | |
	Stimulus	*Response*	*Stimulus*	*Response*
(a)	Cabbage	Pen	Flower	Spark
(b)	Knife	Chimney	Table	River
(c)	Sponge	Trumpet	Bottle	Comb

The patient is given instructions much like those for the paired-associate item of the Wechsler Memory Scale. He is told: 'I am going to read you a list of words, two at a time. Listen carefully, because after I finish I shall expect you to remember the words that go together. For example, if the words were "East–West, Gold–Silver", then when I said the word "Gold" you would, of course, answer (pause) . . . "Silver". Do you understand? Now listen carefully to the list as I read it'.

The examiner allows an interval of about 5 seconds between the pairs of words when reading the list. After the presentation of the list another 5-second interval is allowed. The stimulus words are then presented one by one in random order. Thus, the examiner asks: 'What went with "Flower"?' The patient is then allowed about 10 seconds to reply and if his answer is correct the examiner says, 'That's right'. If the reply is wrong he says, 'No', and supplies the correct association. If no reply is given by the patient within about 10 seconds the correct response is again supplied by the examiner.

The material is presented in this way until the patient gets three consecutive correct responses for each stimulus word or until each stimulus word has been presented 30 times, whichever is sooner. The examiner stops presenting each stimulus as its criterion is reached. Supposing that one pair is learned to the criterion before the other two then the appropriate stimulus word is dropped out and the remaining pairs are simply alternated.

The score on this test is the sum of the number of times the stimulus words are presented before the criterion is reached. Inglis compared a group of elderly patients with obvious memory disorder with a control group matched for age and intelligence. The mean of the group with memory impairment was 59·0 with a standard deviation of 25·06, and the mean of the control group was 13·0, with a standard deviation of 6·16.

References

Abrams R. and Taylor M. A. (1973) Anterior bifrontal ECT: a clinical trial. *Br. J. Psychiatry* **122**, 587–590.

Ackner B., Harris A. and Oldham A. J. (1957) Insulin treatment of schizophrenia: a controlled study. *Lancet* **1**, 607–611.

Ackner B. and Oldham A. J. (1962) Insulin treatment of schizophrenia. A three-year follow-up of a controlled study. *Lancet* **1**, 504–506.

Alanen Y. O. (1968) From the mothers of schizophrenic patients to the interactional family dynamics. In: Rosenthal D. and Kety S. S. (ed.) *The Transmission of Schizophrenia.* Oxford, Pergamon.

Ansari J. M. A. (1976) Impotence: prognosis (a controlled study). *Br. J. Psychiatry* **128**, 194–198.

Arnold M. B. (1961) *Emotion and Personality, Vol. 1.* London, Cassell.

Baker G. H. B. and Brewerton D. A. (1981) Rheumatoid arthritis: a psychiatric assessment. *Br. Med. J.* **282**, 2014.

Barton J. L., Mehta S. and Snaith R. P. (1973) The prophylactic value of extra ECT in depressive illness. *Acta Psychiatr. Scand.* **49**, 386–392.

Bateson G., Jackson D. D., Haley J. and Weakland J. (1956) Toward a communication theory of schizophrenia. *Behav. Sci.* **1**, 251–264.

Benedek-Jaszmann L. J. and Hearn-Sturtevant M. D. (1976) Premenstrual tension and functional infertility. *Lancet* **1**, 1095–1098.

Blackburn R. (1975) An empirical classification of psychopathic personalities. *Br. J. Psychiatry* **127**, 456–460.

Browning J. S. and Houseworth J. H. (1953) Development of new symptoms following medical and surgical treatment for duodenal ulcer. *Psychosom. Med.* **15**, 328–336.

Cameron N. (1944) Experimental analysis of schizophrenic thinking. In: Kasanin J. (ed.) *Language and Thought in Schizophrenia.* Berkeley, University of California Press.

Chodoff P. and Lyons H. (1958) Hysteria, the hysterical personality and hysterical conversion. *Am. J. Psychiatry* **114**, 734–740.

Cobb S. and Rose R. M. (1973) Hypertension, peptic ulcer and diabetes in air traffic controllers. *JAMA* **224**, 489–492.

Coppen A. and Kessel N. (1963) Menstruation and personality. *Br. J. Psychiatry* **109**, 711–721.

Cornish D. B. and Clarke R. V. G. (1975) *Residential Treatment and its Effects on Deliquency.* Home Office Research Studies No. 32. London, HMSO.

Dunham H. W. (1965) *Community and Schizophrenia: an Epidemiological Analysis.* Detroit, Wayne University Press.

Flor-Henry P. (1969) Psychosis and temporal lobe epilepsy: a controlled investigation. *Epilepsia* **10**, 363–395.

Foerster O. and Gagel O. (1933) Ein Fall von Ependymcyste des III Ventrikels. Ein Beitrag zur Frage der Beziehungen psychischer Störungen zum Hirnstamm. (A case of ependymal cyst in the third ventricle: A contribution to the question of the relationships between psychic disturbances and the brain-stem.) *Z. Gesamte Neurol. Psychiat.* **149**, 312–344.

Friedman M. and Rosenman R. H. (1959) Association of specific overt behavior patterns with blood and cardiovascular findings. *JAMA* **169**, 1286–1296.

Fry J. (1964) Peptic ulcer: a profile. *Br. Med. J.* **2**, 809–812.

Goldberg E. M. and Morrison S. L. (1963) Schizophrenia and social class. *Br. J. Psychiatry* **109**, 785–807.

Hage J. and Jensen K. (1975) Propanolol in the treatment of withdrawal symptoms. *Ugeskr. Laeger* **137**, 628–631.

Halmi K. A., Falk J. R. and Schwartz E. (1981) Binge-eating and vomiting: a survey of a college population. *Psychol. Med.* **11**, 697–706.

Heine B. E., Sainsbury P. and Chynoweth R. C. (1969) Hypertension and emotional disturbance. *J. Psychiatr. Res.* **7**, 119–130.

Hudson J. I., Pope H. G., Jonas J. M. and Yurgelun-Todd D. (1983) Family history study of anorexia nervosa and bulimia. *Br. J. Psychiatry* **142**, 133–138.

Insel T. R., Murphy D., Cohen R. M., Alterman I., Kilts C. and Linnoila M. (1983) Obsessive–compulsive disorder. A double-blind trial of Clomipramine and Chlorgyline. *Arch. Gen. Psychiatry* **40**, 605–612.

Kay D. W. K. and Roth M. (1961) Environmental and hereditary factors in the schizophrenias of old age ('late paraphrenia') and their bearing on the general problem of causation in schizophrenia. *J. Ment. Sci.* **107**, 649–686.

Kraepelin E. (1919) *Dementia Praecox and Paraphrenia* (trans. Barclay M.). Edinburgh, Livingstone.

Kraepelin E. (1921) *Manic-Depressive Insanity and Paranoia* (trans. Barclay M.). Edinburgh, Livingstone.

Leonhard K. (1959) *Die Aufteilung der Endogenen Psychosen,* 2nd ed. (The Classification of the Endogenous Psychoses). Berlin, Akadamie.

Maddocks P. D. (1970) A five-year follow-up of untreated psychopaths. *Br. J. Psychiatry* **116**, 511–515.

Mannheim H. (1955) *Group Problems in Crime and Punishment.* London, Routledge & Kegan Paul.

Maxwell R. D. H. (1968) Electrical factors in electroconvulsive therapy. *Acta Psychiatr. Scand.* **44**, 436–448.

Meduna L. J. and McCulloch W. S. (1945) The modern concept of schizophrenia. *Med. Clin. North Am.* **29**, 147.

Merry J., Reynolds C. M., Bailey J. and Coppen A. (1976) Prophylactic treatment of alcoholism by lithium carbonate. *Lancet* **3**, 481–487.

Perris C. (1966) A study of bipolar (manic-depressive) and unipolar recurrent depressive psychoses. *Acta Psychiatr. Scand.* **42**, Suppl. 194.

Perris C. (1975) EEG techniques in the measurement of the severity of depressive syndromes. *Neuropsychobiology* **1**, 16–25.

Rahe R. H. and Arthur R. J. (1978) Life change and illness studies: past history and future direction. *Psychosom. Med.* **40**, 95–98.

Rahe R. H., Romo M., Bennett J. and Siltanen P. (1974) Recent life changes, myocardial infarction and abrupt coronary death. *Arch. Intern. Med.* **133**, 221–228.

Rathod N. H., de Alarcon R. and Thomson I. G. (1967) Signs of heroin usage detected by drug users and their parents. *Lancet* **2**, 1411–1414.

Rees L. (1956) Physical and emotional factors in bronchial asthma. *J. Psychosom. Res.* **1**, 98–114.

Rees L. (1959) The role of allergic and emotional factors in hay fever. *J. Psychosom. Res.* **3**, 234–241.

Rees L. (1964) Physiogenic and psychogenic factors in vasomotor rhinitis. *J. Psychosom. Res.* **8**, 101–110.

Reid W. H., Blowin P. and Schermer M. (1976) A review of psychotropic medications, and the glaucomas. *Int. Pharmacopsychiat.* **11**, 163–174.

Roos R., Gajdusek D. C. and Gibbs C. J. (1973) The clinical characteristics of transmissible Creutzfeldt-Jacob disease. *Brain* **96**, 1–20.

Rosenthal D. and Kety S. S. (ed.) (1968) *The Transmission of Schizophrenia.* Oxford, Pergamon.

Roth M. (1955) Natural history of mental disorder in old age. *J. Ment. Sci.* **101**, 281–301.

Schneider K. (1958) *Psychopathic Personalities* (trans. Hamilton M. W.) London, Cassell.

Singer M. T. and Wynne L. C. (1965) Thought disorder and family relations of schizophrenics: IV Results and implications. *Arch. Gen. Psychiatry* **12**, 201–202.

Slater E. (1938) Zur Erbpathologie des Manisch-depressiven Irreseins. Die Eltern und Kinder von Manisch-Depressiven. (Inheritance of manic-depressive insanity. The parents and children of manic-depressives.) *Z. Gesamte Neurol. Psychiat.* **163**, 1–147.

Slater E. (1966) Expectation of abnormality on paternal and maternal sides: a computational model. *J. Med. Genet.* **3**, 159–161.

Slater E., Beard A. W. and Glithero E. (1963) The schizophrenia-like psychoses of epilepsy. *Br. J. Psychiatry* **109**, 95–150.

Slater E. and Shields J. (1969) Genetical aspects of anxiety. In: Lader M. H. (ed.) *Studies in Anxiety. Br. J. Psychiatry* Special Publication No. 3.

Snaith R. P. (1968) A clinical investigation of phobias. *Br. J. Psychiatry* **114**, 673–697.

Taylor D. C. (1972) Mental state and temporal lobe epilepsy: a correlative account of 100 patients treated surgically. *Epilepsia* **13**, 727–765.

Tyrer P. and Alexander J. (1979) Classification of personality disorder. *Br. J. Psychiatry* **135**, 163–167.

Williams D. (1969) Neural factors related to habitual aggression. *Brain* **92**, 503–520.

Winokur A., March V. and Mendels J. (1980) Primary affective disorder in relatives of patients with anorexia nervosa. *Am. J. Psychiatry* **137**, 695–698.

World Health Organization, Expert Committee on Drug Dependence (1969) WHO Techn. Rep. Ser. 407.

Further reading list

General Works

Arthur R. J. (1971) *An Introduction to Social Psychiatry.* Harmondsworth, Penguin Books.

Crown S. (1981) *Practical Psychiatry, Vol. 1.* London, Northwood Books.

Silverstone T. and Barraclough B. (ed.) (1975) *Contemporary Psychiatry Br. J. Psychiatry.* Special Publications No. 9.

Sullivan H. S. (1954) *The Psychiatric Interview.* London, Tavistock.

The History of Psychological Medicine

Ellenberger H. F. (1970) *The Discovery of the Unconscious.* London, Allen Lane, The Penguin Press.

Wollheim R. (1971) *Freud.* London, Fontana-Collins.

Wyss D. (1966) *Depth Psychology: A Critical History.* London, Allen & Unwin.

Aetiology and General Principles

Mendels J. (1973) *Biological Psychiatry.* New York, Wiley.

Rutter M. (1972) *Maternal Deprivation Reassessed.* Harmondsworth, Penguin Books.

Slater E. and Cowie V. (1971) *The Genetics of Mental Disorders.* New York, Toronto, Oxford University Press.

General Symptomatology

Bickerstaff E. R. (1968) *Neurological Examination in Clinical Practice.* Oxford, Blackwell.

Costello C. F. (ed.) (1970) *Symptoms of Psychopathology: a Handbook.* New York, Wiley.

Eysenck H. J. (ed.) (1973) *Handbook of Abnormal Psychology,* 2nd ed. London, Pitman Medical.

Hamilton M. (ed.) (1974) *Fish's Clinical Psychopathology.* Bristol, Wright.

Hoenig J., Anderson E. W., Kenna J. C. and Blunden R. (1962) Clinical and psychological aspects of the mnestic syndrome. *J. Ment. Sci.* **108,** 541–559.

The Neuroses

Beech H. R. (ed.) (1974) *Obessional States.* London, Methuen.

Bruch H. (1966) *Eating Disorders.* London, Routledge & Kegan Paul.

Freud S. (1959) *The Complete Psychological Works,* Vol. I-XXIV. London, Hogarth Press.

Ladee G. A. (1966) *Hypochondriacal Syndromes.* Amsterdam, Elsevier.

Lader M. and Marks I. M. (1971) *Clinical Anxiety.* London, Heinemann Medical.

Marks I. M. (1969) *Fears and Phobias.* London, Heinemann Medical.

Psychopathic Personalities

Hare R. D. (1970) *Psychopathy: Theory and Research.* New York, Wiley.

Petrilowitsch N. (1966) Psychopathie und Neurose. *Psychiat. Neurol. (Basel)* **152,** 17–27.

Petrilowitsch N. and Baer R. (1967) Psychopathie 1945–1966. *Fortschr. Neurol. Psychiat.* **35,** 617–649.

Psychosomatic Disorders

Claridge G. (1973) Psychosomatic relations in physical disease. In: Eysenck H. J. (ed.) *Handbook of Abnormal Psychology,* 2nd ed., Ch. 19. London, Pitman Medical.

Hamilton M. (1955) *Psychosomatics.* London, Chapman & Hall.

Alcoholism and Drug Addiction

Glatt M. (1982) *Alcoholism.* Sevenoaks, Hodder & Stoughton.

Jellineck E. M. (1960) *The Disease Concept of Alcoholism,* 2nd ed. Newhaven, Hillhouse Press.

Phillipson R. V. (ed.) (1970) *Modern Trends in Drug Dependence and Alcoholism.* London, Butterworths.

Affective Disorders, including Manic-Depressive Disease

Angst J. (1966) *Zur Ätiologie und Nosologie Endogener Depressiver Psychosen.* (The Aetiology and Nosology of Endogenous Depressive Psychoses.) Berlin, Springer. (English translation published in *Foreign Psychiatry,* Spring 1973.)

Angst J. (ed.) (1973) *Classification and Prediction of Outcome of Depression.* Stuttgart, Schattaver.

Kendall R. E. (1968) *The Classification of Depressive Illnesses.* London, Oxford University Press.

Paykel P. S. (ed.) (1982) *Handbook of Affective Disorders.* Edinburgh, Churchill Livingstone.

Perris C. (1966) A study of bipolar (manic-depressive) and unipolar recurrent depressive psychoses. *Acta Psychiatr. Scand.* **42**, Suppl. 194.

Winokur G., Clayton P. and Woodruff R. A. (1969) *Manic-Depressive Illness.* St Louis, Mosby.

Schizophrenia and Paranoid States

Hamilton M. (ed.) (1984) *Fish's Schizophrenia,* (3rd ed.) Bristol, Wright.

Leonhard K. (1979) *The Classification of Endogenous Psychoses,* 5th ed. Chichester, Wiley.

Rosenthal D. and Kety S. S. (ed.) (1968) *The Transmission of Schizophrenia.* Oxford, Pergamon.

Wing J. K. and Brown G. W. (1970) *Institutionalism and Schizophrenia.* London, Cambridge University Press.

Organic States

Benson D. F. and Blumer D. (ed.) (1975) *Psychiatric Aspects of Neurologic Disease.* New York, Grune & Stratton.

Kennedy A. (1949) The organic reaction types. In: Rees J. R. (ed.) *Modern Practice in Psychological Medicine.* London, Butterworths Medical. Reprinted in *Abnormal Psychology* (1967), ed. M. Hamilton. Harmondsworth, Penguin Books.

Lishman W. A. (1978) *Organic Psychiatry.* Oxford, Blackwell Scientific.

Pincus J. H. and Tucker G. J. (1974) *Behavioural Neurology.* London, Oxford University Press.

Sexual Disorders

Bancroft J. (1974) *Deviant Sexual Behaviour.* Oxford, Clarendon Press.

Masters W. H. and Johnson V. E. (1970) *Human Sexual Inadequacy.* London, Churchill.

Treatment and Management

Abrams R. and Essman W. B. (ed.) (1982) *Electroconvulsive Therapy.* New York, Spectrum Publications Inc.

Bandura A. (1969) *Principles and Behaviour Modification.* London, Holt, Rinehart & Winston.
Detre T. P. and Jarecki H. G. (1971) *Modern Psychiatric Treatment.* Philadelphia, Lippincott.
Frank J. D. (1974) Therapeutic components of psychotherapy. *J. Nerv. Ment. Dis.* **159**, 325–342.
Hamilton M. (ed.) (1984) *Fish's Schizophrenia,* 3rd ed. Bristol, Wright.
Kadis A. L. et al. (1974) *Practicum of Group Psychotherapy.* New York, Harper & Row.
Malan D. H. (1963) *A Study of Brief Psychotherapy.* London, Tavistock Publications.
Morgan R. (1974) Industrial Therapy. *Br. J. Hosp. Med.* **11**, 231.
Silverstone T. and Turner P. (1974) *Drug Treatment in Psychiatry.* London, Routledge & Kegan Paul.

Psychiatry and the Law

Bluglass R. (1983) *A Guide to the Mental Health Act 1983.* Edinburgh, Churchill Livingstone.
Gibson E. (ed.) (1975) *Homicide in England and Wales, 1967–1971.* Home Office Study No. 31. London, HMSO.
de Reuck A. V. S. and Porter R. (ed.) (1968) *The Mentally Abnormal Offender.* A Ciba Foundation Symposium. London, Churchill.
Walker N. and McCabe S. (1973) *Crime and Insanity in England.* Volume II: *New Solutions and New Problems.* Edinburgh, University Press.
Whitlock F. A. (1963) *Criminal Responsibility and Mental Illness.* London, Butterworths.

Glossary

The purpose of this glossary is to help the newcomer to psychiatry and those without a medical training. It is not intended to be a psychiatric dictionary. The entries of technical phrases are to be found under the first letter of the first word. For example, 'Primary Gain' is to be found under the letter 'P'—not under the letter 'G'.

Abnormal Personality: A personality with traits which deviate markedly from what is generally accepted as normal. This deviation is a quantitative and not a qualitative one.

Absence: A temporary loss of consciousness due to epilepsy without any convulsive phenomena.

Active Algolagnia: A synonym for sadism (q.v.).

Affect: A sudden accentuation of emotion, which is intense, does not last long, and is often reactive. Also a synonym for mood.

Affective Disorder: Illnesses in which the central symptom is a disturbance of affect.

Agnosia: A failure to recognize a pattern of sensation presented in a given sensory channel. This is due to coarse brain disease. It can be classified according to the sensory channel affected, so that there is visual agnosia, auditory agnosia, tactile agnosia, and so on.

Agoraphobia: A morbid fear of open spaces.

Agraphia: A loss of ability to write in the absence of any disorder of the part of the nervous system responsible for hand movements.

Aim Inhibition: The child eliminates the erotic elements in his attachment to a loved object, but retains the feelings of love and tenderness towards the object. Some gratification of the original cathexis (q.v.) still occurs.

Akathisia: An unpleasant feeling of restlessness accompanied by over-activity which is produced by some phenothiazines.

Akinesia: A state in which the patient shows no voluntary movements.

Alcohol Addiction: This is recognized by the inability to stop drinking once the individual has begun to drink alcohol.

Alcoholism: This term is often used to designate heavy drinkers or alcohol addicts (q.v.). It is best restricted to those persons who have permanent mental or physical defects due to prolonged excessive consumption of alcohol.

Alexia: A loss of ability to read or an inability to learn to read in the absence of any disorder of the visual cortex and the oculomotor apparatus.

Allelomorphs: A pair of genes which determine the inheritance of a particular character.

Alogia: Negative formal thought disorder (see *Formal Thought Disorder*).

Amentia: Sometimes used in Britain as a synonym for mental defect. In German-speaking countries it means a subacute delirious state.

Aminehypothesis: The hypothesis that depressive illness is associated with a functional deficiency of cerebral mono-amines noradrenalin and serotonin.

Amnesia: A loss of memory.

Amnestic Syndrome (Amnestic State): A subacute organic psychiatric state in which the presenting features are difficulty in the registration of new memories, confabulation and complete disorientation for time and place. Comprehension is disordered and there is 'tram-line' thinking. Also called the 'Korsakoff State' or 'Korsakoff Syndrome'.

Anal Eroticism: The enjoyment of the sensations which occur during defecation and the voluntary retention of faeces. According to Freudian theory this occurs in the anal sadistic stage of libidinal development.

Analytical Psychology: The psychological theories of C. G. Jung.

Anankastic Personality (Anankast): The overmeticulous, rigid, precise individual often referred to in Britain as an obsessional personality and in the USA as a compulsive personality. Personalities of this kind may or may not have obsessions and compulsions.

Anorexia: Loss of appetite.

Anorexia Nervosa: A complete loss of appetite in adolescent or young adult females, associated with overactivity, the cessation of menstruation, and fine downy hair over the back.

Anterograde Amnesia: Loss of memory for a period of time, during which the subject is apparently conscious.

Anticathexis: According to Freud some unconscious ideas are likely to produce emotional conflict if they appear in consciousness. Opposing ideas are, therefore, given a charge of instinctual energy in order to keep the troublesome ideas out of consciousness. This process, which forms the basis of repression (q.v.), is anticathexis. (See also *Cathexis.*)

Anxiety: An unpleasant affective state with the expectation but not the certainty of something unpleasant happening.

Anxiety–Elation Psychosis: A cycloid psychosis (q.v.) in which there is either a clinical picture of severe anxiety with ideas of reference or ecstasy with a desire to help others.

Anxiety Hysteria: This term was first used by Freud for a variety of hysteria (q.v.), in which the anxiety was localized to one situation and appeared as a phobia (q.v.). It has also been used by some psychiatrists to describe states in which, unlike classic conversion hysteria, there is a mixture of anxiety and conversion symptoms. It is best regarded as an outmoded term.

Anxiety State: A psychogenic reaction in which a normal person is reacting to severe stress or an abnormal person to mild stress. Marked anxiety may be a presenting symptom in depression, in schizophrenia, or in an organic state.

Aphasia: A central disorder of speech in which the necessary pathways to and from the brain are not disordered. (See *dysphasia.*)

Aphonia: Loss of ability to phonate, so that the subject can only whisper. It is not uncommon in hysteria.

Apophanous Idea: A delusional idea which suddenly appears in consciousness with no previous preparation. It is also known as an autochthonous or sudden delusional idea.

Apophanous Mood: A strange uncanny mood state in which the patient feels that there is something happening around him, but he does not know what it is. A delusional mood.

Apophanous Perception: A new significance is attributed to a perception, usually in the sense of self-reference, in the absence of any emotional or rational cause.

Apophany: A state in which one or more psychological phenomena acquire a new delusional significance, i.e. primary delusional experiences or experiences of significance are occurring.

Archetype: A Jungian term for the psychological expression of an instinct which is to be found in the collective unconscious (q.v.). Also used for collective images which are frequently found in the unconscious.

Asyndetic Thinking: Cameron's term for positive formal thought disorder. (See *Formal Thought Disorder.*)

Athletic Physique: One of Kretschmer's three types of physique, in which there is a marked development of the skeleton and the musculature.

Aura: A sensation or other psychological phenomenon, which occurs immediately before the onset of an epileptic fit.

Autism: A turning away from reality and an excessive indulgence in fantasy thinking.

Autistic Thinking: Excessive fantasy thinking. Also known as dereistic thinking.

Autochthonous Delusion: See *Apophanous Idea.*

Auto-Eroticism: Masturbation (q.v.).

Autonomous Dysthymia: A depressive illness in which the mood is qualitatively changed and in which early morning wakening, diurnal mood variation, and overvalued or delusional ideas associated with the patient's basic worries usually occur. The illness may or may not be provoked by some external event, but once it begins its course it is relatively independent of the causal event and the environment.

Belle Indifférence: Bland indifference in the presence of a hysterical conversion symptom.

Bell's Mania: Acute delirious mania; probably a severe attack of mania with delirium due to exhaustion, malnutrition, drugs, or intercurrent infection.

Bender: Alcoholic jargon for a period of continuous drinking which lasts for a few days and stops because of lack of money or physical exhaustion.

Bestiality: Sexual relations with an animal. Also known as 'erotic zoophilia'.

Binovular Twins: Twins who have developed from different fertilized ova and therefore have different genetic constitutions.

Bisexuality: In psychoanalytic writings this expresses the fact that all human beings have conscious or unconscious feelings for individuals of both sexes. Strictly it means the ability to have sexual experiences with both sexes.

Blackout: In Britain this word usually means a loss of consciousness or a loss of memory. As a technical term it designates a loss of memory occurring after a few drinks of hard liquor, not sufficient to produce drunkenness. This marks the onset of the prodromal stage of alcohol addiction and is also known as a 'palimpsest'.

Body Image: This is the organization of all the sensory input from the body to form an image of 'schema', which acts as a system of reference for all bodily activities.

Bradyphrenia: A slowing down of mental processes, particularly applied to the slow mental activity in post-encephalitics.

Broca's Area: An area at the posterior end of the third left frontal convolution of the brain. Broca claimed that it was responsible for articulation, but it is now believed to be the area of the brain which is responsible for the final organization of the motor aspects of speech.

Bromism: Poisoning with bromides, usually due to the administration of medicines containing bromide. A blood level of 200 mg per 100 ml is associated with bromism in normal subjects, but in elderly patients bromism may occur at blood bromide levels between 100 and 200 mg per 100 ml. It is unusual for blood levels below 100 mg per 100 ml to be associated with symptoms.

Castration Complex: An unconscious group of ideas associated with anxiety and consisting of the fantasy that the penis or clitoris will be removed by the parent of the same sex. This complex arises at the Oedipal stage of libidinal development, when the child has sexual desires for the parent of the opposite sex.

Catalepsy: A synonym for flexibilitas cerea (q.v.).

Cataplexy: A sudden loss of all power of movement and loss of all muscle tone without loss of consciousness. This is often associated with narcolepsy (q.v.).

Catatonia: A variety of schizophrenia in which the outstanding symptoms are disorders of motor behaviour.

Catharsis: Literally 'purgation'. Used in psychiatry for the relief obtained by the intense expression of the emotion associated with an unpleasant experience or a conflict.

Cathexis: Freud suggested that every idea was charged with instinctual energy, which supplied the impetus for the expression of the idea. This attachment of a charge of instinctual energy to an idea is a cathexis.

Chromosome: These are microscopical structures into which the nucleus divides at the beginning of cell division. Later, each chromosome divides into two equal portions. Chromosomes occur in homologous pairs and carry genes (q.v.). Each species has its specific number of chromosomes and in humans this is 46. Since the individual develops from the fusion of two sex cells it is necessary for the number of chromosomes to be halved at some stage in the development of the sex cells. This occurs in a special kind of cell division called 'reduction division' or 'meiosis'.

Clang Associations: Two thoughts are associated on the basis of rhyme or assonance.

Coitus Interruptus: The removal of the penis from the vagina during sexual intercourse, so that the ejaculation occurs outside the vagina. A common but unsafe method of birth control. Freud believed that this gave rise to anxiety.

Coitus Reservatus: Cessation of sexual intercourse before either party has had an orgasm.

Collective Unconscious: The part of the unconscious which Jung considered was not personal to the individual but was a part of the inheritance of the human race.

Coma: A state of unconsciousness due to acute coarse brain disease from which the patient cannot be roused.

Complex: A group of repressed ideas and the affects associated with them.

Compulsion: An act which the patient feels compelled to carry out, although he realizes it is senseless and that he is not being directed by outside influences. (See also *Obsession.*)

Concrete Attitude: Goldstein claimed that this attitude occurred in coarse brain disease and in schizophrenia. The patient is unable to think abstractly and to get away from the concrete aspects of the situation.

Condensation: The fusion of heterogenous elements of thoughts, based on non-logical associations. A feature of the primary process (q.v.), which is seen clearly in dreams and in schizophrenic thinking.

Conditional Reflex: Also incorrectly called a 'conditioned reflex'. A neutral stimulus is regularly applied to an animal just before and during the application of a stimulus which is known to produce an unlearned response. After some time the neutral stimulus is capable of eliciting the response. A conditional reflex has been formed and the previously neutral stimulus has now become a conditional stimulus.

Confabulation: Detailed plastic false memories. These are classically seen in the amnestic state, but also occur in some chronic schizophrenics and appreciation-needing psychopaths.

Confusion: This term is often used somewhat loosely for perplexity or bewilderment. Strictly it should be reserved for those patients who show clear evidence of disorientation for time and place.

Confusional State: A low-grade delirium, usually worse at night and associated with some degree of incoherence. The term 'subacute delirious state' suggested by Mayer-Gross, Slater, and Roth is more appropriate.

Confusion Psychosis: A cycloid psychosis (q.v.), in which there is either a state of excited incoherence or a poverty of speech with perplexity.

Constitution: The total psychological make-up of the individual due to the interaction, up to the time of consideration, of the inherited predispositions, chance physical damage to the brain, and environmental influences.

Conversion Hysteria: The partial solution of a psychological conflict by the conversion of the conflict into a physical or mental symptom.

Coprophagia: Eating faeces. Occurs in young children, idiots, dements, and some deteriorated schizophrenics.

Creutzfeldt-Jakob Disease: A presenile dementia in which lesions occur in the cerebral cortex, the basal ganglia and the motor cells of the spinal cord.

Cunnilingus: The application of the mouth and the tongue to the vulva, clitoris, or anterior vagina.

Curator Bonis: A receiver appointed by a Scottish court to administer the financial affairs of someone who is mentally unfit to do so.

Cycloid Psychoses: A group of recurrent mental disorders in which, although the symptomatology is reminiscent of schizophrenia, complete recovery occurs.

Cyclothymia: Used variously to mean manic-depressive insanity and the mood variation of the cyclothymic personality (q.v.).

Cyclothymic Personality: One of the four types of personality associated with manic-depressive insanity. The mood is elevated for several days or weeks and then is depressed for a similar period, after which a period of elation occurs, and so on.

Delirium: An acute organic psychiatric state in which consciousness is changed in a dream-like way.

Delusion: An unshakeable belief which is out of keeping with the patient's educational, cultural and social background.

Dementia: A permanent loss of intellectual function due to coarse brain disease.

Dementia Praecox: A misleading, out-of-date synonym for schizophrenia (q.v.).

Depersonalization: The subjective experience of a change in the personality whereby it seems unable to make contact with the outside world.

Derealization: The subjective experience of unreality of the environment, although the subject knows that it is real. This usually occurs in association with depersonalization.

Dereistic Thinking: Synonym for autistic thinking (q.v.).

Dipsomania: Recurrent bouts of excessive drinking. These patients are not alcohol addicts, but episodic psychopaths who from time to time are unable to tolerate the tedium of everyday life.

Displacement: The use of an associated word or concept in place of the correct word or concept. This occurs in the primary process (q.v.) and can be seen in neurotic symptom formation, dreams, and schizophrenic thinking.

Dissociation: A mental mechanism which splits off from consciousness some mental contents which are troubling the conscious mind.

Dominant Inheritance: The inherited character appears in the phenotype (q.v.) when only one member of the allelomorphic gene pair which carry the character is present.

Drug Addiction: A psychological or physical dependence on the effects of a drug, which leads to an overpowering need for the drug and to obtaining it by any means.

Dysmnesia Syndrome: A suggested synonym for amnestic syndrome (q.v.).

Dysphasia: Since aphasia (q.v.) literally means an *absence* of speech rather than a disorder of speech, some use the term 'dysphasia' instead.

Dysplastic Physique: A physique which shows some features of all the three basic Kretschmerian types.

Dysthymia: An unpleasant mood state. (See also *Autonomous Dysthymia.*)

Echolalia: The patient automatically repeats the words spoken by the examiner.

Echopraxia: The patient automatically repeats the actions carried out by the examiner.

Ecstasy: A state of exaltation which can be seen in epilepsy, in schizophrenia and in abnormal personalities.

Ego: Freud used this term for that part of the mind whose contents are potentially conscious and which balances the demands made by the real world, the superego (q.v.) and the id (q.v.).

Ego Ideal: The conscious standards which the individual sets himself to achieve.

Ego Psychology: Freud paid little attention to the ego and considered that it derived its psychic energy from the id and superego. Some of his pupils, notably Anna Freud, Hartmann, and Federn, have developed the psychoanalytic theory of the ego, which is usually called 'ego psychology'.

Ejaculatio Praecox: Ejaculation before or immediately after the insertion of the penis into the vagina.

Electroconvulsive Treatment (ECT): An epileptic fit is produced by the passage of an electric current through the head by means of electrodes applied to the temples. Useful in the treatment of depression and depressive and catatonic symptoms in schizophrenia.

Electroplexy: Synonym for electroconvulsive treatment.

Emotion: 'The felt tendency toward anything intuitively appraised as good (beneficial), or away from anything intuitively appraised as bad (harmful). This attraction or aversion is accompanied by a pattern of physiological changes organized towards approach or withdrawal' (Arnold).

Emotional Incontinence: Synonym for lability of affect (q.v.).

Empathy: The ability to feel oneself into the situation of another person.

Endogenous Depression: A depressive illness believed to be due to a constitutional predisposition. Some psychiatrists believe that such illnesses cannot be provoked by external events and that depressions produced in this way are 'reactive' or 'neurotic'. The view taken in this book is that depressive illness can be provoked by psychological trauma, but its subsequent course is independent of the provoking factors. If this is the case the illness, although constitutionally determined, cannot be called 'endogenous'. (See also *Autonomous Dysthymia.*)

Erotogenic Zones: Areas of the body, usually mucocutaneous junctions, which, when stimulated, give rise to erotic feelings. According to psychoanalytic theory the different stages of libidinal development are related to the primacy of a particular erotogenic zone.

Essential Hypertension: A condition in which the blood pressure is permanently raised for no known reason. This is supposed to be a psychosomatic disorder (q.v.).

Euphoria: A mild persistent elevation of mood, usually associated with a sense of bodily well-being known as 'eutonia'.

Exhibitionism: Loosely used by the laity to mean 'showing off'. Technically it is used for the sexual perversion in which sexual pleasure is obtained from exposing the genitals to another person.

Existentialism: A philosophical trend which tries to place the individual in the middle of the world and to derive the meaning of his existence from the individual himself.

Experimental Neurosis: Non-adaptive behaviour produced in animals by presenting them with an insoluble problem or some other frustrating situation. Also called 'animal neurosis'. Similar conditions can be produced experimentally in humans. The relationship of these states to naturally occurring human neurosis is not clear.

Extraversion: Jung divided personalities into two groups; those who turned their psychic energy outwards and made relationships with others very easily, and those who turned their psychic energy inwards and lived more in their inner fantasies. The first type were called 'extraverts', because they turn their psychic energy outwards, while the second group were called 'introverts' (q.v.).

Fellatio: Licking or sucking the penis.

Fetishism: Obtaining sexual pleasure from an inanimate object.

Fixation: Freud described three main stages of infantile sexual development at which conflicts could occur. If a conflict at one of these stages is not fully resolved then fixation is said to have occurred. This is because some of the libido or instinctual energy is fixed at this point which is called the 'fixation point'.

Flexibilitas Cerea: A waxy flexibility, in which the patient allows the examiner to put his body in any position and maintains the new position for 30 seconds or more.

Flight of Ideas: A rapid progress of thought in which the individual elements are not rationally connected, but where their sequence depends on chance association, particularly on rhyming and assonance (see *Clang Associations*). This disorder characteristically occurs in mania but it is occasionally seen in schizophrenia and in organic states.

Folie à Deux: Induced insanity, in which one member of a household, who is aggressive and assertive, develops a paranoid illness which is imposed on a more submissive partner. When the two partners are separated the induced insanity disappears.

Forepleasure: The enjoyment of sexual play before the insertion of the penis.

Formal Thought Disorder: A disorder of conceptual thinking in someone who has previously been able to think conceptually. It may be negative, when the patient is unable to form concepts; or it may be positive, when the patient produces false concepts by means of condensation, displacement, or the misuse of symbols.

Frigidity: The failure of a woman to achieve an orgasm during sexual intercourse.

Fugue: A wandering state which may occur in hysteria or depressive illness.

Functional: This adjective is used by English-speaking physicians to mean that they can find no physical disease and that the illness is therefore psychogenic.

Functional Psychosis: This term is used to designate manic-depressive disease and schizophrenia, since they are both serious mental illnesses in which no physical changes in the brain have so far been found. It is a convenient term, but it must be remembered that the words 'functional' and 'psychosis' cannot be properly defined.

Ganser State (Ganserism): Simulated madness, in which the patient behaves in such a way as a lay person would expect a madman to behave. He gives approximate answers which show that he knows the correct answer. Despite an apparent absence of all knowledge these patients can wash, dress and take care of themselves. Also known as 'hysterical pseudodementia'.

Gene: A hereditary factor present in every cell. Any one inherited character is determined by two genes which form a pair known as allelomorphs.

General Paralysis of the Insane (GPI; General Paresis): A dementia associated with a spastic paralysis of all limbs due to syphilis.

Genotype: The genetic constitution of the individual, as opposed to the phenotype (q.v.), which is the physical expression of the genetic structure.

Gerstmann's Syndrome: Inability to calculate, agraphia, finger agnosia and right-left disorientation due to lesion of the left angular gyrus in the right-handed.

Globus Hystericus: The complaint of a lump in the throat and difficulty in swallowing found in some hysterical patients.

Grandiosity: The patient believes that he is much more important than he really is. This may occur in mania, in schizophrenia and in general paresis.

Guardianship: Most European countries have legal provisions which allow a mentally ill, psychopathic, or mentally defective person to be deprived of his civil rights to some degree. The patient is placed in the care of a guardian in order to prevent him from wasting his resources, being exploited by others, or exposing his dependants to unnecessary hardship.

Hallucination: A perception without an external object.

Hallucinosis: A state in which hallucinations are continuously present.

Hebephrenia: A variety of schizophrenia in which the outstanding feature is the disorder of affective expression.

Hemi-Anaesthesia: A loss of sensation over one half of the body.

Hemiparesis: A weakness on one side of the body.

Hemiplegia: A loss of power in one half of the body.

Heterosexuality: Sexual desires and practices between members of the opposite sexes.

Heterozygote: An individual who has an allelomorphic pair of genes which are dissimilar.

Homosexuality: Sexual desires and practices between members of the same sex.

Homozygote: An individual who has a pair of allelomorphic genes for a given character which are similar.

Hyperkinesia: A state of continuous overactivity of the voluntary muscles.

Hypertension: Raised blood-pressure.

Hypnagogic Hallucinations: Hallucinations occurring as the subject is falling asleep. They may occur in any sense modality but are usually visual or auditory.

Hypnopompic Hallucinations: Hallucinations occurring as the sleeper is waking up.

Hypochondriacal Delusions: Delusions of bodily ill-health.

Hypochondriasis: A state of mind in which the patient believes or is afraid that he has a bodily illness, although there is no evidence to support such ideas.

Hypomania: Mild mania, in which there are euphoria, overactivity and prolixity without any flight of ideas. The patient is usually able to put on a good front for a short period and to rationalize his previous unruly behaviour.

Hypothermia: A body temperature below the normal range.

Hysteria: A mental illness in which the symptoms are unconsciously motivated.

Hysterical Personality: An individual who needs to be appreciated and does not get the necessary appreciation without behaving in an unusual way. As these patients do not necessarily suffer from hysterical illness a better term is 'appreciation-needing personality'.

Hysterical Pseudodementia: A synonym for Ganser state (q.v.).

Iatrogenic Illness: A condition produced by the side-effects of treatment, whether surgical, drug or psychotherapeutic.

Ictal: Appertaining to an epileptic fit.

Ictus: An epileptic fit. This term is not often used in Britain.

Id: The unorganized, instinctual, unconscious part of the mind postulated by Freud.

Identification: This term is used in two ways by psychoanalysts. It can be used for the mental mechanism which operates when the individual takes on the attitudes and ideas of another person, or for the way in which the ego identifies one object with another.

Idiots: Before the Mental Health Act 1959, the legal meaning of this term was: 'Persons so deeply defective in mind from birth, or from an early age, as to be unable to guard themselves against common physical dangers.'

Illusion: A false perception based on an incorrect interpretation of an external stimulus.

Imago: An unconscious organized image.

Incest: Sexual relations between close blood relatives. According to psychoanalytic theory unconscious incest wishes occur in everyone.

Incoherent Thinking: Thought in which no understandable connection between successive thoughts can be found.

Individual Psychology: The psychological theories of Alfred Adler.

Induced Insanity: Synonym for folie à deux (q.v.).

Introjection: The mental mechanism by which an object is incorporated into the mind; rather like the way in which food is incorporated into the body.

Introversion: In psychoanalytic theory this is the turning back of the libidinal energy on to the ego, because an object has been lost and the libido attached to it has been set free. This is the initial stage in a neurosis. In Jungian theory introversion is the attitude of turning in on oneself and living one's own fantasies.

Introvert: A person whose reactions and attitudes are mainly determined by his inner life.

Inversion: A synonym for homosexuality.

Invert: A homosexual; but sometimes used for a male homosexual who has very feminine ways.

Involution: Retrogressive physical and psychological changes occurring in middle life. In women it occurs between 40 and 55 years of age and in men between 45 and 60 years of age.

Involutional Melancholia: A severe depressive illness occurring in the involution; characterized by marked agitation, severe hypochondriasis (especially affecting the bowels) and by delusions of guilt and persecution. Sometimes this term is used very loosely for agitated depressions in middle life.

Isolation: A mental mechanism, particularly seen in obsessional states, in which complexes lose their emotional charge and their ideational associations, so that the idea may appear in consciousness without the emotion, and vice versa.

Jacksonian Epilepsy: The fit begins in one part of the body, usually the thumb or big toe, and spreads through the limb until the whole body is affected and consciousness is lost. This is due to a focal lesion of the part of the brain immediately responsible for motor activity. Also known as 'focal epilepsy'.

Korsakoff's Psychosis: An amnestic syndrome (q.v.) or 'Korsakoff state', together with polyneuritis, usually due to prolonged abuse of alcohol. Korsakoff was a famous Russian psychiatrist who, of course, wrote his name in Cyrillic script. Unfortunately when he wrote in German he transliterated his name in at least two different ways. The spellings 'Korsakov' and 'Korsakow' are to be found in the literature. The spelling given here was used by Korsakoff himself on at least one occasion.

Lability of Affect: The patient suddenly bursts into tears or explodes into laughter as the result of a very slight emotional stimulus, or even in the absence of any obvious emotional stimulus. Sudden weeping is much more common than sudden laughter. This symptom occurs in psychiatric organic states, particularly in arteriosclerotic dementia.

Latency Period: According to Freudian theory infantile sexual development ceases at about 4–5 years of age and is followed by the latency period in which there is little interest in sex. This lasts until the onset of puberty.

Leptosome: The leptosomic or asthenic body-build is the thin bony habitus with poorly developed musculature. Usually the nose is large and the chin recedes, giving rise to the so-called angle profile. Kretschmer, who described this body-build, claimed that it was often found in schizophrenics.

Leucotomy: More correctly, 'prefrontal leucotomy'. A neurosurgical operation in which the fibres connecting the frontal lobes and the thalami are cut.

Libido: Generally used to mean sexual desire and drive. In the Freudian sense it means sexual instinct and the psychic energy associated with it.

Lilliputian Hallucinations: Visual hallucinations in which small human beings or animals are seen.

Lobotomy: An American synonym for leucotomy (q.v.).

Logoclonia: The repeated utterance of parts of a word. This occurs in coarse brain disease, particularly in Alzheimer's disease.

Macropsia: An illusion in which objects appear larger than normal.

Mania: A mental illness characterized by elevated mood, flight of ideas and overactivity.

Mania à potu: Pathological intoxication (q.v.).

Mannerism: A strange stilted execution of a voluntary action or a distortion of a normal posture.

Masochism: Sexual satisfaction obtained from the experience of pain and discomfort.

Masturbation: The subject produces sexual satisfaction by stimulating his own genitals or other areas, e.g. the anus, likely to cause sexual pleasure. Also inaccurately called 'onanism' (q.v.).

Megalomania: A psychosis with delusions of grandeur. A term not much used by English-speaking psychiatrists today.

Mental Disorder: The Mental Health Act 1983 defines this as: 'Mental illness, arrested or incomplete development of the mind, psychopathic disorder, and any other disorder or disability of mind.'

Mental Health Officer: An official of a Scottish local authority who has certain duties laid down by the Mental Health (Scotland) Act 1960.

Mental Impairment: The Mental Health Act 1983 defines this as 'a state of significant impairment of intelligence and social functioning, associated with abnormally aggressive or seriously irresponsible conduct on the part of the person concerned'. Severe mental impairment signifies the same when disabilities are severe.

Mental Welfare Officer: The English equivalent of a Mental Health Officer.

Metapsychology: Freud used this term for what is now usually called 'depth psychology', in order to express his concept that mental functioning depends on factors outside consciousness. It is now used for the psychoanalytic theory which takes into account the dynamics, structure and economics of the mind.

Micropsia: An illusion in which objects appear smaller than usual.

Moral Imbecile: A person with no moral scruples, with or without some degree of mental defect.

Moral Insanity: This term was first introduced by Pritchard to designate that variety of insanity in which there were no delusions. The word 'moral' in the early nineteenth century meant much the same as the word 'psychological' today. By the middle of the nineteenth century the term 'moral insanity' was used to describe persons who would now be called 'psychopaths' and 'alcohol addicts'.

Mutism: Absence of speech from any cause.

Narcissism: Primary narcissim is the first stage of ego organization, in which the child does not differentiate between himself and the environment, so that the world is the child's ego. In secondary narcissism the structure of the mind has fully developed and libido which has been attached to objects is withdrawn from them and becomes attached to the ego.

Narcolepsy: Sudden attacks of irresistible need to sleep.

Negativism: Often used loosely for any refusal of a patient to make personal contact with an examiner or to carry out reasonable requests made by him. Kleist used this term for active resistance to all interference.

Neurasthenia: Literally 'tired nerves'. First applied to neuroses in which the outstanding feature was fatigue. As the complaint of tiredness may be a leading symptom in acute and chronic anxiety states, depressive illness and mild coarse brain disease, it is best avoided, but it can be used on insurance certificates.

Neurone: The cell which forms the basic unit of the nervous system. These cells are capable of being excited by others and transmit the excitation to other neurones.

Neuropsychiatry: A popular term in the USA and in the British Armed Forces in World War II. Both psychiatry and neurology are separate specialties, the former being the more important.

Nihilistic Delusions: The patient believes he is dead and that everything around him is dead or reduced to nothing.

Object: A psychoanalytic term designating a person or thing which is invested with libido and which gratifies instinctual urges.

Object Choice: A selection of an object in the psychoanalytic sense.

Object Libido: The energy of the sexual instinct which is attached to objects.

Obsession: A content of consciousness which cannot be got rid of, although when it occurs it is judged to be senseless or at least as dominating without cause. The essential feature is that this experience occurs against the patient's will, but it is recognized as his *own* thought. A compulsion is the motor expression of an obsession.

Obsessional State: An illness characterized by severe obsessions.

Oedipus Complex: A set of ideas centring around the desire to have sexual relations with the parent of the opposite sex. Oedipus was a king in Greek mythology who unwittingly killed his father and married his mother.

Onanism: Used by German-speaking and psychoanalytic writers as a synonym for masturbation. This shows a lack of Biblical scholarship, for although Onan 'spilled his seed upon the ground' he was indulging in coitus interruptus and not masturbation.

Oral Eroticism: Sexual excitement from stimulation of the lips and mouth.

Organ Neurosis: Used by psychoanalysts as a synonym for psycho-somatic disorders. It has also been used for anxiety states in which the anxiety symptoms have become restricted to one physical system, e.g. cardiac neurosis, in which the anxiety symptoms are held to be due to a cardiovascular disorder.

Orientation: Used in psychiatry to mean that the patient knows who he is, where he is and what time it is. This is referred to as 'orientation for person, place and time'. Loss of orientation is called 'confusion' and occurs in organic states.

Palilalia: A form of perseveration in which a word is repeated with increasing frequency.

Palimpsest: See *Blackout.*

Paraesthesia: Unpleasant tingling sensations.

Paralogia: This term has been used for several different phenomena. Kraepelin used it for 'talking past the point' or *Vorbeireden* (q.v.). Kleist used it for positive formal thought disorder.

Paranoia: Originally meant delusional insanity, but Kraepelin used it for a group of patients who had marked paranoid delusions, but showed little in the way of psychological disorders apart from the delusions.

Paraphasia: A variety of speech disorder in which the subject chooses the wrong word or uses a non-existent one.

Paraphrenia: A schizophrenic illness in which there are marked paranoid delusions and auditory hallucinations without deterioration of personality.

Paresis: Weakness of a muscle or group of muscles.

Parkinsonism: A syndrome due to disorders of the basal ganglia, consisting of rigidity, tremor, a mask-like face and a posture of slight generalized flexion. A reversible Parkinsonism, known as 'pseudo-parkinsonism', is produced by phenothiazines, reserpine, haloperidol, and other neuroleptics.

Passive Algolagnia: A synonym for masochism (q.v.).

Pathogenic: Causative of disease.

Pathognomonic: Characteristic of a given disease.

Pathological Intoxication: A twilight state with extreme violence which occurs after a slight to moderate intake of alcohol in the absence of the signs of drunkenness. The patient has no memory for the episode.

Pathoplastic Factors: Those factors with modify the clinical features and the course of illness and are not directly related to the psychological disorder.

Peptic Ulcer: An ulcer occurring in the stomach, in the first part of the duodenum, or in any place where there is gastric mucosa.

Persona: The part of the mind which the individual presents to the world.

Pfropfhebephrenia (Pfropfschizophrenia): Schizophrenia occurring in a mental defective. Also called 'grafted schizophrenia', which is a direct translation of this German term.

Phallic Phase: The last stage of infantile sexual development when sexual excitement is centred on the genitals.

Phantom Limb: The sensation that the limb is present after it has been amputated. Sometimes very painful.

Phenotype: The total characteristics of an organism which are an expression of its genetic constitution. Because of the dominance of some genes, the presence of genetic modifiers, and chance factors, the genetic constitution can only be partially expressed in the phenotype.

Phobia: A morbid fear. There are three varieties: (1) conditioned phobias which are learned in childhood; (2) obsessional phobias; and (3) hysterical phobias.

Pleasure–Pain Principle: Freud postulated that the id tended to try to avoid pain and to gratify primitive impulses with no consideration for reality.

Post-traumatic Amnesia: Loss of memory following injury to the brain. The duration of this amnesia is directly proportional to the severity of the brain damage.

Primary Delusion: A delusion which cannot be derived from some other psychological event. (See *Apophany.*)

Primary Gain: When a conflict is partly solved by the production of a hysterical conversion symptom there is some relief from anxiety, so that there is a primary gain from the hysterical illness.

Primary Process: The direct expression of the unconscious instinctual drives. It is illogical and disregards space and time.

Process: Schizophrenia produces a sharp break in the natural development of the personality in the same way as an organic process affecting the brain. This has led to the assumption that schizophrenia is due to some organic process affecting the finer mechanisms of the brain. Different authors have claimed that different groups of symptoms are 'process symptoms' indicating an active schizophrenic illness. In American literature the term 'process schizophrenia' is used to indicate schizophrenia which leads to a deterioration of the personality.

Process Course of Illness: The type of schizophrenia which runs a steady downhill course.

Process Schizophrenia: See *Process.*

Prodromas: The initial signs of illness which occur before the pathognomonic signs.

Projection: A mental mechanism whereby repressed unwanted ideas and attitudes are attributed to others.

Projection Test: A test in which incompletely structured material is presented to a patient and he is required to describe what he sees or to construct a story based on the material.

Pseudodementia: See *Ganser State.*

Pseudohallucinations: Hallucinations which lack the lively character of perceptions and can be distinguished from real perceptions.

Pseudologia Fantastica: Fantastic lying by appreciation-needing (hysterical) psychopaths.

Psychic Reality: Reality as it appears to the patient.

Psychoanalysis: Originally a special technique of psychological treatment based on free association. It also means the theories elaborated by Freud and his followers.

Psychogenic: A disorder produced by psychological factors. It should be noted that not all psychogenic disorders are hysterical since this latter term implies the presence of unconscious motivation.

Psychogenic Reaction: A reaction of an individual to psychological trauma. The symptomatology will depend on the personality, the intelligence and the social background of the individual and on the nature of the trauma.

Psychopathic Disorder: This is defined by the Mental Health Act 1983 as a persistent disorder or disability of mind (whether or not including subnormality of intelligence) which results in abnormally aggressive or seriously irresponsible conduct on the part of the person concerned. Promiscuity or immoral conduct, sexual deviance or dependence on alcohol or drugs, by themselves do not fall within the categories of mental disorder.

Psychopathic Personality (Psychopath): Most English-speaking psychiatrists use this term for antisocial individuals who have been emotionally unstable from childhood or adolescence, have a normal intelligence, are only certifiably insane for short periods, lack foresight and fail to learn from punishment. German-speaking psychiatrists tend to regard psychopathic personalities as grossly abnormal people and accept Schneider's definition: 'Abnormal personalities. . . who suffer from their abnormality or cause society to suffer from their abnormality.'

Psychosomatic Disorders: Often used loosely for the physical expression of psychological disorders. It is best restricted to those disorders in which psychological factors appear to play an important part in producing a disorder of the function or the structure of the body. If the disorder is one of function it is not one which is normally associated with emotion and cannot be imagined by the subject.

Pyknic: A physique described by Kretschmer who claimed that it was the commonest body-build among manic-depressives. The head is spheroidal, the face round, the neck short, the thoracic and abdominal cavities are voluminous, and the limbs are well proportioned and rather graceful.

Pyromania: Fire-setting carried out for pleasure.

Rationalization: The production of a rational explanation for an emotionally determined pattern of behaviour.

Reaction: This is used rather loosely for any change in the psychological state which is brought about by external events which do not damage the brain. Jaspers has defined a reactive psychiatric illness as 'one in which there is a clear relation between the illness and the alleged cause; the content of the illness is the same as the cause, and if the cause can be reversed the illness will disappear'.

Reaction Formation: This is a mental mechanism in which unconscious complexes are kept out of consciousness by the presence of the opposite set of ideas in consciousness. For example, unconscious sexual desires may be kept in check by a conscious prudish attitude.

Reactive Depression: This term is used by many English-speaking psychiatrists in a rather ill-defined way. It can mean a state of unhappiness which has occurred as a response to some psychological trauma or, in other words, excessive normal unhappiness. It can also mean a depressive illness which has been provoked by a psychological upset or in which the symptoms fluctuate in response to environmental changes.

Recessive Inheritance: This is when the manifestation of an inherited character does not occur unless members of the given allelomorphic pair of genes are identical. This means that the affected person must receive a similar gene from each parent, so that disorders with a recessive inheritance appear in a sibship and affect one-quarter of the offspring of the union.

Reduction Division: The division of the precursors of the sex cells, ovum and spermatozoon, in which the number of chromosomes is halved.

Regression: This occurs when the organization of the mind passes back to a level corresponding to an earlier stage of development. In psychoanalytic theory this is brought about by introversion (q.v.) of libido, which activates the more primitive levels of function.

Repression: An unconscious mental mechanism which prevents ideas and affects from becoming conscious.

Resistance: The unconscious opposition to free discussion of psychological problems during psychotherapy.

Retrograde Amnesia: Loss of memory for a period preceding an injury to the brain.

Ritual: Compulsions carried out in a rigid set way.

Sadism: A sexual perversion in which sexual enjoyment is obtained from the infliction of pain and degradation on the love object. Also used very loosely to indicate the enjoyment of the physical and psychological suffering of others.

Schizoid: This term means 'resembling schizophrenia' (q.v.), but is particularly used as an abbreviation for 'schizoid personality'. This indicates a shut-in withdrawn person who is more interested in his inner fantasy life than the real world. Kallmann has claimed that the schizoid is the heterozygote for the schizophrenic gene, while the schizophrenic is the homozygote. This is not in accordance with the facts.

Schizophasia: A variety of schizophrenia in which there is gross speech disorder which is often in marked contrast to the intelligence shown by the patient's general behaviour.

Schizophrenia: A group of mental disorders in which there is no coarse brain disease and in which many different clinical pictures can occur. The form and content of the symptoms cannot be understood as arising emotionally or rationally from the affective state, the previous personality, or the current situation, with the proviso that paranoid delusions are not diagnostic of schizophrenia in the absence of other clearly non-understandable symptoms.

Scoptophilia: Sexual enjoyment from watching nude men, women, or children, or from watching normal or perverse sexual activities.

Secondary Gain: The disability produced by a psychological illness may lead to environmental changes which are advantageous to the patient, so that, apart from the primary gain produced by the neurotic solution of the conflict, there is secondary gain due to favourable fortuitous changes in the environment.

Secondary Processes: These are the processes used by the ego to deal with the demands of the real world and to modify the demands made by the instinctual drives. They are therefore based on logical thinking in contrast to the illogical pictorial thinking of the primary process.

Sopor: A state of marked drowsiness in which the patient can make purposeful reactions to some stimuli.

Stupor: A state of motor inactivity usually associated with mutism or diminished verbal responses.

Subconscious: An unsatisfactory synonym for the unconscious (q.v.).

Sublimation: A mental mechanism in which there is a desexualization of the instinctual energy which is then used to support non-sexual drives.

Subnormality: The English legal term for moderate mental defect. It is defined as: 'A state of arrested or incomplete development of mind (not amounting to severe subnormality) which includes subnormality of intelligence and is of a nature or degree which requires or is susceptible to medical treatment or other special care or training of the patient'.

Superego: This is the part of the mind which imposes a moral censorship on the ego. It is formed in childhood by the child taking over what he considers to be the parental attitudes, so that the attitudes of the superego are often very severe and punitive.

Symbolism: An illogical variety of thinking in which symbols are used in a concrete way.

Syndrome: A group of symptoms and signs which tend to occur together and which are probably the expression of a disorder of function produced by one or more disease processes.

Thought Disorder: Sometimes used loosely for formal thought disorder (q.v.); but there are three other forms of thought disorder, namely, disorder of the stream of thought, the possession of thought and the content of thought.

Thyrotoxicosis: Overactivity of the thyroid gland causing overactivity, tremulousness, loss of weight and a hot moist skin. Thought to be a psychosomatic disorder (q.v.).

Transexualism: The delusion that the subject has the mind of the sex opposite to his or her anatomical sex.

Transference: The transference of an emotional attitude towards some important person in the individual's childhood on to someone else with whom the individual comes into contact. This particularly occurs in the treatment situation when the patient identifies the therapist with a parent or parental figure.

Transvestism: Sexual enjoyment from wearing the clothes of the opposite sex.

Traumatic Neurosis: A neurosis occurring after severe physical or psychological trauma. A useless term, best avoided.

Trisomy: Owing to faults in reduction division (q.v.) a germ cell may contain a pair of homologous chromosomes (q.v.) instead of the usual one. If this cell fertilizes or is fertilized by a normal sex cell then the new individual will have three chromosomes instead of the normal pair. This is trisomy, and trisomy of the twenty-first chromosome is responsible for many cases of mongolism, a form of mental defect.

Twilight State: A condition in which there is a restriction of consciousness due to coarse brain disease or anxiety.

Ulcerative Colitis: Ulceration of the lower part of the bowel of uncertain origin. Sometimes claimed to be a psychosomatic disorder (q.v.).

Unconscious: The Freudian unconscious is that part of the mind which cannot normally be made conscious. It is composed of the id (q.v.), a part of the superego (q.v.) and repressed material which has been conscious but has been pushed out of consciousness.

Uniovular Twins: Twins who have developed from the same fertilized ovum which split into two separate parts after the first division. These twins have exactly the same genetic constitution, so that if an inherited defect occurs in one, it should occur in the other.

Urethral Eroticism: Sexual enjoyment from the act of passing urine.

Vorbeireden: Talking past the point.

Voyeurism: A synonym for scoptophilia. (q.v.)

Withdrawal Syndrome: In drug addiction there is a physical change in the nervous system so that the normal functions cannot continue without an adequate intake of the drug. If the drug is withdrawn symptoms appear which are due to the malfunctioning of the nervous system. These symptoms constitute the withdrawal syndrome, which may last for hours or days depending on the nature of the drug and the individual's constitution.

Word Salad: Incomprehensible schizophrenic speech.

INDEX

Abortion Act 1967, 249–50
Abraham K., 188
Abrams R., 216
Abreaction, 222
Ackner B., 18
Adler A., 16, 29–31
Admission to hospital, 203
  compulsory, 229–30
  emergency, 235–6
  informal, 229, 233
  seasonal variation, 7
Adolescent crises, 146
Aetiology, 1–7
Affect, 55
  disorders, 58
Affective psychoses, 113–34
  aetiology, 115–17
  anxiety states (q.v.)
  depression (q.v.)
  heredity, 115
  incidence, 114
  main groups of, 114
  mania (q.v.)
  mixed states, 130–1
  personality, 115
  physical constitution, 115–17
  psychoanalytic theory, 117–18
  reactive factors, 117
  senile, 176–7
After care, 249
Ageing
  psychology of, 175
Agitation
  treatment, 208
Agnosia, 67
Aim inhibition, 26
Akinesia, 63, 140
Alanen Y. O., 136
Alcoholic dementia, 106
Alcoholic hallucinosis, 104
Alcoholics Anonymous, 102
Alcoholism, 100–6
  aetiology, 101
  clinical features, 100–1
  delirium tremens, 103–4

Alcoholism (cont.)
  paranoia, 106
  prognosis, 103
  psychological disorders and, 103–6
  treatment, 101–3
Alexander J., 71
Alexia, agnostic, 65
Algolagnia
  active, 188–9
  passive, 189
Alienation of thought, 45
Alzheimers' disease, 64, 157, 158, 168
  clinical picture, 169
  course, 169
  neurological signs, 169
  pathological changes, 168
Ambivalence, 58
Amenorrhoea, 96
Amentia, 59
Amnesia
  anterograde, 50
  chronic, 159
  hysterical, 81
  organic, 50, 156
  psychogenic, 50
  retrograde, 50, 156
  total, 50
Amphetamine addicts, 155
Amyostatic syndrome, 159
Anal stage, 25
Analytical psychology, 31–3
Animal magnetism, 14–15
Anorexia nervosa, 88–91
  aetiology, 89
  clinical features, 89–90
  depression, 124
  diagnosis, 90
  incidence, 88
  prognosis, 90
  treatment, 91
Ansari J. M. A., 186
Antidepressants, 125–9
Anxiety, 56
  anxiety states (q.v.)
  frigidity and, 188

Anxiety (*cont.*)
impotence and, 185–6
Anxiety states, 76–8, 131–4
acute, 77
affective disorders, as, 131
chronic, 77–8
classification, 76–7
diagnosis, 133
phobic, 78
symptoms, 132–3
treatment, 133–4, 208
Aphasia, 65
amnestic, 65
central, 65
expressive, 66
intermediate, 65
receptive, 65
Apophany, 45–6
Apraxia, 66
Arab world, 9
Archetypes, 32
Aretaeus the Cappadocian, 8
Arnold M. B., 55
Arthur R. J., 92
Asthma, bronchial, 92–3
Asyndetic thinking, 48
Autism, 141
Autistic thinking, 43
Authochthonous ideas, 14
Auto-eroticism, 194
Autoscopy, 39
Avicenna, 9

Baillarger J., 12
Baker G. H. B., 98
Barton J. L., 216
Bateson G., 136
Bayle A. L. J., 12
Behaviour
abnormal patterns, 62–4
disorders, 59–64
goal-directed, 63
immoral, 64
manneristic, 64
subjective experience, 59
Behaviour interpretations, 1
Behaviour therapy, 33–5, 223–4
Belle indifférence, 57, 79
Benedek-Jaszmann L. J., 97
Bennett J., 97
Bernheim H., 15
Bestiality, 193
Bethlem Hospital, 17

Bicêtre, 10
Bini L., 18
Blackburn R., 71
Bleuler E., 14
Bonhoeffer K., 14
Bowlby J., 29
Braid J., 10, 15
Brain damage, 3–4
abnormal personality and, 3
Brain disease, coarse, 3–4
Brain injury, 165–6
acute confusional states, 165–6
amnestic states, 166
dementia, 166
depression, 167
epilepsy, 166
organic states, unequivocal, 166
personality changes, 166
post-concussional syndrome, 167
psychiatric disorders, functional, 167
psychological reactions, 167
schizophrenia, 167
sequelae, 165
subdural haematoma, 166–7
Brain lesions, 37
Brain stem syndromes, 160
Brewerton D. A., 98
Browning J. S., 94
Brutality, 63
Bulimia nervosa, 90
Burckhardt G., 19

Calmeil L. F., 12
Cameron N., 48
Capgras syndrome, 52
Case-taking, 251–8
history, 251–4
psychological examination, 254–8
Catatonia, 13, 141
organic, 156
periodic, 143–4
Carletti Ugo, 18
Charcot J. M., 10, 15
Child
development, 30
position in family, 30
Childbearing
psychological illness in, 7, 173–4
Chlorpromazine, 208
Chodoff P., 69
Christianity, 9
Chynoweth R. C., 97
Circumstantiality, 44

Clang associations, 43
Clarke R. V. G., 75
Classification
    functional psychoses, 22
    organic states, 22
    problems of, 20–22
    psychogenic reactions, 22
Climatic conditions, 7
Clouston T., 175, 225
Clubs for patients, 207
Coarse brain disorders
    Bonhoeffer's theory, 14
    mental disorders, 11, 151–3, 156
Cobb S., 97
Cocaine, 109–10
Coma, 54
Conditioning, 33–5
Confabulation, 51
    expansive, 156
Confusional state, 7, 54, 154
    apathetic, 154
Conolly J., 10
Conrad K., 45
Consciousness
    clouding, 53
    deficiencies, 52–3
    definition, 52
Consciousness disorders, 52–5
    fugues, 54
    organic states, 153–4
    sleep disorders, 54–5
    twilight states, 54
    types of, 53–5
Constitution, 2
    genetic factors, 2
Conversion reaction, 78
Convulsion therapy, 18–19
Cooper D. G., 136
Coppen A., 96
Cornell Medical Inventory, 93
Cornish D. B., 75
Coronary artery disease, 97–8
    epidemiological studies, 97
    paroxysmal tachycardia, 98
    personality theories, 97
Cortico-striato-spinal degeneration,
    171–2
Counter-conditioning, 34
Court reports, 249
Creutzfeldt–Jakob disease, 171–2
    EEG, 172
Criminal responsibility, 242–4
Criminality, 74
    criminal psychopathic instituions, 75
Cyclothymia, 13

Day hospital, 206
Déjà vu, 51, 159
Delaye J. B., 12
Delirium, 54
    acute, 153–4
    senile patients, 181–2
    subacute, 154
Delirium tremens, 103–4
    aetiology, 103
    course, 104
    delirium, 103–4
    prodromal period, 103
    prognosis, 104
    treatment, 104
Delusions, 7, 37
    apophany, 45–6, 138
    autochthonous, 46
    definition, 45
    exhaustion, physical, 7
    grandiose, 47, 139
    guilt, 47
    hypochondriacal, 47, 139
    insanity, 11, 138–9
    memories, 51
    nihilistic, 47
    paranoid, 46–7, 144–5
    persecutory, 47, 138–9
    poverty, 47
    primary, 45–6
    progressive dementia, 157
    secondary, 45, 46
    types of, 46–7
Dementia
    brain injury, 166
    definition, 59
    epilepsy, in, 165
    multi-infarct, 179–81
    paranoides, 13
    praecox, 12, 13, 14, 59, 135
    presenile, 167–73
    progressive, 156–8
    senile, 177–9
Dementia, progressive, 156–8
    aetiology, 157
    behaviour, 158
    definition, 156
    emotions, 158
    epilepsy, 158
    intellectual changes, 157
    memory, 157
    onset, 157
    outcome, 158
    personality, 158
de Paul, St Vincent, 9
Depersonalization, 58

Depersonalization (*cont.*)
  in puerperium depression, 7
Depression, 121–30
  anorexia, 124
  antidepressive drugs, 125–9, 209
  brain injury, 167
  definition, 56
  delusions in, 46–7, 123
  depersonalization, 7, 122
  differential diagnosis, 124–5
  ECT, 125, 129–30
  endogenous, 6
  fatiguability, 124
  guilt, 121–2
  hallucinations, 123
  hypochondriasis, 122–3
  intelligence, 123
  maternal deprivation and, 4
  memory, 123
  mood, 121
  motor activity, 122
  obsession in, 87, 122
  organic disorders, 155
  paranoid, 145
  prognosis, 130
  provoked, 6
  psychoanalytic theory, 117
  psychotherapy, 130
  puerperium, 7
  reactive, 6, 124
  schizophrenia, 124–5
  sleep, 124
  suicide, 123–4
  treatment, 125–30, 209–10
Depressive position, 29
Depressive reactions, 84
Desensitization, systematic, 34
Development
  psychological influences in, 4
Diabetes mellitus, 95
Displacement, 26
Dissociative reaction, 78–9
Divorce, 241–2
Double bind
  impotence and, 186
  schizophrenia, 136
Dreams
  Freud's theory, 28
Drug dependence, 100–12
  alcoholism, 100–6
  barbiturates, 110–11
  benzodiazepines, 110–11
  diagnosis, 108–9
  euphoriants, 109–10
  hypnotics, 111

Drug dependence (*cont.*)
  morphine substitutes, 108
  opiate dependence, 107–8
  psychological theories, 111–12
  sleep deprivation, 55
  social factors, 112
  treatment, 109, 111
Drugs
  affective disorders and, 116–17
  amphetamine, 19
  antidepressive, 125–9, 213–14
  chlorpromazine, 19
  dependence, 100–12
  disulfiram, 102
  euphoriants, 109–10, 127
  hallucinogenics, 110
  haloperidol, 120, 208
  hypnotics, 111, 127, 209
  iproniazid, 20
  lithium, 120, 129
  monoamine oxidase inhibitors, 129, 134
  morphine substitutes, 108
  neuroleptics, 210–13
  opiates, 107–8
  phenothiazines, 19, 120
  psychotomimetic, 214
  psychotropic, 210–14
  reserpine, 19, 116, 212
  sedatives, 127, 207–8
  thymoleptics, 213–14
Drug therapy
  agitation, 208
  anorexia nervosa, 91
  anxiety states, 133–4, 208
  depression, 125–9, 209–10
  excitement, 207–8
  homosexuality, 198
  impotence, 186
  insomnia, 209
  mania, 120–1
  obsessional states, 88
  psychotherapy and, 227
  schizophrenia, 148–9
  sexual perversions, 197
Dunham H. W., 136
Dysmegalopsia, 41–2
Dysmenorrhoea, 96

Echolalia, 61, 141
Echopraxia, 61, 141
Edinburgh School of Psychiatry, 16
Egas, Moniz A. C., 19

Ego, 24, 26, 28
Elation, 56
Electric fish, 18
Electroconvulsive therapy (ECT)
　　agitation, 122
　　contraindication, 217
　　depression, 125, 129–30, 174
　　indications, 217
　　mania, 120–1
　　procedure, 215–16
　　schizophrenia, 149–50
Elliotson J., 15
Ellis H. H., 196
Emotion
　　abnormal expressions, 57–8
　　definition, 55
　　disorders, 55–7
　　schizophrenia, 140
Emotional hyperaesthetic syndrome,
　　154–5
　　chronic, 158
Emotional incontinence, 57
Emotional lability, 57
Enuresis
　　behaviour therapy, 223
Environment, social, 4–5
　　brain damage and, 3
Epilepsy, 8
　　amnesia, 50
　　apophany, 46
　　auras, 163
　　automatism, 163
　　confusional states, 163–4
　　dementia, 165
　　dysthymia, 164
　　environment, 3
　　excitement, 63
　　functional psychosis, 156
　　hallucinations, 39, 41, 164
　　ictal moods, 163
　　paranoia, 164
　　personality changes, 164–5
　　psychiatric disorders in, 163–5
　　psychomotor attacks, 163
　　schizophrenia and, 18, 137, 146
　　temporal lobe personality, 165
　　thought disorders, 44
　　twilight states, 54, 164
　　uncinate fits, 163
Erikson E., 29
Erotic zoophilia, 193
Esquirol J. E. D., 11
Essential hypertension, 97
Excitement, 63, 207
　　sedation, 207–8

Exhaustion, physical
　　confusional states, 7
Exhibitionism, 191–2
　　clinical features, 191–2
　　psychoanalytic views, 192
　　symptomatic, 191
Exogenous paranoid hallucinatory
　　syndrome, 155
Extrovert, 31

Falret J. P., 12
Federn P., 138
Feeling
　　definition, 55
　　disorders, 55–7
Fetishism, 190, 193
　　psychoanalytic theory, 193
Fictive goal, 31
Fish F., 38, 98, 181
Flechsig P., 13
Flexibilitas cerea, 62
Flight of ideas, 43
Flooding, 34
Flor-Henry P., 156
Foerster O., 116
Folie à double forme, 12
Folie circulaire, 12
French School of Psychiatry, 11–12
Freud S., 14, 15–16, 23–9, 31, 79, 92,
　　138, 190,219
Friedman M., 97
Frigidity, 187
　　partial, 187
　　physical causes, 188
　　psychological causes, 188
　　treatment, 188–9
　　varieties, 187
Fromm E., 29
Frontal lobe syndrome, 159
Fry J., 94
Fugues, 54
　　hysterical, 81
Fulton J. F., 19
Functional analysis, 34
Functions (Jung's), 31–2

Gagel O., 116
Galen, 8
Ganser S. J., 81
Ganser states, 81

General paralysis of the insane (GPI), 12, 16, 161–3
  clinical picture, 162
  delusions, 157
  expansive confabulatory syndrome, 156
  frontal lobe lesions, 159
  malaria therapy, 17
  signs and symptoms, 162
  treatment, 162–3
General paresis (*see* General paralysis of the insane)
Genetic constitution, 2
German School of Psychiatry, 12–14
Gerontophilia, 192
Gerstmann's syndrome, 42
Gilbert W. S., 80
Gjessing R., 7, 143
Goldberg E. M., 136
Goltz L., 19
Graves' disease, 95
Griesinger W., 12
Group therapy, 75, 220
Guardianship, 75, 230–1, 233, 236, 239
Gudden B. von, 13
Guilt delusions, 47

Hage J., 107
Hallucinations, 7, 36–41
  autoscopy, 39
  causes, 37
  deep sensation, of, 40
  epilepsy, 39, 41, 164
  exhaustion, physical, 7
  extracampine, 39
  functional, 38
  hearing, 37
  Lilliputian, 39, 42
  mass, 39
  olfactory, 39
  pseudohallucinations, 36
  reflex, 40
  tactile, 40
  taste, of, 39–40
  temporal lobe lesions, 159
  term, introduction of, 11
  thoughts, 38
  true, 37
  vestibular, 40
  visual, 39
  voices, 38
Hallucinatory syndromes, 41

Hallucinosis
  alcoholic, 104
  confusional, 41
  fantastic, 41
  organic, 155
  self-reference, 41
  verbal, 41
Halmi K. A., 90
Haloperidol, 120
Hamilton M., 196
Hanwell Asylum, 10, 11
Harris A., 18
Hartmann E. von, 29
Haslam J., 16
Hay fever, 93–4
Hearn-Sturtevant M. D., 97
Hebephrenia, 13
Hecker E., 12, 13
Heine B. E., 97
Hepatolenticular degeneration, 172–3
  clinical features, 172
  course, 172–3
Herxheimer H., 93
Hill G., 10
Hippocrates, 8
History of psychiatry, 8–22
  ancient world, 8–9
  Britain, in, 16–17
  dark ages, 9
  early Christianity, 9
  mental hospitals, 10
  middle ages, 9
  modern clinical psychiatry, 11–14
  modern psychiatry, 10
  neuroses, theories of, 14–16
  non-restraint movement, 10
  psychotherapy, 14–16
  Renaissance, 9–10
  treatment developments, 17–20
  U.S.A., in, 17
  value of, 8
Homosexuality
  aetiology, 196
  female, 196–7
  impotence and, 186
  Kinsey's scale, 194–5
  male, 194–5
  psychiatric disorders and, 195
  psychoanalytic theories, 196
  social aspects, 197
  treatment, 197–8
Horney K., 29
Houseworth J. H., 94
Hudson J. I., 89
Humoral theory, 8

Huntington's chorea, 9, 61, 170–1
  clinical picture, 171
  course, 171
  EEG, 171
  pathological findings, 170–1
  progressive dementia, 157
Hyperacusis, 42
Hyperemesis gravidarum, 173–4
Hypersomnia, 54
Hypertension, 97
Hyperthyroidism, 95
Hypnosis, 221–2
  techniques, 221
  treatment, 221–2
  value, 222
Hypnotism, 14–15
  term coined, 15
Hypochondria, 47
Hypochondriacal developments, 84
Hysteria, 8
Hysterical reactions, 78–83
  adolescent, 146
  aetiology, 79
  anxiety hysteria, 80
  definition, 78
  Freud's theory, 79–80
  Janet's theory, 79
  prognosis, 83
  psychological theories, 79
  sociological theory, 80
  symptoms, 80–2
  treatment, 83

Id, 23
Identification, 27
Illusions, 36
Impotence
  physical causes, 185
  psychological causes, 185–6
  treatment, 186
  variations of, 185
Incoherence, 44
Individual psychology, 29–31
Infantile sexuality, 16, 24
Inferiority complex, 31
Insanity
  delusion and, 11
Insel T. R., 88
Insomnia, 55
  treatment, 208–9
Institute of Psychiatry, 17
Institutional care
  acute patient, 203–4

Institutional care (cont.)
  admission, reasons for, 203
  chronic patient, 204
  clubs for patients, 207
  community mental health services,
    206–207
  day hospital, 206
  day patients, 205–6
  hospital organization, 204–5
  night patients, 205–6
  psychiatric unit, 206
  rehabilitation, 204
  segregation, 204
  self-government, 205
  sub-acute patient, 204
  therapeutic community, 205
  work, 205
Insulin coma therapy, 18
Intelligence
  definition, 58
  disorders, 59
Introjection, 27
Introversion, 27, 31
Involutional melancholia, 124
Irritable colon syndrome, 94
Isaac Judaeus, 218
Isolation, 27

Jacobsen C., 19
Jacobson F., 223
James I of England, 9
Janet P., 79
Jaspers K., 5, 69, 144
Jensen K., 107
Jordanburn Nerve Hospital, 17
Jung C. G., 14, 16, 31–3

Kahlbaum K. L., 12, 13
Kahlbaum's criteria of disease entity,
  12–13
Kallmann F. J., 196
Kay D. W. K., 176
Kessel N., 96
Kety S. S., 136
Kinsey A. C., 193, 194, 196
Klein M., 28–9, 138
Kleinian views, 28–9
Kleist K., 14, 113
Koch J. L. A., 15
Korsakoff syndrome, 10, 104, 105, 106,
  153
  clinical picture, 105

Korsakoff syndrome (*cont.*)
  prognosis, 105
  treatment, 105
Kraepelin E., 13–14, 17, 113, 130, 135,
    141, 144, 170, 175
Kraft-Ebing R. von, 12
Kretschmer E., 115

Laing R. D., 136
Lange C. G., 6
Latency period, 25
Learning theory, 223
Legal aspects, 228–50
  Abortion Act, 249–50
  admission, compulsory, 229–30
  admission, informal, 229, 233
  after care, 249
  civil law, 241–2
  consent to treatment, 231–2, 238
  court reports, 249
  crime and mental illness, 244–7
  criminal proceeding patients,
    238–40
  criminal responsibility, 242–4
  detention in hospital, 230, 236–7
  divorce, 241–2
  emergency admission, 235–6
  guardianship, 75, 230–1, 233, 236,
    239
  leave of absence, 231
  Lunacy Act 1808, 10
  marriage, 241–2
  Mental Health Act Commission, 235
  Mental Health Act 1983, 229–34
  Mental Health Acts, 228
  Mental Health Review Tribunals, 235
  Mental Health (Scotland) Act 1960,
    235
  mentally abnormal offenders, 232–4
  prison-hospital transfer, 234
  psychiatrist as witness, 244
  restriction orders, 234
  sexual offenders, 247–8
  supervision, 248–9
  testamentary capacity, 241
Leonhard K., 68–71, 72, 113, 142
Leucotomy (lobotomy), 19, 217–18
  complications, 217–18
  indications, 218
  obsessional states, 88
  technique, 217
Lewis A. J., 57
Lewis W. B., 12

Libido
  development, 24–5, 117
  release, 27
Liébault A., 15
Lilliputian hallucinations, 39, 42, 104
Lima A., 19
Lithium, 120, 129, 214
Logoclonia, 61, 64, 169
Lunacy Act of 1808 (England), 10
Lyons H., 69
Lysergic acid diethylamide (LSD), 42

McCulloch W. S., 143
McNaghten D., 244
Macropsia, 41
Maddocks P. D., 74
Magnet reaction, 62
Malaria therapy, 17
Management, 199–203
  complaint definition, 200
  diagnosis, 203
  environment, 201
  individual's assessment, 200–1
  interview, 199–200
  therapeutic situation control,
    201–3
  treatment plan, 203
Mania, 8, 113–14, 146, 155
  behaviour, 118
  bodily changes, 119
  delusional ideas, 119
  differential diagnosis, 119–20
  hallucinations, 119
  mood, 118
  overactivity, 119
  psychoanalytic theory, 117
  speech, 119
  symptoms, 119
  treatment, 120–1
Manic-depression, 3
  movements in, 60
Manic-depressive disease, 113–18
  types of, 113
Manic-depressive insanity, 13
Mannheim H., 75
Marijuana, 110
Marriage
  legal aspects, 241–2
  problems, 202
Masculine protest, 30
Masochism, 190
  psychoanalytic theories, 190–1
Masturbation, 194

Maternal deprivation, 4
depression and, 4
Maudsley H., 17
Maudsley Hospital, 16, 17
Maudsley Personality Inventory, 93, 96
Maxwell R. D. H., 215
Mayer-Gross W., 143
Meduna J. L. von, 18
Mehta S., 216
Melancholia, 8
Memory disorders, 49–52
amnesia, 50
false memories, 51
Korsakoff syndrome, 50, 153
minute memory, 50
misidentification, 52
progressive dementia, 156
recognition distortion, 51
registration failure, 50
recall distortion, 51
recall failure, 51
testing, 256, 257–8
Mendelian recessive condition, 3
Menorrhagia, 96
Menstrual disorders, 96–7
Mental deficiency, 3
Mental Health Acts, 228–34
Mental hospitals, 10–11
admission to, 229–30, 233, 235–6
Mental illness
adoption studies, 3
aetiology, 1–7
age, 6
brain damage, 3–4
causation of, 2
climatic conditions, 7
constitution, 2
cousin marriages, 3
environment, social, 4–5
exhaustion, physical, 7
family histories, 2–3
genetics of, 2–3
operations, 7
physical factors, 6–8
physiological endocrine changes, 6–7
pregnancy, 7
psychological influences, 4
puerperium, 7
seasonal variations, 7
sex, 6
situational stress, 2
stress, 5–6
twin studies, 3
Merry J., 103
Mescaline, 42

Mesmer F. A., 10, 14
Metonyms, 48
Meyer A., 17
Micropsia, 41
Mind
economics of, 25–7
structure of, 23
Minnesota Multiphasic Personality
Inventory, 71
Modelling, 3–5
Modified insulin therapy, 215
indications, 215
technique, 215
Mono-amine oxidase inhibitors (MAOI),
129, 134, 213–4
Monro J., 16
Mood, 56
changes, 56–7
Moral insanity, 16
Morel B. A., 12, 13
Morgagni G. B., 10
Morison Sir A., 16
Morris J. N., 97
Morrison S. L., 136
Mother's influence on child, 4
Motor behaviour, 59–64
abnormal patterns, 62–4
abnormally induced, 61–2
adaptive movements, 60
disorders classification, 59
non-adaptive movements, 60–1
posture disorders, 62
Movements
abnormally induced, 61–2
choreiform, 61
expressive, 60
goal directed, 60
reactive, 60
spontaneous, 60–1
Müller-Hegemann D., 208
Multi-infarct dementia, 179–81
aetiology, 179
clinical features, 179–80
course, 180
diagnosis, 181
prognosis, 180–1
treatment, 181
Münchausen syndrome, 73
Murder, 64
Mutism, 64

Nacht S., 189
Nancy School, 15

Narcissism, primary, 24
Narcoanalysis, 222
Narcolepsy, 54
Necrophilia, 193
Negativism, 63
Neologisms, 49
Neoplasms, cerebral
    psychiatric symptoms, 173
Neuroleptics, 148
Neurosis
    Adlerian theory, 30–1
    character neurosis, 28, 71–2
    compensation, 82
    diagnostic criteria, 20–2
    engagement, 82
    experimental, 19
    Freudian theory, 27–8
    Jungian theory, 32–3
    Klein's theory, 28–9
    learned maladaptive behaviour, 33
    post-Freudian views, 29
    theories of, 14–16
Non-restraint, 10–11, 16

Obedience, automatic, 61
Observational learning, 33–4
Obsession, 44–5
Obsessional reactions, 86–8
    aetiology, 86
    clinical picture, 86–7
    course, 87
    differential diagnosis, 87–8
    treatment, 88
Oedipal conflict, 23, 79, 189, 191
Offenders, mentally abnormal, 232–4
Old age disorders, 174–83
    affective psychosis, 176–7
    classification, 175–6
    delirious states, 181–2
    multi-infarct dementia, 179–80
    paranoid states, 182–3
    senile dementia, 177–8
    statistics, 175
Oldham A. J., 18
Oneiroid state, 141
Oneirophrenia, 143
Operant conditioning, 33–4
Operations
    psychoses and, 7
Opiate dependence, 107–9
    abstinence syndrome, 107–8
    administration of drug, 107
    diagnosis, 108

Opiate dependence (cont.)
    symptoms, 107
    treatment, 109
Oral stage, 24–5, 117
Organ inferiority, 30
Organic states, 151–183
    classification, 153
    coarse brain disease, 151–3
    defect states, 158–60
    dementia, progressive, 156–8
    encephalitis, 161
    general paresis, 161–3
    irreversible, 153, 156–60
    meningitis, 161
    reversible, 153–6

Paedophilia, 192
Palilalia, 61, 64, 169
Parakinesia, 61, 141
Paramnesia, 51
Paranoia, 46–7, 84–6, 144
    alcoholic, 106
    personality, 144–5
Paranoid position, 29
Paranoid states, 144–6
    epilepsy, in, 164
    organic, 145, 155
    senile, 182–3
Parietal lobe syndrome, 159
Paroxysmal tachycardia, 98
Pavlov I., 33, 218
Pavlovian conditioning, 33
Pentamethylenetetrazol (cardiazol), 18
Peptic ulcer, 99
Perception disorder, 36–42
Periodic mental illness, 13
Perplexity, 58
Perris C., 113, 115, 116
Perseveration, 44, 61, 64
Persona, 32
Personality
    abnormal, 68–75
    aggressive, 73
    anankastic, 69
    antisocial, 74
    anxious, 70
    brain injury, 166
    case-taking details, 253–4
    cyclothymic, 70, 115
    dementia, 158
    depressive, 115
    drug addiction, 111
    emotive, 70

Personality (*cont.*)
epilepsy, in, 164–5
epileptoid, 69
hypomanic, 70
hysterical, 69–70
International Classification of
Diseases, in, 71
irritable, 115
Leonhard's classification, 69–71
manic, 115
mixed, 71
multiple, 81
paranoid, 70, 144–5
psychopathic, 72–5
psychosomatic disorders, 92, 94, 97
reactive-labile, 70
role in illness, 225
schizoid, 136
Schneider's list, 71
sociopathic, 73
subdepressive, 70
Personality, abnormal
brain damage and, 3
Petrilowitsch N., 68, 72
Phallic stage, 25
Phantom limb, 42
Phobias, 57
conditioned, 57
obsessional, 57
Phrenitis, 8
Physical disease
causation of, 1–2
Pick's disease, 157, 159, 169
clinical picture, 170
course, 170
neurological signs, 170
pathological changes, 169–70
Pickering G. W., 97
Pinel P., 10, 11, 16
Posture disorders, 62
Predispositions to mental illness, 2
Pregnancy, 7, 173
Premenstrual tension, 6–7, 96–7
behaviour and, 7
Priapism, 187
Prichard J. C., 11, 16
Projection, 26
Prolixity, 44
Provoked depression, 6
Pseudodementia, 81
Psoriasis, 98
Psychoanalysis, 15, 23–9, 219–20
classical technique, 219–20
Jungian, 32, 320
modified, 220

Psychoanalysis (*cont.*)
term usage, 23
Psychoanalytic theory
character neuroses, 71–2
Psychobiology, 17
Psychodrama, 220
Psychogenic reactions, 76–9
Psychological explanations, nature of, 1
Psychological influences
development and, 4
maternal deprivation, 4
parental attitudes, 4
Psychological theories, 1
Psychology
analytical (Jungian), 31–3
empathic, 1
explanatory, 1
individual (Adlerian), 29–31
interpretative, 1
Psychopathy
aetiology, 73–4
characteristics, 72
classification, 72
treatment, 74–5
Psychoses
affective, 113–34
anxiety-elation, 142
confusion, 142–3
cycloid, 142
diagnostic criteria, 20–22
hysterical, 82
motility, 143
Psychosomatic disorders, 92–9
cardiovascular disorder, 97–8
definition, 92
endocrine disorders, 95–7
Freudian view, 92
gastrointestinal disorders, 94
personality theories, 92, 94, 97
respiratory disorders, 92–4
rheumatoid arthritis, 98
skin disorders, 98
Psychotherapy, 218–27
abreaction, 222
alcoholics, 102
anxiety, 133
behaviour therapy, 223
depression, 130
development of, 14–16
drugs in, 227
goals, 225–6
group therapy, 220
hypnosis, 221–2
insight, 225, 226
Jungian, 32, 220

Psychotherapy (*cont.*)
  narcoanalysis, 222
  problem definition, 224
  progress review, 226–7
  psychoanalysis, 219–20
  psychodrama, 220
  psychopaths, 74–5
  relaxation therapy, 223
  resistance, 226
  short term, 224
  suggestion, 221
  supportive, 227
  techniques, 224–6
  temple sleep, 9
  transference, 219
Psychotomimetic drugs, 214
Psychotropic drugs
  classification, 210
  neuroleptics, 210–2
  sedative, 212–4
Puerperium, 7
  depersonalization, 7
  depression, 7, 174
  organic states, 174
  schizophrenia, 7, 137, 174

Quakers, 10

Rahe R. H., 92, 97
Reaction
  formation, 26
  meaning in psychiatry, 5
Reactive illness, 5
  Jasper's criteria, 5–6
Reciprocal inhibition, 34
Rees L., 93
Reformation, the, 9
Regression, 27
Rehabilitation, 204
Reid W. H., 128
Relaxation therapy, 208, 223
Remembering, 49–50 (*see also* Memory
  disorders)
Repression, 26
  failure, 28
Retreat, The, 10, 17
Robertson A., 162
Robertson G. M., 16
Role playing, 35
Romo M., 97
Roos R., 172
Rose R. M., 97

Rosenman R. H., 97
Rosenthal D., 136
Roth M., 175, 176, 179–83

Sacred Disease, 8
Sadism, 189–90
  psychoanalytic theories, 190–1
Sainsbury P., 97
Sakel M., 18
Savage G., 17
Schizo-affective illnesses, 142–3
Schizophrenia, 3, 135–44
  aetiology, 135–8
  aphasia, 65
  autism, 141
  behaviour disorders, 140–1
  brain injury, 167
  brutality, 63
  catatonia, 141
  classification, 141–2
  concept, 135
  consciousness disorders, 141
  course, 147
  delusions, 138–9
  depression, 124–5
  development, 136
  differential diagnosis, 146
  distribution, 4
  echolalia, 61
  echopraxia, 61
  ECT, 149–50
  emotional disorders, 140
  epilepsy and, 18, 137, 146
  grafted, 143
  hallucinations, 37–42, 139
  heredity, 135–6
  mannerism, 64
  memory disorders, 51–2, 141
  metabolism, 137
  moral deterioration, 64
  motor disorders, 140–1
  movements, 60, 141
  nervous system disorders, 137
  neuroleptics, 148–9
  obsession, 87
  origin of term, 14
  paranoid, 145
  paraphrenia, 144
  personality, 136
  precipitation, 137
  prognosis, 147–8
  prophylaxis, 150
  pseudoneurotic, 143

Schizophrenia (*cont.*)
  psychoanalytic theory, 137–8
  puerperium, 7
  social isolation, 136
  special forms, 142–4
  speech disorders, 64, 141
  stupor, 141
  symptomatology, 138–9
  thought disorder, 43–9, 138–9
  treatment, 148–50
  twins studies, 136
  voices, hallucinatory, 139
  writing disorders, 64
Schneider K., 68, 71, 72, 151, 195, 225
Schröder H., 41
Schultz Z., 223
Scoptophilia, 191
Scott R., 9
Scribonius Largus, 18
Seasonal variations
  hospital admission, 7
  suicide, 7
Sedatives, 127, 207–8
Segregation, 204–5
Sejunction, 14
Self-government, in hospital, 205
Senile dementia, 177–9
  aetiology, 177
  diagnosis, 179
  morbid anatomy, 178
  outcome, 179
  psychiatric clinical picture, 178–9
  treatment, 179
Sense deception, 36–41
Sense distortion, 41–2
  bodily sensation, 42
  hearing, 42
  visual, 41
Sensory deprivation, 37
Sexual disorders, 184–98
  classification, 184
  frigidity, 187
  homosexuality, 194–8
  impotence, 185–7
  perversions, 189–94
  priapism, 187
  psychoanalytic theories, 189
  sexual partner deviations, 192–4
  treatment, 197–8
Sexual intercourse (normal), 184
Sexual offenders, 247–8
Shields J., 131
Siltanen P., 97
Singer M. T., 136
Situational stress, 2

Skae D., 16
Skinner B. F., 33
Slater E., 115, 131, 137, 196
Sleep disorder, 54–5
  depression, 124
  hypersomnia, 54
  narcolepsy, 54
  insomnia, 55
  inversion of rhythm, 55
  sleep deprivation, 55
Snaith R. P., 131, 216
Speech disorders, 64
  neurological, 65–7
Stereotypy, 61
Stokvis S., 98
Stress, 5–6
  reaction to, 5–6, 76–8
  significance, 5
  situational, 2
Stupor, 62–3, 82, 140
  organic, 154
Subdural haematoma, 166–7
Sublimation, 26
Suggestion, 37, 221
Suicide, 12
  depression, 123
  management, 200
  pregnancy (rare), 7
  seasonal variations, 7
Sullivan H. S., 29
Sumerian civilization, 9
Superego, 23, 26, 28
Sydenham's chorea, 61
Sydenham T., 10
Symptomatology, 36–67
Symptom complex, 13

Taylor D. C., 165
Taylor M. A., 216
Temple sleep, 9
Temporal lobe symptoms, 159
Testamentary capacity, 241
Therapeutic community, 205
Thought blocking, 44
Thought disorder, 43–9
  attitudes, disordered, and, 49
  classification, 43
  content of thought, 45–7
  form of though, 48–9
  neologisms, 49
  possession of thought, 44–5
  schizophrenia, 138–9
  stream of thought, 43

Thought echo, 38
Thymoleptics, 213–14
Thyroid extract, 150
Tics, 61
Token economy, 34
Torticollis, spasmodic, 61
Transexualism, 194
Transit syndrome, 154–6
Transvestism, 194
Treatment (general), 199–227
  consent to, 231–2
  developments, 17–20
  drugs (*see* Drugs *and* Drug
    therapy)
  management (q.v.)
  physical, 215–18
  psychoanalysis, 219–20
  psychotherapy, 218–19
  symptomatic, 207
Tremor, 60–1
Tuke D. H., 17
Tuke W., 10, 17
Twilight states, 54
  hysterical, 81
  organic, 154
Tyrer P., 71

Unconscious, the, 23, 31, 32
Undoing, 27
Urticaria, 98

Vasomotor rhinitis, 93
Veraguth's sign, 60
Verbigeration, 13, 141
Voices, hallucinatory, 38
Voyeurism, 191
  psychological theories, 191

Wagner-Jauregg J. von, 17
Walther-Büel H., 173
Wernicke, C., 14
Wernicke's encephalopathy, 105–6
  clinical picture, 106
  outcome, 106
  pathology, 106
  progressive dementia, 157
  treatment, 106
Westphal C. F. O., 12
Weyer J., 9
Wieck H., 151
Wikler A., 111
Williams D., 74
Williamson T., 181
Wilson's disease, 172–3
Winokur A., 89
Witchcraft, 9–10
Witness, psychiatrist as, 244
Wolpe J., 223
Work, in hospital, 205
Writing disorders, 64
Wundt W., 13
Wynne L. C., 136